# Addiction in the Older Patient

# Addiction in the Older Patient

EDITED BY MARIA A. SULLIVAN

*and*

FRANCES R. LEVIN

OXFORD
UNIVERSITY PRESS

# OXFORD
UNIVERSITY PRESS

Oxford University Press is a department of the University of Oxford. It furthers
the University's objective of excellence in research, scholarship, and education
by publishing worldwide. Oxford is a registered trade mark of Oxford University
Press in the UK and certain other countries.

Published in the United States of America by Oxford University Press
198 Madison Avenue, New York, NY 10016, United States of America.

Library of Congress Cataloging-in-Publication Data
Names: Sullivan, Maria (Maria A.), 1961- , editor. | Levin, Frances R., editor.
Title: Addiction in the older patient / edited by Maria Sullivan, Frances R. Levin.
Description: Oxford ; New York : Oxford University Press, [2016] | Includes bibliographical references.
Identifiers: LCCN 2016008473| ISBN 9780199392063 (pbk.) | ISBN 9780199392087 (epub) |
ISBN 9780199392070 (U-pdf)
Subjects: | MESH: Substance-Related Disorders | Aged | Substance Abuse Detection |
Behavior, Addictive—therapy
Classification: LCC RC564 | NLM WM 270 | DDC 362.29—dc23
LC record available at http://lccn.loc.gov/2016008473

9 8 7 6 5 4 3 2 1

Printed by Webcom, Inc., Canada

# CONTENTS

# CONTRIBUTORS

**Esra Alagoz, PhD**
Center for Health Enhancement
  Systems Studies
University of Wisconsin–Madison
Madison, Wisconsin

**Francesca L. Beaudoin, MD, MS**
The Alpert Medical School
  of Brown University
Rhode Island Hospital
The Miriam Hospital
Providence, Rhode Island

**Olivera J. Bogunovic, MD**
Ambulatory Services
Partners Addiction Psychiatry
  Fellowship
Department of Psychiatry,
  Harvard Medical School
Boston, Massachusetts
Division of Drug and Alcohol
  Abuse, McLean Hospital
Belmont, Massachusetts

**Christina A. Brezing, MD**
Division on Substance Abuse,
  Department of Psychiatry
Columbia University Medical Center
New York State Psychiatric Institute
New York, New York

**Isis Burgos-Chapman, MD**
Cornell Scott–Hill Health Center
Department of Psychiatry
Yale School of Medicine
New Haven, Connecticut

**Stacy A. Cohen, MD**
Mental Health Center
Pacific Clinics
The Camden Center
Los Angeles, California

**Ilana Crome, MD, FRCPsych**
Keele University
Queen Mary University, London
St George's University, London
Imperial College, London
London, England
South Staffordshire and Shropshire
  Healthcare NHS Foundation Trust
Stafford, England

**Elizabeth Evans, MD**
Division on Substance Abuse
Columbia University
New York Psychiatric Institute
New York, New York

**David Gustafson, Jr., MS**
Center for Health Enhancement
  Systems Studies
University of Wisconsin–Madison
Madison, Wisconsin

**Margaret M. Haglund, MD**
Department of Psychiatry
Cedars Sinai Medical Center
Los Angeles, California

**Kim Johnson, PhD**
Center for Health Enhancement
  Systems Studies
University of Wisconsin–Madison
Madison, Wisconsin

**Anna Terajewicz LaRose, MD**
Boston University Medical Center
VA Boston Healthcare System
Boston, Massachusetts

**Anna Levesque, MD**
Addiction Institute of New York
Mount Sinai West Hospital
New York, New York

**Frances R. Levin, MD**
Division on Substance Abuse
New York State Psychiatric Institute
Columbia University Medical Center
New York, New York

**Roland C. Merchant, MD, MPH, ScD**
Department of Emergency Medicine
  and Epidemiology
Brown University
Providence, Rhode Island

**Larissa J. Mooney, MD**
Ronald Reagan UCLA
  Medical Center
Resnick Neuropsychiatric Hospital
UCLA Medical Center, Santa Monica
Los Angeles, California

**Edward V. Nunes, MD**
National Institute on Drug Abuse
Department of Psychiatry
Columbia University Medical Center
New York, New York

**Andrew Quanbeck, PhD**
Center for Health Enhancement
  Systems Studies
University of Wisconsin–Madison
Madison, Wisconsin

**Rahul Rao, MD, MSc**
South London and Maudsley
  NHS Foundation Trust
Visiting Researcher, Institute
  of Psychiatry
London, England

**John Renner, Jr., MD**
Boston University School
  of Medicine
VA Boston Healthcare System
Boston, Massachusetts

**Kevin Sevarino, MD, PhD**
Yale University School of Medicine
New Haven, Connecticut
Newington Mental Health
Connecticut VA Healthcare System
Newington, Connecticut

**Maria A. Sullivan, MD, PhD**
Columbia University
New York, New York
Clinical Research and
   Development, Alkermes, Inc.
Waltham, Massachusetts

**Louis A. Trevisan, MD**
Department of Psychiatry
Yale School of Medicine
VA Connecticut Healthcare System
Newington, Connecticut

**Arthur Robin Williams, MD, MBE**
Division of Substance Abuse
Columbia University Department
   of Psychiatry
New York State Psychiatric Institute
New York, New York

CHAPTER 1

# Introduction

*Maria A. Sullivan and Frances R. Levin*

## Scope of the Problem

Alcohol and drug use among older or elderly patients has received relatively little attention, either as a clinical focus, or as a research initiative, to date. This apparent neglect of a critical cohort of affected individuals may be partly explained by prevailing cultural biases among both family members and practitioners, which serve to minimize the perceived extent of the scope of the problem among older adults. Ageism contributes to a pattern of underdiagnosis, in that behavior considered a problem in younger adults does not engender the same urgency for care in older adults (SAMHSA 1998). Primary care physicians as well as specialists do not routinely address or screen older adults for substance use disorders (SUDs) (Rothrauff et al. 2011). But it is also important to recall that evidence for best treatment practices in this older population is lacking, since most clinical research trials specifically exclude older participants. The vast majority of studies exclude individuals older than 65, and indeed, many trials exclude anyone age 60 or older. Thus, our ability even to identify SUDs in the older population relies on extrapolation from younger cohorts. At present, the field of addiction treatment is lacking in data on the clinical presentation and course of illness in older individuals. In particular, we are in need of both sensitive diagnostic instruments and specific prevention and treatment strategies focused on the characteristics of older adults with SUD.

The problem of limited clinical knowledge regarding the phenomenology of alcohol and substance use disorders in later life is rendered more acute by the changing demographics of the U.S. population. Over the next decade, the cohort of aging adults will continue to grow at a rapid rate—and this will pose a significant challenge for the field of addiction treatment. It is estimated that the number of individuals age 65 or older will grow from 40 million in 2010 to 55 million in 2020 (U.S. Census Bureau 2009). And by 2030, there will be about 72.1 million older adults (representing 19.3% of the total population). This considerable increase in older adults will constitute almost a doubling since 2008 (United States Census Bureau 2008). Moreover, the cohort of aging adults is continuing to use alcohol and psychoactive prescription medications at a higher rate than previous generations did (Blow and Barry 2012). For instance, about 50% of adults aged 65 and older and about 25% of individuals over 85 years old drink alcohol (Caputo et al. 2012). Thus, a considerable proportion of the aged 65+ population are at potential risk for the development of alcohol use disorder (AUD). This risk is heightened by the increased effects of ethanol on the central nervous system in the elderly, for whom reduced activity of gastric and liver antidiuretic hormone (ADH) leads to the elevation of blood alcohol levels by up to 25% (Lieber 2005).

Along with alcohol, prescription drugs are the most frequently abused substance by older Americans (Weintraub et al. 2002). Approximately one-third of all prescription drugs in the United States are used by older (age 65+) adults (National Institute on Drug Abuse [NIDA] 2005). Polypharmacy is also common among older adults, who tend to have multiple underlying medical disorders (Ballentine 2008). It is estimated that a rising proportion of older adults will experience prescription SUD because of the aging cohort, and increased accessibility of prescription drugs (Dowling et al. 2008).

Varying definitions of "older adult" appear in the literature, ranging from 50+ years to 65+ years old. The broader age-based definition of older adults reflects the fact that, among individuals with SUDs, there is an accelerated rate of biological aging to a higher medical burden. Furthermore, up to 30% of older patients hospitalized medically and up to 50% of those hospitalized psychiatrically present with AUDs (Blazer and Wu 2009). Yet, for many older adults, a diagnosis of addiction is missed. Accurate assessment of the prevalence of AUD and SUD among older adults in the community is, in fact, hampered by a number of factors.

## Challenges to Identifying Addictive Disorders in Older Adults

The misuse of alcohol or other substances is often a hidden phenomenon, because family members, friends, and employers are not available to notice the types of changes in behavior or personality by which AUD or SUD is frequently identified in younger persons (Johnson 1989). Retirement effectively eliminates the observational aspects of relationships with co-workers and supervisors (Boeri et al. 2008). Alcohol or substance use disorders in the older adult may also be difficult to identify because many screening instruments measure the presence of legal, social, and work-related problems (Zimberg 1984, Johnson 1989). In addition, older adults are often reluctant to seek help for addiction because of the perception of its stigma and shame, which is stronger among older individuals than among younger persons (Oslin et al. 2005).

Another factor that often confounds clinicians is the co-occurrence of multiple medical problems in older patients. Concurrent neurological, cardiac, or gastrointestinal disorders can mimic or mask the acute effects of alcohol or other substances, as well as the withdrawal syndromes associated with alcohol, benzodiazepines, stimulants, or opioids. The 2005–2007 National Survey on Drug Use and Health (NSDUH) found that, among 10,015 respondents aged 50–64 years and 6,289 respondents older than 65 years, "diagnostic orphans" among middle-aged and elderly community adults showed an elevated rate for both binge drinking and the non-medical use of prescription drugs, requiring attention from healthcare providers (Blazer and Wu 2011). Thus, alcohol or prescription misuse in older adults is often missed when strict diagnostic (*Diagnostic and Statistical Manual of Mental Disorders*, 5th Ed. [DSM-5]) criteria for alcohol or substance use disorders are invoked. This text will highlight some of the risk factors and signs of addictive disorders in older individuals that are frequently overlooked.

## Risk Factors in Older Age, and Projected Trends

The National Survey on Drug Use and Health (NSDUH 2004) found that, of individuals aged 50 or older, 12.2% were heavy drinkers, 3.2% were binge drinkers, and 1.8% used illicit drugs. The 2005–2006 NSDUH revealed a relatively high level of binge drinking in men (14%) and women (3%) over the age of 65 years (Blow 1998). Historically, the use of illicit drugs has been relatively rare in older adults. Based on the 2004 NSDUH, among individuals aged 50+ years, 1.8% used illicit drugs (Office on Applied Statistics [OAS] 2005, Huang 2006, Colliver et al. 2006). But by 2020, use of any illicit drug by this cohort is estimated to increase from 2.2% (1.6 million) to 3.1% (3.5 million), and nonmedical use of prescription drugs (opioids, sedatives, tranquilizers, and stimulants) is projected to increase from 1.2% (911,000) to 2.4% (2.7 million). Analysis of the Baby Boom generation in the National Health and Nutrition Examination Survey (NHANES 2012) data found that this cohort is continuing to maintain a higher level of alcohol consumption than did previous older-age cohorts. Moreover, the NSDUH (2012) found that past-month illicit drug use in the aged 55–59 group increased by 50%, from 4.1% (2010) to 6.0% (2011) (Substance Abuse and Mental Health Services Administration [SAMHSA] 2012). In addition to lifetime marijuana use, recent use has continued to rise over the last decade (National Institue on Alcohol Abuse and Alcoholism [NIAAA] 2015). It is expected that the problems of morbidity and mortality related to illicit SUDs will also continue to increase.

Several studies have identified social isolation or loneliness as a risk factor for psychotropic drug misuse among older persons (Jinks et al. 1990, Nubukpo and Clement 2013). Other risk factors for the development of psychoactive medication misuse include: (1) being female, (2) having a history of a psychiatric disorder or a prior SUD, (3) higher levels of psychosocial distress, and (4) poorer functioning (Simoni-Wastila and Yang 2006, Jinks et al. 1990). Additionally, symptoms of pain, anxiety, or sleep disturbance (Patterson et al. 1999, Schonfeld et al. 2009) increase the likelihood of psychoactive prescription misuse.

## Treatment Considerations

There is a substantial body of evidence that motivational brief interventions, delivered by a variety of healthcare providers, can reduce at-risk drinking, alcohol misuse or alcohol consumption among both younger (Babor et al. 1992, Fleming et al. 1997, Wallace et al. 1988) and older adults (Fleming et al. 1999, Lin et al. 2010, Moore et al. 2011). Lin and colleagues found that early reductions in at-risk alcohol use were associated with the following: older adults' concerns about risks, reading educational materials, and the perception of physicians providing advice to reduce drinking. Two large-scale effectiveness studies have examined the implementation of such brief intervention trials in older adults: the Primary Care Research in Substance Abuse and Mental Health for the Elderly study (PRISM-E; Oslin et al. 2006) and the Brief Intervention and Treatment for Elders (Florida BRITE) project (Schonfeld et al. 2010). These two trials identified several barriers to implementation of these brief interventions: (1) stigma from the perspective of older patients; (2) lack of training for healthcare professionals in screening and brief interventions; (3) chronic medical conditions in older adults, which may make it more difficult to identify the role of AUD or SUD in decreased functioning or quality of life; and absent or low reimbursement for providing this service (Blow and Barry 2012).

Certain modifications to a standard pharmacotherapy regimen may need to be made when treating older adults. For instance, detoxification from alcohol or drugs may need to be carried out over a longer period of time (Johnson 1989), and the incidence of medical (e.g., myocardial ischemia, arrhythmias, orthostatic hypotension) and neurological (e.g., delirium tremens, dizziness, seizures) problems is higher in elderly patients than in their younger counterparts (Letizia and Reinbolz 2005). Unfortunately, insurance carriers, including Medicare, do not always recognize that physiological needs of aging patients may require that they remain hospitalized for a longer period of time (Douglass 1984). In addition, detoxification regimens may need to be adjusted to avoid overmedicating-withdrawal symptoms. And disulfiram (Antabuse) is not recommended in older adults, many of whom have cardiac arrhythmias or pulmonary disease, because of the risk of adverse effects (Lamy 1988, Council on Scientific Affairs 1996). On the other hand, difficulties with memory may recommend the use of a monthly long-acting injectable formulation of naltrexone (Vivitrol), in preference to the oral form often used in younger individuals seeking treatment for AUD (Caputo et al. 2012).

And finally, special services for older adults are largely unavailable at present. Using nationally representative cross-sectional data from 346 private substance treatment centers, Rothrauff et al. (2011) found that only 18% provided age-specific services. In both inpatient and outpatient settings, older adults can be expected to relate more readily to groups of their peers who have experienced similar challenges, such as loss of spouse, contraction of social network, loss of physical vigor, and declining cognitive and sexual function. An expert panel commissioned by SAMHSA (1998) offered specific SUD treatment approaches with older adults. These include: engaging in nonconfrontational treatment; focusing on (re)building self-esteem; teaching skills to cope with depression, loneliness, and loss; focusing on (re)building social networks; tailoring content and pace of presentation toward older adults; hiring staff who are interested in and experienced with working with older adults; and providing linkages with medical services and community-based services. Rothrauff et al. (2011) also recommend wraparound services to address older adults' special needs, such as inadequate availability of primary care, housing assistance, and transportation to and from treatment.

## Conclusions

The incidence of alcohol and substance use disorders in older adults is fairly high and certainly underestimated. Addictive disorders in middle-aged and older patients are often undetected in the clinical setting and rarely examined from a research perspective. Symptoms of AUD or SUD overlap with those of other medical conditions prevalent in this population, and the kinds of distress engendered by SUDs in later life frequently evade detection on standardized assessments of work or social functioning. Older patients themselves are often reluctant to reveal SUDs because of the shame and stigma associated with addiction, which is heightened in this generational cohort.

The field of addiction treatment has for too long overlooked the needs of older adults struggling with addictive disorders. An emerging literature on tailored treatments for this population suggests the benefits of brief interventions, cognitive-behavioral therapy, and age-specific treatment services in both the inpatient and outpatient settings. Given the opportunity to benefit from these treatments, older patients have the capacity to demonstrate outcomes at least as successful as those in younger individuals.

The goal of this book is to review the evidence-based literature on addiction in the older patient. We will examine each of the major classes of substances, both prescribed and illicit, and offer guidelines for the accurate assessment and effective treatment of alcohol and substance use disorders in this vulnerable and rapidly growing population. We will consider diagnostic challenges that arise from cultural or practitioner bias against older patients, as well as medically related or atypical presentations of alcohol or substance use disorders in older adults, including unique challenges faced by older women challenged by addiction. And we will explore the role for both traditional and technology-based screening and brief interventions, as well as the importance of developing and implementing effective treatment strategies tailored to the needs of an older population. It is our hope that clinicians will find this text useful in helping them identify individuals at risk for, or actively engaged in, addictive disorders, and that the recommendations set forth here may help frame and guide clinical interactions with older patients who could benefit from timely treatment interventions in this domain. Above all, this book is offered as a practical handbook of useful clinical information to aid clinicians in increasing their awareness of, attention to, and skills in assessing and treating, addiction in our older patients.

# References

Babor T, Grant M. Project on identification and management of alcohol-related problems. *Report on Phase II: a randomized clinical trial of brief interventions in primary health care.* Geneva: WHO; 1992.

Ballentine NH. Polypharmacy in the elderly: maximizing benefit, minimizing harm. *Crit Care Nurs Q* 2008;31(1):40–45.

Blazer DG, Wu LT. The epidemiology of alcohol use disorders and subthreshold dependence in a middle-aged and elderly community sample. *Am J Geriatr Psychiatry* 2011;19(8):685–694.

Blow F. Substance abuse among older adults. Treatment Improvement Protocol (TIP) Series 26. Center for Substance Abuse Treatment Substance Abuse Among Older Adults, DHHS Publication No. (SMA) 98–3179, Rockville, MD 1998.

Blow FC, Barry KL. Alcohol and substance misuse in older adults. *Curr Psychiatry Rep* 2012;14:310–319.

Caputo F, Vignoli T, Leggio L, Addolorato G, Zoli G, Bernardi M. Alcohol use disorders in the elderly: a brief overview from epidemiology to treatment options. *Exper Gerontol* 2012;47:411–416.

Colliver JD, Compton WM, Gfroerer JC, Condon T. Projecting drug use among aging baby boomers in 2020. *Ann Epidemiol* 2006;16(4):257–265.

Council on Scientific Affairs, American Medical Association. Alcoholism in the elderly. *JAMA* 1996;275:797–801.

Division P, ed. Projections of the population by age and sex for the United States: 2010 to 2050 (NP2008-T12). In P. Division, ed., U.S. Census Bureau, Suitland, MD; 2008.

Douglass R. Aging and alcohol problems: opportunities for socioepidemiological research. In M. Galanter, ed., *Recent developments in alcoholism*. New York: Plenum Press; 1984:251–266.

Dowling GJ, Weiss SR, Condon TP. Drugs of abuse and the aging brain. *Neuropsychopharmacology* 2008;33(2):209–218.

Fleming MF, et al. Brief physician advice for problem drinkers—a randomized controlled trial in community-based primary care practices. *JAMA* 1997;277:1039–1045.

Huang B. et al. Prevalence, correlates, and comorbidity of non-medical prescription drug use and drug use disorders in the United States: results of the National Epidemiological Survey on alcohol and related conditions. *J Clin Psychiatry* 2006;67:1062–1073.

Jinks MJ, Raschko TT. A profile of alcohol and prescription drug abuse in a high-risk community-based elderly population. *Ann Pharmacother (DICP)*, 1990;24:971–975.

Johnson KK. How to diagnose and treat chemical dependency in the elderly. *J Gerontol Nurs* 1989;15(12):22–26.

Lamy P. Actions of alcohol and drugs in older people. *Generations* Summer 1988, 32–36.

Letizia M, Reinbolz M. Identification and managing acute alcohol withdrawal in the elderly. *Geriatr Nurs* 2005;26:176–183.

Lieber CS. Metabolism of alcohol. *Clin Liver Dis* 2005;9:1–35.

Lin JC, et al. Determinants of early reductions in drinking in older at-risk drinking in primary care. *J Am Geriatr Soc* 2010;58:227–233.

Moore AA, Blow FC, Hoffing M, et al. Primary care based intervention to reduce at-risk drinking in older adults: a randomized controlled trial. *Addiction* 0000;106(1):111–120.

National Health and Nutrition Examination Survey (NHANES): Analytic Guidelines, 2011–2012. Centers for Disease Control and Prevention, Atlanta, GA. Available at http://www.cdc.gov/nchs/data/nhanes/analytic_guidelines_11_12.pdf. Accessed on April 17, 2016.

National Institute on Drug Abuse (NIDA). NIDA Community Drug Alert Bulletin 2005. Available at http://archives.drugabuse.gov/PrescripAlert/. Accessed on April 17, 2016.

National Institute on Alcohol Abuse and Alcoholism (NIAAA). *Older Adults*. 2015. Retrieved from http://www.niaaa.nih.gov/alcohol-health/special-populations-co-occurring-disorders/older-adults. Accessed on March 30, 2015.

Nubukpo C, Clement JP. Medical drug abuse and aging. *Geriatr Psychol Neuropsychiatr Vieil.* 2013;11(3):305–315.

Office of Applied Studies. Results from the 2003 National Survey on Drug Use and Health Services Administration. DHHS Publication No. (SMA) 04-3964. NSDUH Series H-25, Rockville, MD; 2004.

Office of Applied Statistics (OAS). The DASIS Report: Older adults in substance abuse treatment. OAS; 2005. Available at http://OAS.samhsa.gov/2k7/olderTX/olderTX.cfm. Accessed on April 17, 2016.

Oslin DW, Slaymaker VJ, Blow FC, Owen PL, Colleran C. Treatment outcomes for alcohol dependence among middle-aged and older adults. *Addict Behav* 2005;30:1431–1436.

Patterson TL, Jeste TV. The potential impact of the baby-boom generation on substance abuse among elderly persons. *Psychiatr Serv* 1999;50:1184–1188.

Rothrauff TC, Abrahan AJ, Bridge BE, Roman PM. Substance abuse treatment for older adults in private centers. *Subst Abus* 2011;32(1):7–15.

Schonfeld L, et al. Screening and brief intervention for alcohol and other substances: The Florida BRITE project. *Gerontologist* 2010;50:496.

Schonfeld L, et al. Screening and brief prevention for substance misuse among older adults: The Florida BRITE Project. *Am J Public Health* 2009;99:1–7.

Simoni-Wastila L, Stickler G. Risk factors associated with problem use of prescription drugs. *Am J Geriatr Pharmacother* 2004;4:380–394.

Substance Abuse and Mental Health Services Administration. Results from the 2011 National Survey on Drug Use and Health Services Administration. 2012. Available at http://www.samhsa.gov/data/sites/default/files/Revised2k11NSDUHSummNatFindings/Revised2k11NSDUHSummNatFindings/NSDUHresults2011.htm. Accessed on April 17, 2016.

Substance Abuse and Mental Health Services Administration/Center for Substance Abuse Treatment. Substance abuse among older adults. Treatment Improvement Protocol (TIP) Series 26. 1998. Available at http://www.ncbi.nlm.nih.gov/books/NBK64419/. Accessed on April 17, 2016.

United States Census Bureau. Table 12. Projections of the Population by Age and Sex for the United States: 2010 to 2050. (NP2008-T12), Population Division, U.S. Census Bureau; Release Date: August 14, 2008.

Wallace P, Cutler S, Haines A. Randomized controlled trial of general-practitioner intervention in patients with excessive alcohol consumption. *BMJ* 1988;297:663–668.

Weintraub E, Weintraub D, Dixon L, Delananty J, et al. Geriatric patients on a substance abuse consultation service. *Am J Geriatr Psychiatr* 2002;10(3):337–342.

Zimberg S. Diagnosis and management of the elderly alcoholic. In: Atkinson R, ed., *Alcohol and drug abuse in old age*. Washington, DC: American Psychiatric Press; 1984:24–33.

CHAPTER 2

# Recognizing Addiction in Older Patients

*Anna Levesque and Edward V. Nunes*

## Introduction

Substance use disorder (SUD) is often perceived as a problem affecting mainly adolescent or younger adults. However, its increasing prevalence in the geriatric population represents a significant public health concern (Simoni-Wastila et al. 2006, Han et al. 2009). Various factors, such as widowhood, divorce, isolation, poor health status, depression, and anxiety, may predispose older adults to initiate or to persist in using psychoactive substances (Taylor et al. 2012, Aira et al. 2008, Jinks et al. 1990, St. John et al. 2009, Brennan et al. 1990, Fink et al. 1996). According to the 2012 National Survey on Drug Use and Health (NSDUH), 2% of people 65 and older reported alcohol dependence or abuse (SAMHSA 2013a). In addition, nearly 22% of American older adults report using at least one psychoactive medication, and it is estimated that there will be a 100% increase in medication misuse between 2001 and 2020 in this population (1.2–2.4%) (Simoni-Wastila et al. 2005, Colliver et al. 2006). An increasing number of older patients report addiction treatment, and emergency department visits related to SUDs, further indicative of this growing problem (SAMHSA 2010). Although alcohol and psychoactive medication are the substances most frequently used among the elderly, the prevalence of illegal drug use is increasing with the aging of the baby-boomer generation, who are more likely than previous generations to bear the risk factor of having experimented with illicit drugs in their youth (Koechl et al. 2012).

Recognizing the signs of SUDs in elderly is not always easy, as they may manifest in subtle and confusing ways. Clinical indicators interpreted as warning signs of substance use in younger patients (for example, cognitive impairments, unsteadiness of gait, insomnia, or social isolation) are symptoms that may be indicative of other common medical or psychiatric problems frequently encountered among aging adults, making diagnosis more challenging (Mulinga 1999, Lang et al. 2007). Social stereotypes, such as the false assumption that older adults do not suffer from SUDs, may also contribute to misidentification of such conditions by decreasing suspicion by families and of healthcare providers (Naik et al. 1994). As a result, the problem often remains unrecognized by doctors and family members, preventing patients from receiving appropriate treatment. In addition, most clinical screening and diagnosis tools were designed and validated for younger populations and are not always adapted to the elderly, which also limits problem recognition (Aalto et al. 2011, .O'Connell et al. 2004, Graham 1986).

With age, metabolism of alcohol and other substances is slower, leading to higher blood levels and stronger effects. Pharmacodynamics of alcohol and other substances may also change with age. Misrecognition of SUDs in the elderly is especially concerning, given that older individuals are more vulnerable to suffering serious complications from their use. Concerns of family and friends are the most common causes for elderly patients seeking consultation for SUDs (Finlayson et al. 1988). Primary care providers also play a key role in the prevention, screening, and treatment of such disorders. Increasing families' and healthcare providers' awareness of the different ways SUDs can present in older adults could significantly improve health outcomes in this population.

DIAGNOSIS OF SUBSTANCE USE DISORDER

*The Diagnostic and Statistical Manual of Mental Disorders* (DSM) includes the criteria most widely used in North America to diagnose SUDs. In the fifth edition (DSM-5), "Substance Use Disorder" is defined as a problematic pattern of substance use leading to clinically significant impairment or distress, as manifested by two or more of the 11 criteria listed in Box 2.1, within a 12-month period (APA 2013). SUD is classified as mild, moderate, or severe according to the number of fulfilled criteria.

These criteria have lower sensitivity in geriatric populations, as some of the diagnostic criteria do not apply well to older patients (Blow et al. 2014). For example, metabolic changes associated with aging result in higher sensitivity to the effects of substances such as alcohol, benzodiazepine, and opioid following lower consumption amounts (Vogel-Sprott et al. 1984, Vestal et al. 1977, Atkinson 1990, Greenblatt et al. 1991, Greenblatt et al. 1982, Moore et al. 2007, Blow 1998). Hence, an older patient with a problematic pattern of substance consumption may not necessarily spend a great deal of time in activities related to substance use and may not develop tolerance or withdrawal, as

---

**Box 2.1  Diagnostic Criteria for Substance Use Disorder According to the 5th Edition of the DSM (APA 2013)**

1. The substance is often taken in larger amounts or over a longer period than was intended.
2. There is a persistent desire or unsuccessful efforts to cut down or control substance use.
3. A great deal of time is spent in activities necessary to obtain the substance, use the substance, or recover from its effects.
4. There is a craving, or a strong desire or urge, to use the substance.
5. Recurrent substance use results in a failure to fulfill major role obligations at work, school, or home.
6. Substance use is continued despite persistent or recurrent social or interpersonal problems caused or exacerbated by the effects of the substance.
7. Important social, occupational, or recreational activities are given up or reduced because of substance use.
8. There is recurrent substance use in situations in which it is physically hazardous.
9. There is continued substance use despite patient's knowledge of having a persistent or recurrent physical or psychological problem that is likely to have been caused or exacerbated by the substance.
10. Tolerance develops, as shown by a diminished effect when using the "usual" amount, or a need for increasing amounts to achieve the desired effect.
11. Withdrawal symptoms follow efforts to quit.

---

**Mild** = Two to three symptoms; **Moderate** = Four to five symptoms; **Severe** = Six or more symptoms

---

suggested in the DSM-5 criteria. For example, an older patient might present with a pattern of drinking that has not changed over the years, and that was not a problem when he was younger. Thus, there do not appear to be escalation of use, tolerance, withdrawal, or loss-of-control features. However, the patient may have substantial alcohol-related impairments (e.g., insomnia, gastrointestinal [GI] problems, or interpersonal problems) that might erroneously be attributed to other medical or psychiatric conditions. Also, the elderly may show fewer of the behavioral disturbances or social "red flags" typically found in younger adults with addictions (Graham 1986). Therefore, criteria regarding reduced activities and failure to fulfill obligations may not apply to retired patients with a decreased baseline level of daily activities. Alternative definitions, such as hazardous drinking and medication misuse, may be more helpful in identifying patients with less severe problematic patterns of substance use that do not fulfill SUD diagnostic criteria (Fink et al. 1986, WHO 1992, SAMHSA 2013b). Or, a patient may simply present with a medical condition (e.g., GI distress, insomnia) that is being caused or exacerbated by alcohol or another substance without a use disorder per se (e.g., if the patient is able to cut down or quit upon advice from the physician without difficulty).

## Alcohol

### NORMAL ALCOHOL METABOLISM

There are multiple pathways involved in alcohol metabolism, each of which creates metabolites that contribute to its toxicity. Alcohol is first metabolized into acetaldehyde, mainly by the enzyme alcohol dehydrogenase (ADH) located in the stomach and in the liver (Auty et al. 1977, Kaplowitz et al. 2007). To a lower extent in non-chronic users, enzymes from the cytochrome P4502E1 located in the liver are also involved in this reaction (Lieber 2004). The acetaldehyde generated from this first reaction is then metabolized into acetate through the action of acetaldehyde dehydrogenase (ALDH), an enzyme located in the liver.

Following its ingestion, alcohol metabolism starts in the stomach, where there is a significant amount of ADH (Auty et al. 1977). Remaining alcohol is slowly absorbed from the stomach, and then, more rapidly, from the small intestine. Once it enters the bloodstream, alcohol is directed throughout the portal vein to the liver, where the majority of the metabolism takes place. The first phase of alcohol metabolism that follows ingestion and absorption from the digestive system is called the *first-pass metabolism*, which eliminates about 10% of the absorbed alcohol (Weathermon et al. 1999). Residual alcohol from the first-pass metabolism is redistributed into the body and eventually returns to the liver, where metabolism is subsequently repeated. First-pass metabolism is less efficient in women, who have lower amounts of ADH in the stomach than men do, leading to higher levels of circulating alcohol following the ingestion of an equivalent amount (Frezza et al. 1990, Thomasson 1995).

### ALCOHOL METABOLISM IN THE ELDERLY

Aging modifies the metabolism and distribution of alcohol through different mechanisms, in addition to increasing the sensitivity of certain organs to its toxicity. Those physiological changes are clinically meaningful because they have an impact on clinical presentation, screening, diagnosis, and treatment of alcohol use disorder (AUD) in this population.

The amount of ADH enzymes in the stomach naturally decreases with aging (Seitz et al. 1993). Common medical conditions found among the elderly, such as atrophic gastritis and *Helicobacter pylori*, also reduce the amount of gastric ADH, as these conditions are associated with the reduction in the number of mucosal cells containing the enzymes (Thuluvath et al. 1994). The quantity of ADH is further compromised in older women, who already have a lower baseline gastric level of ADH than men (Frezza et al. 1990, Thomasson 1995). This decline in the available number of metabolic enzymes reduces first-pass metabolism efficacy, which in turn leads to higher blood alcohol levels compared to those in younger adults following an equivalent consumption. Reduced hepatic blood flow has been observed in older adults, but it is unclear whether or not it contributes to the decline of first-pass metabolism (Moore et al. 2007, Seitz et al. 2007, Durnas et al. 1990). Aging also causes an increase in the proportion of body fat and a decrease in the proportion of body water (Vogel-Sprott et al. 1984, Vestal et al. 1977). Given that alcohol is mostly distributed in the aqueous space, alcohol volume of distribution decreases with aging, hence increasing blood concentration (Vogel-Sprott et al. 1984, Vestal et al. 1977). Furthermore, increased central nervous system sensitivity to the effect of alcohol has been described among older adults (Moore et al. 2007). The cumulative effect of those changes may lead older adults to experience marked intoxication symptoms following the ingestion of amounts of alcohol that would be judged safe among younger adults, making the screening and the diagnosis of problematic alcohol use more challenging.

## CLINICAL PRESENTATION

Recognizing AUD in the elderly is particularly challenging because many of the associated symptoms are similar to those of other medical conditions frequently encountered among older adults. In addition, alcohol intake may exacerbate preexisting health problems or contribute to the onset of common diseases in the elderly population (Moore et al. 2007). Hence, it is essential for clinicians to maintain a high level of suspicion when assessing older adults, as symptoms evocative of AUD can easily be confused with common geriatric conditions. Screening for AUD should be performed when older patients present with deterioration of a chronic disease, new onset of a condition potentially associated with alcohol use, deterioration or new onset of a cognitive or a psychiatric disorder, or decreased effectiveness of a pharmacological treatment (Moore et al. 2007, Caputo et al. 2012). In the following paragraphs, different possible clinical presentations of AUD among the elderly will be discussed.

Heavy alcohol intake has toxic effects on different organs of the digestive system. It is estimated that about 90–100% of chronic heavy drinkers eventually develop alcoholic fatty liver, 30% develop alcoholic steatohepatitis, and 10–20% ultimately develop cirrhosis (Meier et al. 2008). Given certain modifications in alcohol distribution and metabolism, older adults are more likely to suffer from alcoholic liver disease (ALD) and to experience complications such as portal hypertension, ascites, and esophageal varices (Seitz et al. 2007, Potter et al. 1987). Although the clinical presentation of ALD is similar to that encountered in a younger population, older adults more frequently report general malaise and anorexia (Woodhouse et al. 1985). The risk of upper GI bleeding is higher among older alcohol users, given the lower number of parietal cells associated with aging, a change that predisposes them to gastritis and ulcers (Menninger 2002). Furthermore, AUD is a common cause of acute and chronic pancreatitis, chronic diarrhea, and electrolyte imbalances (Bode et al. 2003, Kristiansen et al. 2008).

Consumption of large quantities of alcohol can lead to malnutrition, including primarily depletion of folic acid, vitamin B-6 (pyridoxine) and vitamin B-1 (thiamine), due to poor dietary intake and decreased nutrient absorption (Bode et al. 2003, Cabre et al. 2001, Fonda et al. 1989, Vech et al. 1975). Folic acid deficiency is found among 60–80% of alcoholics and can cause macrocytic anemia and intestinal malabsorption (Markowitz et al. 2000). There are rare complications of pyridoxine depletion, including peripheral neuropathy, stomatitis, glossitis, cheilosis, irritability, confusion, and depression (Markowitz et al. 2000, Cook et al. 1997). Deficiencies in thiamine occur in 30–80% of chronic drinkers and can lead to peripheral neuropathies, cardiomyopathies, and Wernicke-Korsakoff syndrome (Markowitz et al. 2000, Thomson et al. 1987). A triad of oculomotor abnormalities, ataxia, and delirium is characteristic of Wernicke's encephalopathy. If it remains untreated, this condition can progress to Korsakoff's syndrome, a dementia that is characterized by anterograde and retrograde amnesia and confabulation. Data on the role of alcohol in the development of dementia are mixed (Moriyama et al. 2006). The prevalence of dementia is estimated to be five times higher among the elderly with chronic alcohol use than among non-drinkers (Caputo et al. 2012). Also, about 25% of people with dementia have a comorbid AUD (Oslin et al. 1998). A direct neurotoxic effect of alcohol is thought to be associated with brain atrophy and overall cognitive impairments, although this concept remains under debate (Moriyama et al. 2006). Aging reduces the number of brain cells in the basal ganglia, the neocortex, the reticular activating system, and the hippocampus—leading to higher risk of delirium during intoxication or withdrawal from alcohol (Menninger 2002). In the clinical context of acute confusion in the elderly, it is important to consider delirium tremens among the differential diagnosis, as it is a potentially life-threatening condition.

Although light alcohol intake has been shown to have some cardiovascular benefits (Ronksley et al. 2011), chronic heavy drinking can deleteriously impact various risk factors of cardiovascular disease, increasing risk for hypertension, glucose metabolism abnormalities, and truncal obesity with increased waist circumference (Caputo et al. 2012). Older adults suffering from AUD are also at higher risk of stroke and of dilated cardiomyopathy, which may lead to ventricular dysfunction and heart failure (Piano 2002).

Alcohol use also impacts the endocrine system, notably through alterations in the hypothalamic-pituitary axis (Caputo et al. 2012). High cortisol levels have been described among chronic alcohol users, causing pseudo-Cushing syndrome, whose clinical presentation is hardly distinguishable from that of the primary form of Cushing (Newell-Price et al. 2006). Alcohol also inhibits antidiuretic hormone, which leads to increased diuresis that can exacerbate or cause incontinence problems (Menninger 2002). In addition, AUD is associated with poorer control of diabetes, and it may also increase risk of hypoglycemia due to an inhibition of gluconeogenesis (Moore et al. 2007, O'Keefe et al. 1997, Yki-Jarvinen et al. 1988).

AUD is a significant risk factor for accidents, falls, and bone fractures in the geriatric population (Caputo et al. 2012). Consequences of drinking such as confusion, ataxia, balance problems, orthostatic hypotension, neuropathies, and myopathies predispose patients to accidents and falls (Moore et al. 2007, Blow 1998). In addition, lower bone density is common among older patients with AUD, especially when it is combined with other risk factors for osteoporosis (i.e., tobacco smoking), leading to increased risks of fractures (Bikle et al. 1985, Israel et al. 1990).

Alcohol is a dose-dependent risk factor for the development of multiple tumors, including those of the oropharynx, larynx, esophagus, liver, colon, rectum, prostate, and breast (Thun et al. 1997, Zhu et al. 2014, Gong et al. 2009). Chronic alcohol consumption also significantly reduces the level of T and B lymphocytes, leading to an increased susceptibility to infectious diseases (Girard et al. 1987). Bacterial pneumonia or reactivation of latent tuberculosis can be consequences of a decline in the immune system. Finally, alcohol consumption in the elderly often leads to suboptimal control of chronic diseases such as hypertension, diabetes, gout, or epilepsy because of poor compliance with treatment and directly deleterious effects of alcohol on these diseases (Moore et al. 2007, Blow 1998, Kerr et al. 1990).

## PSYCHIATRIC COMORBIDITIES

Older adults with any SUD have high rates of comorbid psychiatric disorders, estimated between 21% and 66% (Blow et al. 2014). Predominant psychiatric diagnoses in the elderly are depressive disorders, generalized anxiety disorder, alcohol dependence, dementia, and bipolar disorders (Seby et al. 2011). SUD and mental health disorders have a dynamic effect on one another, as substance use increases the risk of experiencing symptoms of mental illness, which in turn can lead to substance use as a form of self-medication (USDHHS 2010). In addition, both SUD and other mental illnesses can be caused by overlapping factors such as genetic vulnerabilities and early exposure to trauma (USDHHS 2010).

Many seniors report drinking in response to psychosocial triggers such as loneliness or depressed mood (Schonfeld et al. 1991). Depression is not a normal consequence of aging, and it is a frequently missed diagnosis in the geriatric population, given atypical presentations that are often confused with comorbid health problems such as cognitive impairment (Steffens et al. 2000, Koenig et al. 1992). Risk factors for depression in the elderly include female gender, social isolation, widowhood, divorce, low socioeconomic status, medical comorbidities, chronic pain, functional impairment, and cognitive impairment (Cole et al. 2003). Chronic drinking negatively affects mood, and depressed patients have been found to improve their mood after they stop drinking, compared to patients who continue to drink (Caputo et al. 2012). In addition, studies in adults demonstrated that AUD increases the risk of suicide (Hall et al. 1999). When combined, alcohol, depression, and anxiety disorders are responsible for about 70% of cases of suicide in the elderly (Caputo et al. 2012).

Sleep disorders may also lead to the development of late-onset AUD and may cause relapse in abstinent former drinkers (Blow 1998). Alcohol can temporarily facilitate falling asleep, but this effect rapidly fades with chronic use (Roehrs et al. 2001). Hence, long-term alcohol intake may cause difficulty falling asleep and decrease the ability to remain asleep (Blow 1998). Sleep disorder that is related to alcohol is a common clinical presentation. The sedative effects of alcohol facilitate falling asleep, but as the alcohol blood level decreases, there is a rebound of arousal and anxiety, resulting in waking in the middle of the night (middle insomnia). In this setting, cessation of alcohol can significantly improve sleep.

## COMBINATION OF ALCOHOL WITH MEDICATION

It is estimated that 19% of the Americans aged 65 or older occasionally combine medication and alcohol, which can potentially lead to dangerous interactions and suboptimal treatment of medical conditions (Substance Abuse and Mental Health Services Administration [SAMHSA] 2013). The metabolism of alcohol as well as multiple prescription drugs involves a microsomal enzyme from the cytochrome P4502E1 (CYP2E1) located in the liver. CYP2E1 contributes to the metabolism of barbiturates, warfarin, phenytoin, some narcotics, some benzodiazepines, propranolol, acetaminophen, isoniazid, phenylbutazone, methotrexate, tolbutamide, isoniazid, and HAART drugs (Moore et al. 2007). Among occasional drinkers, concomitant use of alcohol with these drugs creates a competition for metabolism, which slows down their elimination. The subsequent rise in the blood concentration of the medication can lead to adverse reactions and drug toxicity. In contrast, chronic alcohol consumption increases the amount of CYP2E1 enzyme in the liver, which then accelerates the metabolism of those drugs (Seitz et al. 2007). This enhanced metabolism often reduces the therapeutic efficacy of the drugs. It can also lead to hepatotoxicity through the accumulation of harmful metabolites. This is the case with acetaminophen, isoniazid, phenylbutazone, and methotrexate, which should be prescribed very cautiously in patients with AUD (Moore et al. 2007).

Moreover, alcohol can exacerbate adverse effects from certain pharmacological treatments. For example, combining alcohol intake with ASA, nonsteroidal anti-inflammatory drugs (NSAIDs), or clopidogrel (an inhibitor of platelet receptors used to prevent clotting) increases the risk of GI bleeding (DeSchepper et al. 1978, Deykin et al. 1982). Symptomatic hypotensive episodes can be a consequence of combining alcohol with anti-hypertensive medication (Lieber 1991). Also, sedation and confusion can occur when combining alcohol with psychoactive medications such as benzodiazepines, antihistamines, sedatives, antidepressants, anticonvulsants, muscle relaxants, or barbiturates (Moore et al. 2007, Linnoila et al. 1990, Adams 1995). Finally, patients using alcohol with certain antibiotics inhibiting the aldehyde dehydrogenase (ALDH) (aldehyde dehydrogenase) enzyme in the liver (e.g., certain cephalosporins), may experience a reaction of flushing, nausea, and vomiting secondary to a toxic accumulation of acetaldehyde (Kitson 1987).

## LABORATORY FINDINGS

Medical assessments of older adults often include a thorough physical examination, laboratory testing, and other forms of diagnostic studies. Different incidental findings can be suggestive of chronic alcohol consumption and may help orient the diagnosis toward AUD. In addition, certain laboratory test-ing can be used as adjunctive screening tools for AUD, although the primary screening tool remains self-report (Babor et al. 1989, Maisto et al. 1985).

Several anomalies can be found in the complete blood count (CBC) of chronic alcohol users. Macrocytosis, an increase in the mean corpuscular volume (MCV) of the red blood cells, can develop after a sustained intake of 80 grams of alcohol per day (Bode et al. 2003, Girard et al. 1987, Savage et al. 1986). Before concluding that macrocytosis is due to alcohol intake, it is important to rule out other possible causes, such as vitamin $B_{12}$ and folate deficiencies, liver problems, hypothyroidism, myelodysplastic syndrome, and the use of certain medications. However, the presence of liver disease and of low $B_{12}$ and folate levels does not exclude a concomitant AUD, as these are common complications of chronic alcohol use. Anemia is another common consequence of chronic alcohol use and can result from direct alco-hol toxicity or from alcohol-related complications, such as liver disease, GI bleeding, and vitamin $B_{12}$ and folate deficiencies (Girard et al. 1987, Savage et al. 1986).Moreover, alcohol is the most common cause of thrombocyto-penia (decreased platelets count), which is found in up to 80% of alcoholic patients (Girard et al. 1987(Girard et al. 1987). Thrombocytopenia can be a consequence of direct alcohol toxicity or of complications from chronic alcohol use such as hypersplenism caused by liver cirrhosis. Alcohol-induced thrombocytopenia rarely reaches platelet levels lower than 10,000/microL. Leukopenia is observed in about 8% of hospitalized alcoholic patients (Girard et al. 1987).

Certain findings on liver function tests may also be suggestive of AUD. Aspartate aminotransferase (AST) and alanine aminotransferase (ALT) el-evation may indicate hepatocellular destruction from alcohol toxicity. As for gamma-glutamyl transferase (GGT), it may reach levels up to 300–1000 IU/L in chronic drinkers (Cohen 1988). Albumin deficiency, increased bilirubin, and elevated international normalized ratio (INR), a measure of clotting time, can result from liver dysfunction, reflecting a more advanced stage of the dis-ease. The prevalence of albumin depletion increases with aging and is found in about 17% of the elderly with alcohol dependence, compared to 3% of younger adults with alcohol dependence (Caputo et al. 2012).

Electrolyte disorders are also common findings among patients suffering from AUD. Loss of appetite, vomiting, reduced water intake, and decreased water and sodium absorption in the intestine predispose drinkers to hypo-natremia and dehydration (Bode et al. 2003). Furthermore, deficiencies in calcium, magnesium, and phosphorus may result from decreased intake and malabsorption (Knochel 1977, Leevy et al. 2005).

AST, MCV, GGT and carbohydrate-deficient transferrin (CDT) have been proposed as useful biomarkers for AUD screening (Table 2.1). Due to its low specificity, AST is a poor screening tool when used alone (Allen et al. 2003). However, it can be meaningful when combined with ALT, since a ratio of AST/ALT greater than 2 is rarely found in other pathologies than AUD, hence strongly suggesting this diagnosis. AST quickly returns to normal levels following sobriety, which makes it an interesting tool to assess relapse in chronic drinkers. Alcohol-related AST elevation increases with aging, with abnormal levels found in 56% of older chronic drinkers compared to 42% of those under 65 (Caputo et al. 2012).

MCV increases with chronic heavy alcohol intake. MCV is moderately useful in AUD screening as it has a rather low sensitivity. Given the long lifespan of a red blood cell, MCV can remain elevated up to four months after initiation of sobriety, which makes it a poor tool to detect relapse (Mundle et al. 1999). Increased MCV levels are found in about 44% of older adults with

*Table 2.1*  **Characteristics of Different Biomarkers Used to Screen for Alcohol Use Disorders**

| Biomarker* | Return to normal levels in abstinence | Advantages | Disadvantages | Effect of aging |
|---|---|---|---|---|
| **AST** | 7 days | Good indicator of relapse<br><br>Easily available | Low specificity (improved when combined to ALT) | Increases the prevalence of abnormal results |
| **MCV** | 4 months | Easily available | Low sensitivity | Increases the prevalence of abnormal results |
| **GGT** | 2–6 weeks | High sensitivity<br><br>Easily available | Low specificity | Not affected |
| **CDT** | 2–4 weeks | High specificity | Poor availability | Not affected |

Modified from Allen et al. 2004.

*AST = aspartate transferase; MCV = mean corpuscular volume; GGT = gamma-glutamyl transferase; CDT = carbohydrate-deficient transferrin.

alcohol dependence, compared to a prevalence of 17% among their younger counterparts (Caputo et al. 2012).

Among all tests, GGT has the best sensitivity to detect AUD. Increased levels of GGT are found in approximately 75% of persons diagnosed with alcohol dependence, and it can remain elevated for two to six weeks after a return to sobriety (Allen et al. 2003). GGT has a low specificity for AUD, and elevated levels can be found in a wide variety of medical conditions, including obstructive liver disease, pancreatic disease, chronic obstructive pulmonary disease, and diabetes. The use of certain medications such as phenytoin and barbiturates can also lead to increased GGT levels.

When used as a single marker, CDT is the most informative laboratory screening tool, with a sensitivity of 60–70% and a specificity of 80–90% (Allen et al. 2003, Mundle et al. 1999). Abnormal levels of CDT develop following consumption of approximately 60 g of alcohol per day for two to three weeks and typically return to normal after two to four weeks of abstinence (Allen et al. 2003). Combining CDT with GGT offers an optimal screening capacity with a sensitivity of 90% and a specificity of 80–90% (Mundle et al. 1999). Neither CDT nor GGT is influenced by aging (Mundle et al. 1999). Unfortunately, CDT is still not usually available in routine clinical practice, although it has been used as a research tool to provide an objective measure of alcohol-use outcome to complement self-report. It is important to remember that, although biomarkers can be helpful to orient a diagnosis, they cannot be used to rule out an alcohol problem, as a substantial proportion of patients with AUD do not present these findings.

## RECOMMENDATIONS AND DIAGNOSIS

Older adults are more vulnerable to deleterious consequences of alcohol consumption. Thus, the National Institute on Alcohol Abuse and Alcoholism (NIAAA) proposed specific drinking guidelines for adults over 65 years old, recommending a maximum of seven drinks per week, with no more than three drinks on any single occasion (NIAAA 1995, NIAAA 2014). A Consensus Panel endorsed the limit of seven drinks per week and recommended a stricter maximum of two drinks on any single occasion (Blow 1998). These amounts should possibly be further reduced for women and in the case of concomitant medication use (Blow 1998). Given that 60–78% of older adults are estimated to take one or more prescription or non-prescription medications, the safe quantity of alcohol consumption for older adults should be determined on a case-by-case basis (Chrischilles et al. 1992).

Some of the diagnostic criteria proposed by the DSM-5 (see Box 2.1) are not applicable to older adults, who are less likely to experience some of the biological, psychological, and social consequences frequently encountered in younger adults with AUD (Blow et al. 2014, Atkinson 1990, Blow 1998). This lack of relevance of some diagnostic criteria to the geriatric population represents a barrier to appropriate diagnosis of certain individuals who do not meet a diagnostic threshold, despite potentially harmful drinking practices. The concept of *hazardous drinking*, defined as a potentially harmful pattern of drinking that can precipitate or exacerbate medical conditions, complicate treatments, and cause adverse reactions to drugs, may be more appropriate in older adults (Fink et al. 1996, SAMHSA 2013, Fink et al. 2002). Hence, when screening for alcohol problems in the elderly, it is important that clinicians not limit their diagnostic consideration to AUD as defined by the DSM-5, but also keep in mind the possibility of less severe types of problematic drinking patterns that also require interventions, such as hazardous drinking.

## SCREENING

Screening for AUD should be part of older adults' annual medical examination. Since problematic drinking can emerge between annual assessments, it is also recommended to screen elders reporting any symptoms suggestive of problematic drinking, in addition to those facing significant life transitions such as a bereavement or separation (Blow 1998). The screening process should begin with a few brief pre-screening questions to quickly rule out individuals for whom further assessment is not required. Pre-screening can start by asking the following question: "Do you drink alcohol, including beer, wine, or distilled spirits?" Patients answering affirmatively should be asked the three following questions:

1. On average, how many days per week do you drink alcohol?
2. On a typical day when you drink, how many drinks do you have?
3. What is the maximum number of drinks you had on any given occasion during the last month? (NIAAA 1995)

Individuals whose alcohol intake exceeds NIAAA or experts panel recommendations (i.e., more than seven drinks per week or more than two or three drinks on any single occasion), those taking medications that can potentially interact with alcohol, and those with medical or psychiatric comorbidities that may be exacerbated by alcohol intake should undergo further screening.

Several self-reported tools have been developed to screen patients for possible AUD. Although most screening tools were initially tested among younger adults, some were validated specifically in geriatric populations. The CAGE (4-item questionnaire; an acronym for these questions, as detailed below), the Alcohol Use Disorders Identification Test (AUDIT), the Michigan Alcoholism Screening Test–Geriatric (MAST-G) and its shortened version, the SMAST-G, are the four main instruments used among older patients (Ewing 1984, Blow et al. 1992, Saunders et al. 1993). Results from psychometric studies assessing the performance of those screening instruments in older populations vary widely, according to factors such as clinical setting, cultural elements, patient characteristics, and the prevalence of AUD in study populations (O'Connell et al. 2004).

The CAGE questionnaire is the screening tool most frequently used in adults, with the advantages of being simple to administer and easy to memorize as an acronym for the questionnaire is based on the content of the following four questions:

1. Have you felt the need to **C**ut down on your drinking?
2. Have people **A**nnoyed you by criticizing your drinking?
3. Have you ever felt **G**uilty about drinking?
4. Have you ever felt you needed a drink first thing in the morning (**E**ye-opener) to steady your nerves or to get rid of a hangover? (Ewing 1984)

The full questionnaire can be administered in less than a minute, and it can be formulated either to detect lifetime or recent and current AUD (Ewing 1984). In younger adults, a positive response to two or more questions is suggestive of problematic alcohol consumption and requires a more in-depth assessment. The CAGE is less sensitive in the geriatric population, and using a cut-off of one positive answer increases the instrument's sensitivity, at the expense of decreasing its specificity (Conigliaro et al. 2000). Median sensitivity and specificities of 66.5% and 89% were drawn from validation studies conducted in different geriatric populations and using a cut-off of two yesses (O'Connell et al. 2004). Buchsbaum and colleagues have demonstrated that decreasing the cut-off to one affirmative response yielded a sensitivity of 86% and specificity of 78% (Buchsbaum et al. 1992).

The MAST-G is a 24-item questionnaire following a yes/no format that can be administered in approximately five minutes. It was developed to detect AUD specifically in elderly patients (Blow et al. 1992). Positive answers to five questions or more leads to AUD detection with high estimated sensitivity (50–95%) and specificity (78–96%) (O'Connell et al. 2004, Blow et al. 2014). The SMAST-G is a shorten version containing ten questions that can be administered in approximately three minutes, with a score of 2 or more suggesting AUD (Blow et al. 1998). Both versions were found to be robust screening instruments in the elderly population (O'Connell et al. 2004).

The AUDIT is a ten-item questionnaire that can be administered in less than five minutes to detect individuals with hazardous and harmful drinking (Saunders et al. 1993). This screening tool includes three questions addressing the quantity and the frequency of drinking, and seven questions assessing specific AUD criteria in addition to consequences of alcohol consumption. A maximal score of 40 points can be obtained, and a cut-off of eight or more positive answers is used to detect unhealthy drinking among adult populations (Reinert et al. 2007). This instrument is less sensitive among the elderly, as it uses recommendations made for younger adults in term of safe amounts of drinking. It also considers the patient's capacity to fulfill social responsibilities that may not correspond to older adult's realities. Thus, a cut-off of five or more positive answers has been suggested in the geriatric population to obtain both sensitivity and specificity of greater than 85% (Aalto et al. 2011).

All those instruments are valid choices to detect alcohol problems in the geriatric population. However, while the CAGE, the MAST-G, and the SMAST-G questionnaires are useful for detecting more severe alcohol problems, they may fail to identify moderate drinkers whose medical, social, or psychiatric condition may be affected by small amounts of alcohol. A questionnaire such as the AUDIT, using a decreased cut-off score, is a useful tool for identifying hazardous drinking among older adults. When the diagnosis remains unclear, it may be necessary to assess the consequences of alcohol use more extensively, taking into accounts the patient's medication, comorbid health conditions, and psychosocial situation. It can also be helpful to gather additional information from relatives, especially for patients with poor insight or impaired cognitive functioning. Finally, the use of biomarkers in combination with self-report screening may help diagnose AUD with accuracy (Kalapatapu et al. 2010).

## PATTERNS OF ALCOHOL USE DISORDER

Two different patterns of AUD, defined as *early* or *late onset*, have been identified and are associated with different patient characteristics. Patients with early onset AUD start experiencing problem drinking at a younger age and maintain a disrupted pattern of alcohol consumption as they grow older. This category accounts for about two-thirds of the elderly suffering from AUD and is more frequently associated with psychiatric comorbidities and with a family history of alcoholism (Liberto et al. 1995). Physical comorbidities such as severe liver damage are also more common in this groups, as these individuals are exposed to toxic effects of alcohol over prolonged periods of time (Liberto et al. 1995). Patients with late-onset AUD develop problematic drinking behaviors later in their life, often in response to a major stressor event such as a retirement, a divorce, a death, or a change in health status (Liberto et al. 1995, Hurt et al. 1988, Finlayson et al. 1988). Overall, these patients tend to have a higher education and socioeconomic levels and to have better general health condition than those with early onset AUD. They also tend to have less severe AUD, associated with better prognoses when adequately identified and treated (Blow 1998, Liberto et al. 1995). However, recognizing patients suffering from late-onset AUD is more challenging, as they often present with fewer and less severe symptoms, which may lead to missed diagnosis and inadequate management (Blow 1998). Hence, it is important for clinicians to maintain high levels of suspicion toward subtle symptoms potentially suggestive of AUD, especially when assessing elders facing significant life stressors.

## Prescription Medications

Medication misuse is a significant problem among the elderly, partly explained by their high exposure to prescription psychoactive drugs. It is estimated that 25% of older adults take at least one psychoactive medication with a potential for abuse (Simoni-Wastila et al. 2006). Elders also tend to have taken psychoactive drugs over longer periods of time than their younger counterparts, which increases the risk of misuse (SAMHSA 2013). Medication misuse can consist in following inappropriate directions for use (i.e., dose, frequency, duration, indication) or in combining the medication with other drugs, potentially leading to adverse effects or interactions. Medication misuse in the elderly is often unintentional. It can result from a patient's misunderstanding of proper intake directions or from a provider's inadequate prescription, such as psychoactive medication prescribed over a too long period of time or to treat a problem for which it is not recommended (SAMHSA 2013). Unfortunately, unintended medication misuse can progress to an SUD, as defined by the DSM-5. Older women with poorer health conditions are at higher risk of developing a problematic pattern of medication use (Blow 1998).

Prescribing psychoactive substances to older patients should be done very carefully. Providers should regularly reassess the treatment indication and verify that patients are following proper directions of use. They should also avoid prolonging treatments past the necessary and recommended periods of time. Fortunately, most states have a database informing clinicians about the combination of controlled medications prescribed for every single patient. As most potentially addictive medications are included in those databases, they represent important screening tools and should be consulted every time a clinician writes a prescription for a controlled medication. To rule out dangerous combinations of drugs, it is also recommended to contact pharmacies and different providers involved in a patient's care to obtain a complete list of medications and to better coordinate treatment. Finally, communication with relatives can be very useful, especially in cases of patients suffering from cognitive impairment.

## BENZODIAZEPINES

Quality of sleep decreases with age, and insomnia is a complaint reported by up to 40% of adults aged 65 and older (Alessi et al. 2011). Aging modifies the natural architecture of sleep, decreases total deep sleep time, and increases the number of awakenings (Ohayon et al. 2004, Haimov et al. 1997, Feinsilver et al. 1993). Anxiety is also a common problem reported by the elderly, and it may be exacerbated by different life stressors associated with aging. Together, insomnia and anxiety represent 95% of the reasons for benzodiazepine prescriptions in the elderly (Blow 1998). Sedatives are the prescription medications most frequently misused in the geriatric population, with a prevalence of intake estimated between 20% and 25% among North American community-dwelling older adults (Voyer et al. 2010, Voyer et al. 2009). A Canadian study of 2,785 randomly selected adults aged 65 and older found a rate of benzodiazepine dependence around 9.5%, defined according to the DSM-IV criteria (Voyer et al. 2010). Similar results were found among 140 patients attending a psychogeriatric clinic, with a benzodiazepine dependence rate of 11.4% (Holroyd et al. 1997).

Benzodiazepines are very effective for treating anxiety and insomnia when used intermittently or regularly over short periods of time. However, tolerance to all effects of benzodiazepines can develop following prolonged regular use, at variable rates and to different degrees. Tolerance to the hypnotic effect tends to develop more rapidly than to the anxiolytic effect (Schneider-Helmert 1988). In many cases, benzodiazepines are used over prolonged periods of time to suppress anxiety and insomnia induced by withdrawal states (Longo et al. 2000).

Older adults are particularly vulnerable to the cognitive and psychomotor effects of benzodiazepines (Pomara et al. 1985, Reidenberg et al. 1978, Pomara et al. 1984). Given the increased proportion of body fat associated with aging, lipid-soluble drugs such as benzodiazepines have a larger volume of distribution, which leads to a longer effect of the medication and to higher risk of substance accumulation and intoxication (Greenblatt et al. 1991, Moore et al. 2007). In addition, the hepatic oxidative metabolic pathways involved in most benzodiazepine metabolism are often impaired in older adults. The use of short-acting benzodiazepines that are metabolized through glucuronidation rather than through the liver oxidative pathway, such as oxazepam and loraz-epam, is safer among elders as it decreases the risk of medication accumulation leading to adverse reactions.

Identifying sedative misuse is challenging, as the clinical presentation is often subtle and there is no consensus regarding diagnosis definition (Rouleau et al. 2003, Reid et al. 1997). As for other substances, the diagnosis of "Sedative Use Disorder" proposed by the DSM-5 possibly lacks sensitivity among the elderly (Blow et al. 2014). Some authors have proposed definitions of benzodiazepine misuse that target prolonged use rather than symptoms of addiction (Rouleau et al. 2003, Whitcup et al. 1987, Morgan et al. 1988). The length corresponding to prolonged use of benzodiazepine has been defined as varying between 30 and 135 days, according to different authors (Egan et al. 2000, Tamblyn et al. 1994).

Risk factors for developing sedative misuse include older age, female gender, polymedication, and comorbid physical and mental illnesses (Llorente et al. 2000). Multiple psychiatric, cognitive, and physical symptoms can be suggestive of benzodiazepine misuse. The combined sedative and muscle re-laxant effects of benzodiazepines can lead to decreased motor coordination and ataxia, increasing the risk of falls and fractures (Rouleau et al. 2003, Leipzig et al. 1999). Anterograde amnesia, confusion, and delirium are fre-quent consequences of benzodiazepine use in the elderly (Rouleau et al. 2003, Larson et al. 1999, Foy et al. 1995). Sedative-induced cognitive impairment may closely mimic symptoms of dementia. Although it has been shown that benzodiazepine intake can worsen symptoms of preexisting dementia such as Alzheimer's disease, data are mixed regarding the possible causal effect of ben-zodiazepines on the development of dementia (Bedard 2003).

Withdrawal from benzodiazepines can be very distressing and potentially dangerous. It is important to recognize patients who are physically dependent on benzodiazepines, and to avoid their sudden discontinuation. For exam-ple, when older patients are hospitalized for medical conditions or following surgeries, clinicians should be careful to maintain standing doses of benzo-diazepines when patients have been taking benzodiazepines for a prolonged period of time. Symptoms of withdrawal include restlessness, anxiety, insom-nia, irritability, tremors, GI upset, increased heart rate, increased blood pres-sure and body temperature, and in more extreme cases, delirium and seizure (Blow et al. 2014).

Patients receiving benzodiazepine prescriptions should have regular visits in order to reassess the need for such pharmacotherapy and to verify proper medication use. Efforts should be made to try alternative approaches, such as cognitive-behavioral therapy for sleep, and an antidepressant for anxiety and depression. Importantly, patients should be educated about the risks of chronic benzodiazepine use and participate in an informed decision-making process with their physician.

## OPIATES

Chronic pain is common among aging patients. For example, it has been estimated that persistent pain affects up to 50% of nursing home residents aged 65 and older (Won et al. 2004). Long-term opiate analgesia is generally not a first-line option for management of chronic, non-malignant pain. However, it is also recognized that it may be a valuable therapeutic modality in some cases of persistent non-cancer pain, especially when alternative approaches such as physical therapy, physical activity, and co-analgesic medication (e.g., acetaminophen, NSAIDs, antidepressants, or anti-seizure medication) are either insufficient or contraindicated (Stewart et al. 2012). In such case, patients may benefit from chronic opioid analgesic treatment, and clinicians should monitor them closely for signs of dose escalation or adverse effects.

Similarly to benzodiazepines, opiate use in the elderly is rarely hidden, as these medications are generally obtained legally through physician prescriptions (Kalapatapu et al. 2010). Older adults are more sensitive to the effects of opioids, and they are more likely to experience adverse reactions, even with small doses of medication (Blow 1998). Such adverse effects of opioid use include sedation, constipation, nausea, impaired balance, hyperalgesia, cognitive impairment, delirium, and respiratory depression. Opioid withdrawal may present with restlessness, dysphoria, nausea, vomiting, muscle aches, tearing, yawning, diarrhea, fever, and insomnia.

Aberrant behaviors such as escalating doses, early requests for medication refills, and seeking prescriptions from multiple doctors are highly suggestive of medication misuse. However, it is important to distinguish pseudo-addiction (the adoption of aberrant behavior secondary to poorly controlled pain) from a true addiction (Kalapatapu et al. 2010). Indeed, it is expected that patients with unrelieved pain may increase their analgesic use and ask for more medication in order to decrease their suffering. Discerning between these two clinical scenarios is not always easy, and different tools have been developed to help detect opioid use disorder among patients with persistent pain (see Table 2.2).

## ILLICIT DRUGS

Little information is available regarding illicit substances' use in the elderly. Only recently, as this problem has become more apparent with the aging of the baby boom generation, has more attention been focused on screening and

*Table 2.2* **Examples of Screening Tools in the Assessment of Opioid Abuse in Patients with Persistent Pain**

| Screening Tool Name | Length | Time | Assessment |
|---|---|---|---|
| Pain Assessment and Documentation Tool (PADT) (Passik et al. 2004) | 41 items | 10 minutes | Assesses patients' progress and response to opioid treatment for chronic pain. |
| Prescription Drug Use Questionnaire (PDUQ) (Compton et al. 1998) | 42 items | 20 minutes | Identifies opioid abuse and dependence in chronic pain patients. |
| Screener and Opioid Assessment for Patients with Pain (SOAPP) (Akbik et al. 2006) | 14 items | 8 minutes | Helps determine the level of monitoring a chronic opioid patient may require. |
| Current Opioid Misuse Measure (COMM) (Butler et al. 2007) | 17 items | 10 minutes | Identifies aberrant behaviors associated with misuse of opioid medications. |
| Opioid Risk Tool (ORT) (Webster et al. 2005) | 10 items | 1 minute | Assesses the risk to develop aberrant opioid-related behaviors based on known risk factors for abuse and dependence. |

Table modified from Kalapatapu et al., 2010.

intervention in the elderly (Dinitt et al. 2011). Cannabis—marijuana—is the illicit drug most frequently used in the geriatric population (Colliver et al. 2006, Dinitto et al. 2011). It is estimated that the number of American adults aged 50 years and older using illegal drugs will reach 3.5 million in 2020, including 3.3 million cannabis users (Colliver et al. 2006). Those numbers may be underestimated, as older people have a greater tendency to under-report illicit substance use (Rockett et al. 2006).

Despite the favorable effect of cannabis to stimulate appetite among cancer patients, and a few putative health benefits such as pain reduction and anti-epileptic properties, cannabis use can also lead to several adverse medical consequences. For example, chronic cannabis use can cause cognitive deficits that can mimic or exacerbate cognitive impairments associated with aging (Taylor et al. 2012). Sustained cannabis use can also cause or exacerbate anxiety disorders (Williamson et al. 2000). Smoked cannabis irritates the airways and is associated with increased respiratory symptoms that can exacerbate or mimic chronic obstructive pulmonary disease (COPD), including cough, sputum production, and wheezing (Tetrault et al. 2007). In addition, smoked cannabis contains numerous carcinogens that possibly predispose to lung cancer (Wu et al. 1988, Sridhar et al. 1994). Importantly, cannabis intoxication increases pulse and cardiac output, which may pose risks for cardiovascular events in older patients with coronary artery disease (Ghuran et al. 2000, Jones 2002). Factors associated with cannabis use in the elderly include a level of education less than completion of high school, a past history of other illegal substance use, and cannabis use before the age of 16 (Colliver et al. 2006).

Although most older cocaine users have a past history of cocaine use disorder in younger age, some case reports have described individuals with no history of SUD who started using cocaine in later life (Kausch 2002). A study comparing patterns of consumption between older and younger cocaine users found no difference in the amount of cocaine used according to age (Kalapatapu et al. 2011). This finding is worrying, as older adults may be at higher risk of severe complications of cocaine use. It is well known that cocaine increases the risks of cardiomyopathy, arrhythmia, stroke, coronary artery aneurysm formation, aortic dissection, and myocardial ischemia or infarction, which are particularly dangerous for elders already suffering of comorbid cardiovascular problems (Schwartz et al. 2010, Maraj et al. 2010). In addition, imaging studies have identified more white-matter lesions among older cocaine users than in younger individuals, which could possibly explain the increased incidence of cognitive deficits seen among older individuals chronically using cocaine (Bartzokis et al. 1999).

## Conclusion

In conclusion, like younger patients, older adults are vulnerable to SUDs. Aging affects the pharmacokinetics and pharmacodynamics of alcohol and other addictive drugs in such a way as to create vulnerabilities that are unique to the geriatric population. As the general population ages, clinicians will see older patients more frequently and will need to be alert to the presentation and risks of substance misuse and SUDs in the elderly. Some elderly patients will have a history or alcohol or other SUDs dating to their younger years, and may present with what is a continuation of this early-onset problem. Others may develop an alcohol or other SUD later in life, with no prior history. Finally, some patients may begin to experience adverse effects from a stable level of alcohol, substance, or medication use that had not previously been a problem, due to reduced metabolism or increased sensitivity of the system to alcohol with advancing age. Multiple barriers to recognizing SUDs in the elderly impede appropriate diagnosis and treatment. It is therefore critical for families, physicians, and other individuals involved in older adults' care to remain aware of subtle and atypical ways in which SUD can present. Regular systematic screening is recommended, using tools validated in the geriatric population. Prescribing psychoactive substances to older patients should always be done very carefully. Physicians should provide individualized education regarding the impact of psychoactive substances on aging patients' health. Increased awareness of SUD can significantly improve the quality of care offered to older adults.

# References

Aalto M, Alho H, Halme JT, Seppa K. The Alcohol Use Disorders Identification Test (AUDIT) and its derivatives in screening for heavy drinking among the elderly. *Int J Geriatr Psychiatry* 2011;26(9):881–885.

Adams WL. Interactions between alcohol and other drugs. *Int J Addict* 1995;30(13–14): 1903–1923.

Aira M, Hartikainen S, Sulkava R. Drinking alcohol for medicinal purposes by people aged over 75: A community-based interview study. *Fam Pract* 2008;25(6):445–449.

Akbik H, Butler SF, Budman SH, Fernandez K, Katz NP, Jamison RN. Validation and clinical application of the Screener and Opioid Assessment for Patients with Pain (SOAPP). *J Pain Symptom Manage* 2006;32(3):287–293.

Alessi C, Vitiello MV. Insomnia (primary) in older people. *BMJ Clin Evid* 2011;Oct 11; 2011. pii: 2302.

Allen JP, Sillanaukee P, Strid N, Litten RZ. National Institute on Alcohol Abuse and Alcoholism (NIAAA), *Biomarkers of heavy drinking*. 2003. Available at http://pubs.niaaa. nih.gov/publications/assessingalcohol/biomarkers.htm (page consulted on 10/10/14).

American Psychiatric Association. *Diagnostic and Statistical Manual of Mental Disorders, Fifth Edition* (DSM-5). Arlington, VA: American Psychiatric Association; 2013.

Atkinson RM. Aging and alcohol use disorders: diagnostic issues in the elderly. *Int Psychogeriatr/IPA*, 1990;2(1):55–72.

Auty RM, Branch RA. Pharmacokinetics and pharmacodynamics of ethanol, whiskey, and ethanol with n-propyl, n-butyl, and iso-amyl alcohols. *Clin Pharmacol Ther* 1977;22(2):242–249.

Babor TF, Kranzler HR, Lauerman RJ. Early detection of harmful alcohol consumption: comparison of clinical, laboratory, and self-report screening procedures. *Addict Behav* 1989;14(2):139–157.

Bartzokis G, Beckson M, Hance DB, et al. Magnetic resonance imaging evidence of "silent" cerebrovascular toxicity in cocaine dependence. *Biol Psychiatry* 1999;45(9):1203–1211.

Bedard, M.-A. [Benzodiazepines: consequences on memory in the elderly]. *Sante Mentale au Quebec* 2003;28(2):23–41.

Bikle DD, Genant HK, Cann C, Recker RR, Halloran BP, Strewler GJ. Bone disease in alcohol abuse. *Ann Intern Med* 1985;103(1):42–48.

Blow F. (1998). TIP 26: Substance Abuse among Older Adults: Treatment Improvement Protocol (TIP) Series 26. Center for Substance Abuse Treatment. Rockville, MD: Substance Abuse and Mental Health Services Administration (US).

Blow FC, Gillespie BW, Barry KL, Mudd SA, Hill EM. Brief screening for alcohol problems in the elderly populations using the Short Michigan Alcoholism Screening Test–Geriatric Version (SMAST-G). *Alcohol Clin Exper Res* 1998;22(Suppl):131a.

Blow FC. Browerarry KJ, Schulenberg JE, Demo-Dananberg LM, Young JP, Beresford TP. The Michigan Alcoholism Screening Test–Geriatric Version (MAST-G): a new elderly-specific screening instrument. *Alcohol Clin Exper Res* 1992;16(372pp).

Blow FC, Barry KL. Treatment of older adults. In RF Ries, DA Fiellin, SC Miller, R Saitz, eds., *The ASAM principles of addiction medicine,* 5th ed. Hagerstown, MD: Wolters Kluwer Health; 2014:541–554.

Bode C, Bode JC. Effect of alcohol consumption on the gut: best practice and research. *Clin Gastroenterol* 2003;17(4):575–592.

Brennan PL, Moos RH. Life stressors, social resources, and late-life problem drinking. *Psychol Aging* 1990;5(4):491–501.

Buchsbaum DG, Buchanan RG, Welsh J, Centor RM, Schnoll SH. Screening for drinking disorders in the elderly using the CAGE questionnaire. *J Am Geriatr Soc* 1992;40(7):662–665.

Butler SF, Budman SH, Fernandez KC, et al. Development and validation of the Current Opioid Misuse Measure. *Pain* 2007;130(1–2):144–156.

Cabre E, Gassull MA. Nutritional aspects of liver disease and transplantation. *Curr Opin Clin Nutr Metab Care* 2001;4(6):581–589.

Caputo F, Vignoli T, Leggio L, Addolorato G, Zoli G, Bernardi M. Alcohol use disorders in the elderly: a brief overview from epidemiology to treatment options. *Exper Gerontol* 2012;47(6):411–416.

Caputo F, Vignoli T, Leggio L, Addolorato G, Zoli G, Bernardi M. Alcohol use disorders in the elderly: a brief overview from epidemiology to treatment options. *Exper Gerontol* 2012;47(6):411–416.

Chrischilles EA, Foley DJ, Wallace RB, et al. Use of medications by persons 65 and over: data from the established populations for epidemiologic studies of the elderly. *J Gerontol* 1992;47(5):M137–M144.

Cohen S. Alcoholism in the elderly. *Can Fam Physician* 1988;34, 723–731.

Cole MG, Dendukuri N. Risk factors for depression among elderly community subjects: a systematic review and meta-analysis. *Am J Psychiatry* 2003;160(6):1147–1156.

Colliver JD, Compton WM, Gfroerer JC, Condon T. Projecting drug use among aging baby boomers in 2020. *Ann Epidemiol* 2006;16(4):257–265.

Compton P, Darakjian J, Miotto K. Screening for addiction in patients with chronic pain and "problematic" substance use: evaluation of a pilot assessment tool. *J Pain Symptom Manage* 1998;16(6):355–363.

Conigliaro J, Kraemer K, McNeil M. Screening and identification of older adults with alcohol problems in primary care. *J Geriatr Psychiatr Neurol* 2000;13(3):106–114.

Conigliaro J, Kraemer K, McNeil M. Screening and identification of older adults with alcohol problems in primary care. *J Geriatr Psychiatr Neurol* 2000;13(3):106–114.

Cook CC, Thomson AD. B-complex vitamins in the prophylaxis and treatment of Wernicke-Korsakoff Syndrome. *Br J Hosp Med* 1997;57(9):461–465.

DeSchepper PJ, Tjandramaga TB, De Roo M, et al. Gastrointestinal blood loss after diflunisal and after aspirin: effect of ethanol. *Clin Pharmacol Ther* 1978;23(6):669–676.

Deykin D, Janson P, McMahon L. Ethanol potentiation of aspirin-induced prolongation of the bleeding time. *N Engl J Med* 1982;306(14):852–854.

Dinitto DM, Choi NG. Marijuana use among older adults in the U.S.A.: user characteristics, patterns of use, and implications for intervention. *Int Psychogeriatr* 2011;23(5):732–741.

Durnas C, Loi CM, Cusack BJ. Hepatic drug metabolism and aging. *Clin Pharmacokinet* 1990;19(5):359–389.

Egan M, Moride Y, Wolfson C, Monette J. Long-term continuous use of benzodiazepines by older adults in Quebec: prevalence, incidence and risk factors. *J Am Geriatr Soc* 2000;48(7):811–816.

Ewing JA. Detecting alcoholism. The CAGE questionnaire. *JAMA* 1984;252(14):1905–1907.

Feinsilver SH, Hertz G. Sleep in the elderly patient. *Clin Chest Med* 1993;14(3):405–411.

Fink A, Hays RD, Moore AA, Beck JC. Alcohol-related problems in older persons: determinants, consequences, and screening. *Arch Intern Med* 1996;156(11):1150–1156.

Fink A, Tsai MC, Hays RD, et al. Comparing the Alcohol-Related Problems Survey (ARPS) to traditional alcohol screening measures in elderly outpatients. *Arch Gerontol Geriatr* 2002;34(1):55–78.

Finlayson RE, Hurt RD, Davis LJ, Jr., Morse RM. Alcoholism in elderly persons: a study of the psychiatric and psychosocial features of 216 inpatients. *Mayo Clin Proc* 1988;63(8):761–768.

Fonda ML, Brown SG, Pendleton MW. Concentration of vitamin B6 and activities of enzymes of B6 metabolism in the blood of alcoholic and nonalcoholic men. *Alcohol Clin Exper Res* 1989;13(6):804–809.

Foy A, O'Connell D, Henry D, Kelly J, Cocking S, Halliday J. Benzodiazepine use as a cause of cognitive impairment in elderly hospital inpatients. *J Gerontol Ser A Biol Sci Med Sci* 1995;50(2):M99–106.

Frezza M, di Padova C, Pozzato G, Terpin M, Baraona E, Lieber CS. High blood alcohol levels in women: the role of decreased gastric alcohol dehydrogenase activity and first-pass metabolism. *N Engl J Med* 1990;322(2):95–99.

Ghuran A, Nolan J. Recreational drug misuse: issues for the cardiologist. *Heart (Br Cardiac Soc)*, 2000;83(6):627–633.

Girard DE, Kumar KL, McAfee JH. Hematologic effects of acute and chronic alcohol abuse. *Hematol Oncol Clin N Am* 1987;1(2):321–334.

Gong Z, Kristal AR, Schenk JM, Tangen CM, Goodman PJ, Thompson IM. Alcohol consumption, finasteride, and prostate cancer risk: Results from the Prostate Cancer Prevention Trial. *Cancer* 2009;115(16):3661–3669.

Graham K. Identifying and measuring alcohol abuse among the elderly: serious problems with existing instrumentation. *J Stud Alcohol* 1986;47(4):322–326.

Greenblatt DJ, Harmatz JS, Shapiro L, Engelhardt N, Gouthro TA, Shader RI. Sensitivity to triazolam in the elderly. *N Engl J Med* 1991;324(24):1691–1698.

Greenblatt DJ, Sellers EM, Shader RI. Drug therapy: drug disposition in old age. *N Engl J Med* 1982;306(18):1081–1088.

Haimov I, Lavie P. Circadian characteristics of sleep propensity function in healthy elderly: A comparison with young adults. *Sleep* 1997;20(4):294–300.

Hall RC, Platt DE, Hall RC. Suicide risk assessment: A review of risk factors for suicide in 100 patients who made severe suicide attempts. Evaluation of suicide risk in a time of managed care. *Psychosomatics* 1999;40(1):18–27.

Han B, Gfroerer JC, Colliver JD, Penne MA. Substance use disorder among older adults in the United States in 2020. *Addiction* 2009;104(1):88–96.

Holroyd S, Duryee JJ. Substance use disorders in a geriatric psychiatry outpatient clinic: prevalence and epidemiologic characteristics. *J Nerv Ment Dis* 1997;185(10):627–632.

Hurt RD, Finlayson RE, Morse RM, Davis LJ, Jr. Alcoholism in elderly persons: medical aspects and prognosis of 216 inpatients. *Mayo Clin Proc* 1988;63(8):753–760.

Israel Y, Orrego H, Holt S, Macdonald DW, Meema HE. Identification of alcohol abuse: thoracic fractures on routine chest X-rays as indicators of alcoholism. *Alcohol Clin Exper Res* 1980;4(4):420–422.

Jinks MJ, Raschko RR. A profile of alcohol and prescription drug abuse in a high-risk community-based elderly population. *DICP: Ann Pharmacother* 1990;24(10):971–975.

Jones RT. Cardiovascular system effects of marijuana. *J Clin Pharmacol* 2002;42(11 Suppl), 58S–63S.

Kalapatapu RK, Paris P, Neugroschl JA. Alcohol use disorders in geriatrics. *Int J Psychiatr Med* 2010;40(3):321–337.

Kalapatapu RK, Sullivan MA. Prescription use disorders in older adults. *Am J Addict* 2010;19(6):515–522.

Kalapatapu RK, Vadhan NP, Rubin E, et al. A pilot study of neurocognitive function in older and younger cocaine abusers and controls. *Am J Addict* 2011;20(3):228–239.

Kaplowitz N, Than TA, Shinohara M, Ji C. Endoplasmic reticulum stress and liver injury. *Semin Liver Dis* 2007;27(4):367–377.

Kausch O. Cocaine abuse in the elderly: a series of three case reports. *J Nerv Ment Dis* 2002;190(8):562–565.

Kerr D, Macdonald IA, Heller SR, Tattersall RB. Alcohol causes hypoglycaemic unawareness in healthy volunteers and patients with type 1 (insulin-dependent) diabetes. *Diabetologia* 1990;33(4):216–221.

Kitson TM. The effect of cephalosporin antibiotics on alcohol metabolism: A review. *Alcohol (Fayetteville)*, 1987;4(3):143–148.

Knochel JP. The pathophysiology and clinical characteristics of severe hypophosphatemia. *Arch Intern Med* 1977;137(2):203–220.

Koechl B, Unger A, Fischer G. Age-related aspects of addiction. *Gerontology* 2012;58(6): 540–544.

Koenig HG, Blazer DG. Epidemiology of geriatric affective disorders. *Clin Geriatr Med* 1992;8 (2):235–251.

Kristiansen L, Gronbaek M, Becker U, Tolstrup JS. Risk of pancreatitis according to alcohol drinking habits: a population-based cohort study. *Am J Epidemiol* 2008;168(8): 932–937.

Lang I, Guralnik J, Wallace RB, Melzer D. What level of alcohol consumption is hazardous for older people? Functioning and mortality in U.S. and English national cohorts. *J Am Geriatr Soc* 2007;55(1):49–57.

Larson EB, Kukull WA, Buchner D, Reifler BV. Adverse drug reactions associated with global cognitive impairment in elderly persons. *Ann Intern Med* 1987;107(2):169–173.

Leevy CM, Moroianu SA. Nutritional aspects of alcoholic liver disease. *Clin Liver Dis* 2005;9(1):67–81.

Leipzig RM, Cumming RG, Tinetti ME. Drugs and falls in older people: A systematic review and meta-analysis: I. Psychotropic drugs. *J Am Geriatr Soc* 1999;47(1):30–39.

Liberto JG, Oslin DW. Early versus late onset of alcoholism in the elderly. *Int J Addict* 1995;30(13–14):1799–1818.

Lieber CS. Hepatic, metabolic and toxic effects of ethanol: 1991 update. *Alcohol Clin Exper Res* 1991;15(4):573–592.

Lieber CS. The discovery of the microsomal ethanol oxidizing system and its physiologic and pathologic role. *Drug Metab Rev* 2004;36(3–4):511–529.

Linnoila M, Stapleton JM, Lister R, et al. Effects of single doses of alprazolam and diazepam, alone and in combination with ethanol, on psychomotor and cognitive performance and on autonomic nervous system reactivity in healthy volunteers. *Eur J Clin Pharmacol* 1990;39(1):21–28.

Llorente MD, David D, Golden AG, Silverman MA. Defining patterns of benzodiazepine use in older adults. *J Geriatr Psychiatr Neurol* 2000;13(3):150–160.

Longo LP, Johnson B. Addiction: Part I. Benzodiazepines—Side effects, abuse risk and alternatives. *Am Fam Physician* 2000;61(7):2121–2128.

Maisto SA, O'Farrell TJ. Comment on the validity of Watson et al.'s "Do alcoholics give valid self-reports?" *J Stud Alcohol* 1985;46(5):447–453.

Maraj S, Figueredo VM, Lynn & Morris D. Cocaine and the heart. *Clin Cardiol* 2010;33(5):264–269.

Markowitz JS, McRae AL, Sonne SC. Oral nutritional supplementation for the alcoholic patient: a brief overview. *Ann Clin Psychiatr* 2000;12(3):153–158.

Meier P, Seitz HK. Age, alcohol metabolism and liver disease. *Curr Opin Clin Nutr Metab Care* 2008;11(1):21–26.

Menninger JA. Assessment and treatment of alcoholism and substance-related disorders in the elderly. *Bull Menninger Clin* 2002;66(2):166–183.

Moore AA, Whiteman EJ, Ward KT. Risks of combined alcohol/medication use in older adults. *Am J Geriatr Pharmacother* 2007;5(1):64–74.

Morgan K, Dallosso H, Ebrahim S, Arie T, Fentem PH. Prevalence, frequency, and duration of hypnotic drug use among the elderly living at home. *BMJ (Clin Res Ed)*, 1988;296(6622):601–602.

Moriyama Y, Mimura M, Kato M, Kashima H. Primary alcoholic dementia and alcohol-related dementia. *Psychogeriatrics* 2006;6(3):114–118.

Mulinga JD. Elderly people with alcohol-related problems: where do they go? *Int J Geriatr Psychiatry* 1999;14(7):564–566.

Mundle G, Ackermann K, Munkes J, Steinle D, Mann K. Influence of age, alcohol consumption and abstinence on the sensitivity of carbohydrate-deficient transferrin, gamma-glutamyltransferase and mean corpuscular volume. *Alcohol Alcoholism (Oxford),* 1999;34(5):760–766.

Naik PC, Jones RG. Alcohol histories taken from elderly people on admission. *BMJ* 1994;308(6923):248.

National Institute on Alcohol Abuse and Alcoholism (NIAAA). *Older adults.* US Department of Health and Human Services, National Institute of Health; 2014. At http://www.niaaa.nih.gov/alcohol-health/special-populations-co-occurring-disorders/older-adults (consulted on 10/5/14).

National Institute on Alcohol Abuse and Alcoholism. (1995). *The physicians' guide to helping patients with alcohol problems.* NIH Pub. No. 95–3769. Rockville, MD: National Institute on Alcohol Abuse and Alcoholism; 2014.

Newell-Price J, Bertagna X, Grossman AB, Nieman LK. Cushing's syndrome. *Lancet* 2006;367(9522):1605–1617.

O'Connell H, Chin A-V, Hamilton F, et al. A systematic review of the utility of self-report alcohol screening instruments in the elderly. *Int J Geriatr Psychiatry* 2004;19(11):1074–1086.

O'Keefe SJ, Marks V. Lunchtime gin and tonic a cause of reactive hypoglycaemia. *Lancet* 1977;1(8025):1286–1288.

Ohayon MM, Carskadon MA, Guilleminault C, Vitiello MV. Meta-analysis of quantitative sleep parameters from childhood to old age in healthy individuals: developing normative sleep values across the human lifespan. *Sleep* 2004;27(7):1255–1273.

Oslin D, Atkinson RM, Smith DM, Hendrie H. Alcohol related dementia: proposed clinical criteria. *Int J Geriatr Psychiatry* 1998;13(4):203–212.

Passik SD, Kirsh KL, Whitcomb L, et al. A new tool to assess and document pain outcomes in chronic pain patients receiving opioid therapy. *Clin Ther* 2004;26(4):552–561.

Piano MR. Alcoholic cardiomyopathy: incidence, clinical characteristics, and pathophysiology. *Chest* 2002;121(5):1638–1650.

Pomara N, Stanley B, Block R, et al. Adverse effects of single therapeutic doses of diazepam on performance in normal geriatric subjects: relationship to plasma concentrations. *Psychopharmacology* 1984;84(3):342–346.

Pomara N, Stanley B, Block R, et al. Increased sensitivity of the elderly to the central depressant effects of diazepam. *J Clin Psychiatr* 1985;46(5):185–187.

Potter JF, James OF. Clinical features and prognosis of alcoholic liver disease in respect of advancing age. *Gerontol* 1987;33(6):380–387.

Reid MC, Anderson PA. Geriatric substance use disorders. *Med Clin N Am* 1997;81(4):999–1016.

Reidenberg MM, Levy M, Warner H, et al. Relationship between diazepam dose, plasma level, age, and central nervous system depression. *Clin Pharmacol Ther* 1978;23(4):371–374.

Reinert DF, Allen JP. The Alcohol Use Disorders Identification Test: an update of research findings. *Alcohol Clin Exper Res* 2007;31(2):185–199.

Rockett IR, Putnam SL, Jia H, Smith GS. Declared and undeclared substance use among emergency department patients: a population-based study. *Addiction* 2006;101(5):706–712.

Roehrs T, Roth T. *Sleep,* Sleepiness, sleep disorders and alcohol use and abuse. *Sleep Med Rev* 2001;5(4):287–297.

Ronksley PE, Brien SE, Turner BJ, Mukamal KJ, Ghali WA. Association of alcohol consumption with selected cardiovascular disease outcomes: a systematic review and meta-analysis. *BMJ* 2011;342, d671.

Rouleau A, Proulx C, O'Connor KP, Belanger C, Dupuis G. [Benzodiazepine use in the elderly: state of the knowledge]. *Sante Mentale au Quebec* 2003;28(2):149–164.

Saunders JB, Aasland OG, Babor TF, de la Fuente JR, Grant M. Development of the Alcohol Use Disorders Identification Test (AUDIT): WHO collaborative project on early detection of persons with harmful alcohol consumption—II. *Addiction* 1993;88(6):791–804.

Savage D, Lindenbaum J. Anemia in alcoholics. *Medicine* 1986;65(5):322–338.

Schneider-Helmert D. Why low-dose benzodiazepine-dependent insomniacs can't escape their sleeping pills. *Acta Psychiatr Scand* 1988;78(6):706–711.

Schonfeld L, Dupree LW. Antecedents of drinking for early- and late-onset elderly alcohol abusers. *J Stud Alcohol* 1991;52(6):587–592.

Schwartz BG, Rezkalla S, Kloner RA. Cardiovascular effects of cocaine. *Circulation* 2010;122(24):2558–2569.

Seby K, Chaudhury S, Chakraborty R. Prevalence of psychiatric and physical morbidity in an urban geriatric population. *Ind J Psychiatry* 2011;53(2):121–127.

Seitz HK, Egerer G, Simanowski UA, et al. Human gastric alcohol dehydrogenase activity: effect of age, sex, and alcoholism. *Gut* 1993;34(10):1433–1437.

Seitz HK, Stickel F. Alcoholic liver disease in the elderly. *Clin Geriatr Med* 2007;23(4):905–921, viii.

Simoni-Wastila L, Yang HK. Psychoactive drug abuse in older adults. *Am J Geriatr Pharmacother* 2006;4(4):380–394.

Simoni-Wastila L, Zuckerman IH, Singhal PK, Briesacher B, Hsu VD. National estimates of exposure to prescription drugs with addiction potential in community-dwelling elders. *Subst Abuse* 2005;26(1):33–42.

Sridhar KS, Raub WA, Jr., Weatherby NL, et al. Possible role of marijuana smoking as a carcinogen in the development of lung cancer at a young age. *J Psychoact Drug* 1994;26(3):285–288.

St John PD, Montgomery PR, Tyas SL. Alcohol misuse, gender and depressive symptoms in community-dwelling seniors. *Int J Geriatr Psychiatry* 2009;24(4):369–375.

Steffens DC, Skoog I, Norton MC, et al. Prevalence of depression and its treatment in an elderly population: the Cache County Study. *Arch Gen Psychiatr* 2000;57(6):601–607.

Stewart C, Leveille SG, Shmerling RH, Samelson EJ, Bean JF, Schofield P. The management of persistent pain in older persons. *J Am Geriatr Soc* 2012;60(11):2081-6.

Substance Abuse and Mental Health Services Administration (SAMHSA). *Drug-related emergency department visits involving pharmaceutical misuse and abuse by older adults. In the Dawn Report.* Rockville, MD: Substance Abuse and Mental Health Services Administration; 2010.

Substance Abuse and Mental Health Services Administration (SAMHSA). *Behavioral health barometer: United States 2013.* HHS Publication No. Sma-13-4796. Rockville, MD: Substance Abuse and Mental Health Services Administration; 2013a.

Substance Abuse and Mental Health Services Administration (SAMHSA). *Older Americans' behavioral health, Issue Brief 5: prescription medication misuse and abuse among older adults.* Rockville, MD: Substance Abuse and Mental Health Services Administration; 2013b.

Tamblyn RM, McLeod PJ, Abrahamowicz M, et al. Questionable prescribing for elderly patients in Quebec. *CMAJ* 1994;150(11):1801–1809.

Taylor MH, Grossberg GT. The growing problem of illicit substance abuse in the elderly: a review. *Prim Care Companion CNS Disord* 2012;14(4): PCC.11r01320.

Tetrault JM, Crothers K, Moore BA, Mehra R, Concato J, Fiellin DA. Effects of marijuana smoking on pulmonary function and respiratory complications: a systematic review. *Arch Intern Med* 2007;167(3):221–228.

Thomasson HR. Gender differences in alcohol metabolism: physiological responses to ethanol. *Recent Dev Alcohol* 1995;12:163–179.

Thomson AD, Jeyasingham MD, Pratt OE, Shaw GK. Nutrition and alcoholic encephalopathies. *Acta Medica Scand Suppl* 1987;717:55–65.

Thuluvath P, Wojno KJ, Yardley JH, Mezey E. Effects of *Helicobacter pylori* infection and gastritis on gastric alcohol dehydrogenase activity. *Alcohol Clin Exper Res* 1994;18(4):795–798.

Thun MJ, Peto R, Lopez AD, et al. Alcohol consumption and mortality among middle-aged and elderly U.S. adults. *N Engl J Med* 1997;337(24):1705–1714.

US Department of Health and Human Services, National Institute on Drug Abuse. *Comorbidity; Addiction and Other Mental Illnesses, 2010*, NIH Publication Number 10-5771; 2010. Available at http://www.drugabuse.gov/publications/research-reports/comorbidity-addiction-other-mental-illnesses/letter-director (consulted on 4/18/16).

Vech RL, Lumeng L, Li TK. Vitamin B6 metabolism in chronic alcohol abuse the effect of ethanol oxidation on hepatic pyridoxal 5'-phosphate metabolism. *J Clin Invest* 1975;55(5):1026–1032.

Vestal RE, McGuire EA, Tobin JD, Andres R, Norris AH, Mezey E. Aging and ethanol metabolism. *Clin Pharmacol Ther* 1977;21(3):343–354.

Vogel-Sprott M, Barrett P. Age, drinking habits and the effects of alcohol. *J Stud Alcohol* 1984;45(6):517–521.

Voyer P, Preville M, Cohen D, Berbiche D, Beland S-G. The prevalence of benzodiazepine dependence among community-dwelling older adult users in Quebec according to typical and atypical criteria. *Can J Aging* 2010;29(2):205–213.

Voyer P, Preville M, Roussel M-E, Berbiche D, Beland S-G. Factors associated with benzodiazepine dependence among community-dwelling seniors. *J Commun Health Nurs* 2009;26(3):101–113.

Weathermon R, Crabb DW. Alcohol and medication interactions. *Alcohol Res Health* 1999;23(1):40–54.

Webster LR, Webster RM. Predicting aberrant behaviors in opioid-treated patients: preliminary validation of the Opioid Risk Tool. *Pain Med* 2005;6(6):432–442.

Whitcup SM, Miller F. Unrecognized drug dependence in psychiatrically hospitalized elderly patients. *J Am Geriatr Soc* 1987;35(4):297–301.

Williamson EM, Evans FJ. Cannabinoids in clinical practice. *Drugs* 2000;60(6):1303–1314.

Won AB, Lapane KL, Vallow S, Schein J, Morris JN, Lipsitz LA. Persistent nonmalignant pain and analgesic prescribing patterns in elderly nursing home residents. *J Am Geriatr Soc* 2004;52(6):867–874.

Woodhouse KW, James OF. Alcoholic liver disease in the elderly: presentation and outcome. *Age Ageing* 1985;14(2):113–118.

World Health Organization (WHO). *ICD-10 Classification of Mental and Behavioural Disorders: Clinical Descriptions and Diagnostic Guidelines 1992; 10th Revision*. Geneva, Switzerland: World Health Organization; 1992.

Wu TC, Tashkin DP, Djahed B, Rose JE. Pulmonary hazards of smoking marijuana as compared with tobacco. *N Engl J Med* 1988;318(6):347–351.

Yki-Jarvinen H, Koivisto VA, Ylikahri R, Taskinen MR. Acute effects of ethanol and acetate on glucose kinetics in normal subjects. *Am J Physiol* 1988;254(2 Pt 1):E175–E180.

Zhu JZ, Wang YM, Zhou QY, Zhu KF, Yu CH, Li YM. Systematic review with meta-analysis: alcohol consumption and the risk of colorectal adenoma. *Aliment Pharmacol Ther* 2014;40(4):325–337.

# CHAPTER 3

# Brief Interventions for Substance-Use Disorder in Older Patients

*Roland C. Merchant and Francesca L. Beaudoin*

## Introduction

Substance misuse among older adults consists of a spectrum of alcohol, to-bacco, and drug use problems, which can range in severity from any use, and it can be a problem simply due to the harmful nature of the substance itself (e.g., smoking), or to abuse or dependence. Substance-misuse brief interventions for older adults consist of an array of structured interventions that have the common features of relative brevity and a short course, although the focus, purpose, length, number, and frequency of the intervention sessions can vary. Substance-misuse brief interventions are intended to serve as a prelude to appropriate follow-up care, although the optimal treatment is yet unknown for older adults with substance misuse. In general, the level of intervention is commensurate with the severity of the substance misuse or risky behavior: brief intervention alone, brief intervention leading to brief treatment, or intensive treatment (Babor et al. 2011).

Brief interventions are an attempt to intercede with older adults who might not otherwise access substance-misuse resources. They can provide an initial link to care for individuals whose substance misuse has not been recognized or has been undertreated. The potential goals of substance-misuse brief interventions for older adults include: reduction in the use or misuse of substances; cessation of their use; reduction in their harmful or risky use, such as binge behaviors; reduction or elimination of the negative consequences of use or misuse, e.g., behavioral problems, social or emotional consequences, or medical/physiological consequences; facilitation of entry into treatment; or re-engagement in care.

The efficacy and effectiveness of substance-misuse brief interventions for older adults remains to be established definitively, although there is some evidence suggesting its value, particularly for alcohol misuse. Although research on brief interventions in general has been increasing, few studies have evaluated the impact of brief interventions for substance misuse among older adults. Accordingly, there is less evidence on the effectiveness and implementation of substance-misuse brief interventions among this growing population. This chapter provides an overview of brief interventions for substance misuse among older adults, a review of research examining the effectiveness of these interventions among this population, and suggestions for research strategies on this topic.

## Screening and Selection of Older Adults for Substance-Misuse Brief Interventions

To date, there are few data to guide the selection of which older adults should receive brief interventions directed at substance misuse. Nevertheless, brief interventions represent the first step after a screening procedure that identifies a substance-misusing older adult who could benefit from help and encouragement to reduce or eliminate substance misuse. Evidence is lacking to address the question of whether brief interventions should be the first level of care that substance-misusing older adults receive, although they usually are considered to be a prelude to further care. In addition, it remains to be determined how brief interventions should best be incorporated into other substance-misuse approaches (e.g., case-management models; individual, family, or group counseling; medication-based therapies; cognitive-behavioral therapy; admission to inpatient or intensive outpatient treatment programs; self-help groups; etc.) (Wu et al. 2011, Kuerbis et al. 2014, Simoni-Wastila et al. 2006). In some circumstances, it may be more appropriate to begin with these other approaches instead of a brief intervention.

An underlying premise of screening is that individuals whose substance-use problem is not receiving attention or who are at risk of problems will be identified. Screening also is used to identify misuse that may not be evident or immediately recognized by clinicians; i.e., misuse that was not apparent from their actions, history, or self-report of problems. Screening could be performed among those whom the clinician suspects might have, or at least be at risk for, a substance problem. As such, the goals of screening might be to uncover hidden problems (i.e., non-targeted screening among "asymptomatic" persons) or to motivate those with suspected problems to recognize them and receive an intervention ("targeted" screening). Screening is often incorporated into brief interventions in a stepwise approach known as "screening, brief intervention, and referral to treatment (SBIRT)." SBIRT encompasses a logical framework: identifying persons using/misusing substances, conducting a brief intervention of some type for those who use/misuse substances, and then securing, or at least recommending, longer-term care when appropriate (Babor et al. 2011). An acronym helpful for remembering the entire process of screening, conducting a brief intervention, and facilitating referral to as-needed further treatment is the "5 A's": Ask (screening), Advise (recommendations), Assess (evaluations), Assist (interventions), and Arrange (securing appropriate treatment). It is a reasonable consideration that selecting older adults for brief interventions should be based, not only on substance misuse history, but also on other factors, such as demographic characteristics, personality attributes or traits, types of substances used/misused, characteristics or severity of substance use/misuse, motivation to change, and previous substance-misuse treatment history. However, there are no studies to date incorporating these factors into the screening and selection for brief interventions for substance-misusing older adults.

There are many other scenarios during which substance using/misusing older adults may be "selected" for a brief intervention: they seek care themselves (self-selected); they are identified by family, friends, clinicians, or others as having a substance use/misuse problem; they are recognized as having a problem based on a financially, legally, medically, or socially negative consequence; or they are screened for use/misuse in other settings such as the community or a judiciary circumstance. In addition, self-recognition of the need for treatment, desire and motivation for treatment, social and other supports, and resources available should affect the type and nature of the brief intervention. The success of non-targeted and targeted screening is affected by factors such as their motivation to change, denial or self-recognition of problems, and severity of use/misuse. It is not yet known, particularly for older adults, if brief intervention needs to be tailored to these two different goals of screening. That is, should a brief intervention after a screening process among "asymptomatic" or unrecognized substance using/misusing older adults be different from the approach used for those whose problems are suspected or recognized by their clinician? Future research may address this question.

Optimal screening methods for substance use/misuse among older adults have not been established. Few screening instruments have been assessed for this population (Wu et al. 2011, Kuerbis et al. 2014, Simoni-Wastila et al. 2006, St. John et al. 2010, Kalapatapu et al. 2010). The accuracy of screening instruments for older adults necessarily depends on their associated metric of assessment. Typical "gold standard" measures for substance-misuse screening instruments are diagnostic criteria for substance abuse or dependence, such as recommended by the *Diagnostic and Statistical Manual of Mental Disorders, Fifth Edition* (DSM-5) (Wu et al. 2011, Simoni-Wastila et al. 2006, APA 2013). However, some of the diagnostic criteria depend on age-related behaviors that are not applicable to older adults, such as the impact of substance misuse on employment. Accordingly, older adults whose health and life are being affected negatively in other ways by substance misuse might not meet criteria in screening instruments developed for younger populations (Kuerbis et al. 2014, Simoni-Wastila et al. 2006, Kalapatapu et al. 2010, Blow et al. 2012). Moreover, the utility of brief interventions might be constrained if the type, nature, or format of a substance-misuse brief intervention selected for an older adult depends on screening instruments that are not appropriate for older adults. Instead, age-appropriate criteria for substance-misuse interventions, commensurate with the goals of screening (e.g., identifying misuse; at-risk, hazardous, problematic, or unhealthy use; and not just dependence), might be a better option (Kuerbis et al. 2014, Simoni-Wastila et al. 2006, Blow et al. 2013).

The goals of screening, the target population, and the setting in which screening instruments are employed, should influence the choice of screening instruments as well as decisions regarding the type and focus of subsequent brief interventions. Questions to consider include: Is the goal to identify those potentially at risk, those with undiagnosed substance misuse, or individuals with severe substance-use disorder who might need more intensive care? What type of brief intervention is planned, and what is the goal of the brief intervention to follow the screening? Will the brief intervention be accompanied by the initiation of pharmacological therapies? How will the features of the screening instrument (e.g., length, performance parameters, and format) fit with the planned interventions?

The performance parameters of the screening instrument (e.g., sensitivity, specificity, predictive value) in the population and setting in which it is administered may determine who receives an intervention and the success of those interventions. For example, a one-time screening initiative launched at a community outreach setting would be likely to involve a brief screening instrument that matches the characteristics of the population screened, is responsive to the limitations of the screening process, and is commensurate with the format and focus of the planned brief intervention. Choice of a screening instrument in this situation would take into account factors such as the short time allotted for screening, the conduct of screening and interventions in a non–substance use/misuse context, the likelihood that the population screened has a low prevalence of substance misuse and is not seeking treatment, and the high probability that limited opportunities for capture and assured linkage to care can occur in this situation. On the other hand, a screening initiative in a primary care clinic could be conducted over multiple visits and might involve a population with a higher prevalence of substance misuse. Such an intervention could be delivered in the context of medical care, and probably would afford more opportunity to ensure follow-up care. A different screening instrument of greater length, capturing more details of use/misuse, including an evaluation of the severity of use, might be more appropriate in this context. One recent study found that, among older adult at-risk drinkers, the benefits of a patient–provider educational intervention were most prominent for patients who received physician discussions; these findings suggest that provider counseling is a critical component of primary care–based interventions (Barnes et al. 2016).

## Format of Substance-Misuse Brief Interventions for Older Adults

There is a variety of possible formats for substance-misuse brief interventions in older adults (Blow et al. 2012). These include a range of breadth, intensity, intent, and length of interventions—from brief advice and brief conversations, to multi-session brief interventions that could resemble formal, longer-term substance-misuse treatment sessions. The distinctions among brief advice, conversations, and multi-session interventions can often be blurred. In general, brief *advice* involves a directed conversation that informs the recipient about next steps (e.g., enrollment in a smoking cessation class). A brief *conversation* involves a discussion about their desire to, opportunities for, steps towards, and motivations to change. A brief *intervention* implies a longer, more structured discussion in which the person conducting the intervention (hereinafter referred to as "the interventionist," who could be a clinician or non-clinician trained to conduct interventions) addresses the concerns of the recipient, emphasizing their motivation to change or to seek further treatment (Babor et al. 2011).

"Brief advice" implies a predominantly unidirectional interaction (interventionist to recipient), involving transmission of information and perhaps resources on how to change their behavior or seek further treatment. "Brief conversation" suggests that a limited dialogue between the interventionist and recipient occurs. An assessment is conducted or the results of an assessment are reviewed, consequences of misuse are discussed, information about interest in and need for change is exchanged, or advice about and usually referral to appropriate resources are provided. Some might reserve the term *brief intervention* for more structured interactions between the interventionist and recipient, which can be one to several sessions in length and vary in frequency (Babor et al. 2011). Brief interventions commonly include several features:

1. An assessment of the substance misuse and its negative consequences;
2. Feedback about the misuse and its negative consequences;
3. Information or education about misuse, negative consequences, and options for reduction of misuse;
4. Advice about elimination of misuse and treatment needs and resources; and often
5. Provision of self-help or other relevant materials (Babor et al. 2011, St John et al. 2010).

As expected, the role of the interventionist, setting, and goal of the brief intervention dictate its format. The goals could be to screen and identify persons who need further treatment and link them to care, or to provide the initial steps of that care. For example, a primary care physician might engage his/her patient in a brief conversation about the negative consequences of alcohol misuse during a routine primary care visit; a community outreach worker might offer brief advice about quitting smoking to an older adult screened during a health fair; or a mental health care provider in an assisted living facility might offer a series of sessions to older adults on prescription drug-use reduction as part of a pain-management program. As noted in these examples, the goals of the intervention program, the skills and resources of the individual or group conducting the program, the setting, the time allotted, and the ability to link to additional services affect the format of the planned interventions.

The theoretical underpinnings of brief advice, conversations, and interventions naturally vary according to their goals, format, and content (e.g., cognitive-behavioral therapy, supportive therapy models, health belief models, etc.). A popular cornerstone of many brief interventions is motivational interviewing or motivational enhancement therapy (Kuerbis et al. 2014). Motivational interviewing is considered to be a client-centered, nonjudgemental approach that aims to enhance the individual's intrinsic motivation by exploring and resolving their ambivalence to change. Motivational interviewing can be applied to other problems (e.g., weight loss or medication adherence), but it often is used the context of substance misuse (Cooper 2012). As such, it can be viewed as the vehicle by which the interventional content is delivered. Unfortunately, there is limited evidence of the efficacy or effectiveness of motivational interviewing or motivational enhancement therapy as a delivery mode for substance-misuse brief interventions for older adults (Kuerbis et al. 2014).

# Content of Substance-Misuse Brief Interventions for Older Adults

The optimal content of substance-misuse interventions for older adults has not yet been determined. Brief interventions typically include any of the following: assessments of the recipient's interest in and motivations to change substance-misuse behaviors and receive help; a review of the history use/misuse and their negative consequences; identification of their future goals for health, activities, interests, relationships, or finances; evaluations of the substance misuse (potentiators, triggers, extent, frequency, and negative consequences of the misuse); personalized reflection and feedback about use or misuse and its negative consequences; provision of normative data regarding use/misuse or recommended levels of use (e.g., no use, or defining "moderate use"); education about misuse, its negative consequences, and treatment options; discussions about current or their prior attempts to change their substance misuse and treatment received; review of the pros and cons of use/misuse and iteration of reasons to reduce or quit use/misuse; creation and negotiation of change plans to decrease/eliminate/avoid use and seek alternatives to use; discussion about plans to assist with situations that might lead to substance use/misuse and interfere with the change plans; and assistance with as-needed linkage to appropriate subsequent resources and care (Kuerbis et al. 2014, St. John et al. 2010, APA 2013, Cooper 2012). A popular framework for brief interventions is the FRAMES model, which involves these components: *Feedback* about risk is given; *Responsibility* for change is placed with the intervention recipient; *Advice* is provided for changing behavior; a *Menu* of change options is offered; *Empathic* and motivational styles are used by the interventionist; and *Self-efficacy* is emphasized (Blow et al. 2012).

Formal evaluations may be used as a tool to facilitate the brief interventions. These evaluations measure the extent of their substance misuse, negative consequences of substance misuse, treatment history, and their motivation to change. These assessments might utilize standardized instruments, which could be self-, provider-, or interventionist-administered. Depending on their length and scope, they might precede the intervention as part of a screening process, occur after the identification of someone with a positive screen, or be incorporated in the brief intervention itself. The type of evaluation chosen should fit with the goals of the intervention, context, and setting. There are some notable challenges with utilizing formal evaluations using standardized instruments among older adults. Few, if any, of these instruments were developed and tested among older adults, so their validity in this population is less uncertain (Wu et al. 2011, Simoni-Wastila et al. 2006, Kalapatapu et al. 2010,

Blow et al. 2012). Furthermore, given that many older adults might not fit current formal diagnostic criteria for substance abuse or dependence, which is the standard some instruments are based on, these instruments might underestimate the extent of, or fail to identify, problems unique to this population (Wu et al. 2011, Kuerbis et al. 2014, Blow et al. 2012). Although growing in popularity as efficient and potentially nonjudgemental approaches to substance-misuse evaluations, it should be noted that computer-based or written self-administered instruments might be difficult for older adults with decreased visual acuity or inexperience with computers (Wu et al. 2011).

Aging and its unique interplay with substance misuse probably influences older adults' experience and reports about their substance use, such as patterns of use; cognitive and physical impairments that interfere with recall and reports of use/misuse and adverse effects of use/misuse; physiological responses to substances that might have an impact on the tolerance, withdrawal, and discontinuation of substance misuse; and adverse effects noted even at lower levels of use. On the other hand, shame about the misuse and concerns about the consequences of admitting problems (e.g., loss of housing)—particularly to a healthcare provider in a perceived judgemental or authoritative role—might also lead to denial and false statements about the misuse when interviewer-administered instruments are used (Wu et al. 2011). Because of these challenges, older adults may require a broader exploration of substance use/misuse during brief interventions than is currently available from standardized instruments developed for younger populations.

Assessments focused on behaviors, symptoms, and the negative consequences of substance misuse, as well as education about these elements, may warrant the inclusion of age-specific content for brief interventions for older adults, different from those for other populations (Kalapatapu et al. 2010, Cooper 2012). However, this need and its impact are not well studied. In general, there is limited direct evidence guiding substance-misuse brief interventions for older adults about acceptable standards of use, even for some commonly used substances (e.g., alcohol), although it is generally recommended for most substances that acceptable levels of use for older adults should be set at lower levels than for younger adults, or that abstinence should be recommended (Kuerbis et al. 2012, St. John et al. 2010, Blow et al. 2002, 2012). Less is known about the health effects and the negative consequences of use for this population than for younger adults. For most substances, symptoms and signs of misuse and its negative consequences are derived from generations of experience, observations, and reports of use of these substances; clinical and laboratory research; and observational studies, much of which is extrapolated from investigations involving younger adults. Despite the limited direct evidence on this topic, it is probably true that the physiological effects of most of these substances and their consequences (behavioral, cognitive, emotional, or physical) are affected by the aging process (Wu et al. 2011, Kuerbis et al. 2014, Simoni-Wastila et al. 2006, Kalapatapu et al. 2010, Blow et al. 2000, Han et al. 2009). Yet, it is not yet known how best to incorporate this information into brief interventions, nor how effective this inclusion might be for this population. Further research is needed on the effectiveness of education on these matters when it is included in brief interventions. However, it seems reasonable and advisable to offer information about the harmful effects of used/misused substances, their potential for greater harm among older adults due to the effects of aging and its impact on metabolism, the hazards of using substances simultaneously, and their potential adverse effects on prescribed and over-the-counter medications.

## Contextual Issues Impacting Substance-Misuse Brief Interventions for Older Adults

The age range for those who might be considered to be "older adults" is quite broad, perhaps over 50 years, depending on the starting age chosen. Furthermore, older adults are not a homogeneous population, especially in regard to age, and this lack of homogeneity can impact the content, format, and delivery of substance-misuse brief interventions. Chronological age and physiological aging are among the contextual issues that might impact the design, delivery, and effectiveness of substance-misuse brief interventions for older adults. There are no known age-related milestones that impact substance misuse and, logically, their interventions. Aging, along with life changes of all types, probably affects one's priorities and outlook regarding recognition or denial of substance use and misuse, as well as one's interest in and motivation to change.

Being part of an age group also implies membership in a cohort that could reflect cultural, educational, and social views as well as life experiences. Period effects or experiences relevant to patients' perceptions include eras in which substance misuse might have been considered either normative or aberrant behavior, variable periods of access to substances, and changing beliefs about substance use/misuse (e.g., advertisement campaigns about alcohol and tobacco, variations in access and popularity of substances and their use, increases in public health concerns about smoking, etc.) (St. John et al. 2010). Such age cohort or period effects probably have an impact on substance-misuse brief interventions for older adults in many ways. People born from 1945 to 1965 and reared in the United States, the cohort known as "baby boomers," have many distinguishing behavioral, educational, experiential, and social distinctions from preceding and succeeding generations. Although not a homogeneous group, baby boomers, particularly compared to their older peers, might have a more permissive or at least a different view of what is considered acceptable or healthy vs. unacceptable or unhealthy behaviors concerning substance use (Kuerbis et al. 2014). Also, in comparison to prior generations, this age cohort has a greater likelihood of a history of use and misuse of substances, more use of a variety of substances, including psychoactive drug use, more experience with previous substance-misuse treatment, and in turn a greater likelihood of accruing physiological dependence and negative consequences of substance misuse (e.g., medical conditions related to long-term alcohol, smoking, and drug use) (Wu et al. 2011, Kuerbis et al. 2014, St. John et al. 2010, Kalapatapu et al. 2010, Blow et al. 2012, Han et al. 2009). Another contextual factor related to age cohort is the types of substances used or misused (Wu et al. 2011, Kuerbis et al. 2014, St. John et al. 2010, Blow et al, 2012, Blazer et al. 2009). For older adults born before 1945, alcohol and smoking are the predominant substances used/misused. Illicit drug use is less common among that age cohort. Polysubstance use/misuse is more common among the baby boomer cohort, as is psychoactive drug use/misuse and prescription drug use/misuse (Wu et al. 2011, Blow et al. 2012, Han et al, 2009, Blazer et al. 2009). Therefore, brief interventions for baby boomers for substance misuse might require approaches that de-emphasize social mores, address polysubstance use and misuse, and explore lifelong and current negative consequences and prior treatment in more depth. In contrast, brief interventions for persons born before 1945 might focus more on concerns about shame regarding substance misuse/use, single substance use/misuse, and explore social mores as motivators for change.

Related to birth cohort and aging is the contextual issue of the onset of use and misuse (Wu et al. 2005, St. John et al. 2010). The interventional needs of early-onset users of substances are likely to differ in many ways from those of late-onset users. Early-onset users typically have longer substance-use histories and consequent, concurrent, or exacerbating psychiatric problems, medical problems, and comorbidities (Wu et al. 2011). The precipitating reasons for use and misuse and continued reasons for use and misuse also might differ from the reasons of those who began substance use/misuse later in life. Late-onset users may be using/misusing because of medical or social changes that developed in later life (e.g., chronic pain syndromes, severe medical problems, changes in social supports, divorce, separation, death of spouses or significant others, etc.) (Wu et al. 2011, Kuerbis et al. 2014). Their use/misuse may stem from a recent life change that is ongoing and still contributing to the use/misuse, or perhaps from a previous change that was a precipitant. Late-onset users might not be cognizant of this precipitant, or could be reluctant to discuss it (e.g., post-traumatic stress from a severe event). Older adults whose coping with stress, tension, or life changes involves avoidance of tackling these issues may turn to alcohol or drugs later in life to manage their problems (Kuerbis et al. 2014). Brief interventions for older adults require flexibility in how to either uncover precipitating causes for late-onset users, or devoting more time to concurrent problems that exacerbate and perpetuate use among early-onset users.

Another age-related factor that probably influences interest and motivation to change and response to brief interventions is the life perspective of older adults who use/misuse substances (Kuerbis et al. 2014, Kalapatapu et al. 2010). Younger adults typically are perceived as "forward-viewing" about their life—thinking about what is ahead—while older adults are "backward-viewing"—reflecting on their life experiences. A foreshortened view of the future might inhibit one's motivation to reduce substance use, affect one's self-efficacy to change use, and limit one's engagement in changing behaviors that one believes help cope with the physical and mental limitations of aging (Kuerbis et al. 2014). Interventionists might explore with older adults which perspective they primarily hold, and adapt the brief intervention accordingly. For example, "forward-viewing" brief interventions might focus on their motivations to change in anticipation of future events (e.g., the birth of a grandchild, upcoming family gatherings, retirement), while "backward-viewing" might reflect on negative consequences of misuse, social mores from youth, role models for change, and other aspects from earlier life experiences.

Regardless of the age cohort of the recipient, brief interventions for substance-misusing older adults need to be responsive to polysubstance use and misuse of all forms. Brief interventions should explore other substances used concomitantly, such as alcohol with smoking, alcohol with prescription benzodiazepines, over-the-counter medications with alcohol and/or drugs, and illicit drugs with alcohol. This exploration could include self-awareness or directed reflection on how polysubstance increases usage or misuse of primarily abused substances, increases the effects of these substances, and leads to more frequent or severe negative consequences of use/misuse. Recipients of brief interventions for substance use/misuse might prefer to prioritize the substances they seek to reduce, or eliminate use, out of a concern of failure from trying to change too many habits at once. However, recognition that these habits are synchronous and must be addressed simultaneously for success could be a point of education and encouragement and construction of appropriate change plans in brief interventions.

Previous experience with substance-misuse treatment is an important issue to screen for and consider, especially with older adults who may have had multiple exposures to various treatment programs. Such older adults are likely to be fully aware of the hazards of their misuse and may already be familiar with standard treatment approaches. Experience might breed contempt for brief interventions from the perspective that they are "too simplistic," they did not work for them previously, or that older patients "have heard it before." Older individuals might harbor a sense of hopelessness about their misuse, marked by beliefs that they are "incurable." Strategies during the brief intervention might include challenging patients to chart ways to address their misuse that draw from prior successes and focus more on linkage to care and longer-term treatment.

Change in family and marital or relationship status is an important contextual factor for substance misuse and should be addressed in brief interventions for older adults (Cooper 2012). The loss of support from others can prompt or intensify substance misuse because of grief, depression, and anxiety. Similarly, substance use may replace the loss of activities that previously were shared and enjoyed. Older adults over time experience changes in their relationships with others due to births, deaths, marriages, divorces, and the beginning and endings of other relationships with significant others, friends, colleagues, and family members. Relationships with adult children, siblings, and parents change over time. Geographic separation from adult children who are more independent and perhaps not living nearby might engender a loss of a sense of purpose among their parents/guardians. By contrast, adopting the caregiver role for siblings, parents, relatives, in-laws, or others might lead to fears about the future. Loss of the usual social supports from time devoted to engaging in the caregiver role, or conversely, feelings of being overwhelmed by the caregiver role, can be contributing factors. Changes in relationships with former friends and colleagues as well as their illnesses and deaths can reduce social support and opportunities for shared activities and lead to social isolation. Any of these changes in relationships might lead to the initiation or escalation of substance misuse, as well as concomitant anxiety and depression, and a downward spiral of increasing social isolation and more substance misuse. Substance-misuse interventions for older adults may require independent or guided investigation to the impact of changes in relationships on substance misuse, social isolation as a potentiator of substance misuse, as well as the challenge of creating new social supports and mitigating the impact of social isolation.

For many older adults, substance use and misuse is interrelated with chronic medical conditions and psychological problems (St. John et al. 2010, Blow et al. 2002, Han et al. 2009). Substance misuse can interact synergistically with concomitant medical, psychological, and cognitive problems that worsen all of their negative effects. It also can be difficult to discern whether negative consequences (e.g., frequent falls) are related more to substance misuse or to medical, psychological, or cognitive problems. These problems also can mask the existence or severity of the substance misuse (Blow et al. 2000). Medical and psychological problems might be treated or untreated, or substances could be misused as substitutes for medical or mental health treatment ("self-medication"). Medical problems could be current, or could be a result of functional decline from prior ailments, such as disabilities from prior acute events (e.g., myocardial infarction, intracranial hemorrhage, cancer). Depression and anxiety are common problems, and might be more prominent among older adults as they face changes in their lifestyle and routines. Many older adults turn to substance misuse as a coping strategy for these stressors of later life, and they may fear feelings of helplessness without the use of substances to face them. Brief interventions for this population should involve investigation of the role of medical and psychological problems that initiated, potentiated, or are exacerbating current substance misuse, which may not be recognized by the recipient. As such, addressing coping mechanisms, referral to services, encouraging seeking treatment, and constructing change plans that incorporate these aspects can be essential to the success of brief interventions for older adults with these problems. Continued use/misuse in the context of medical or psychological conditions that are made worse by substance use/misuse (e.g., viral hepatitis with concomitant alcohol misuse) probably will require evaluation of medical histories; education, inviting self-awareness, and providing feedback during the brief intervention; investigating reasons for misuse (e.g., untreated or undertreated chronic pain, anxiety, depression, insomnia, etc.); and incorporating medical and mental health treatment–seeking strategies in the change plan.

Cognitive decline as a result of the aging process, medical problems, social isolation, reduced mental and physical stimulation, as well as accrued effects of substance misuse, are important contextual considerations for substance-misuse interventions for older adults (Wu et al. 2011, Kalapatapu et al. 2010, Cooper 2012). Cognitive decline can affect one's memory and attention, which could manifest as lack of recall about use/misuse history, unintentional denial of substance misuse and its negative consequences, and problems with completing formal screening use/misuse instruments (Wu et al. 2011). Cognitive decline may also impair insight into substance misuse as a problem, or the recognition of negative consequences related to misuse. In addition, the content, rate, and pace of brief interventions may need to be modified for older adults with cognitive decline. Repetition and review of elements of the brief intervention (e.g., change plans), shorter and more frequent sessions, and a slower pace might be necessary. Referral for formal neurocognitive assessments, involvement of caregivers, review of prescription medications, and referral for social services can be considered as integrated components of the brief intervention.

Medical and psychological problems and cognitive decline typically are related to social isolation, which is a common feature of substance misuse among older adults (Kuerbis et al. 2014, Simoni-Wastila et al. 2006, Cooper 2012). Ill health, disabilities, depression, and anxiety can lead to decreased mobility and activity levels and avoidance of social engagement. Social isolation can be related to loss of social supports and reduced income, as well as changes in life roles (e.g., retirement, caregiving of infirmed spouses and family) and changes in housing (e.g., movement to assisted living arrangements) (St. John et al. 2010, Cooper 2012). Older adults might view substance misuse when alone as more appropriate than witnessed behaviors (St. John et al. 2010). They may also be more likely to engage in substance use/misuse when alone out of shame and stigma, perhaps related to social mores from their upbringing and culture. Interventionists should address the likelihood of social isolation as a precipitant and potentiator of substance misuse. They should be alert to the possibility that shame and stigma may make older adults reluctant to admit to and to address their misuse (Simoni-Wastili et al. 2006, St. John et al. 2010, Blow et al. 2000). Emphasis on a need for assistance and the desire for better health can support a milieu for acceptance of change. Education during the intervention should include the hazards of substance use/misuse, particularly when they are feeling isolated, its perpetuation of social isolation, and challenges in overcoming resistance to change patterns of use—particularly while social and other reinforcers are sometimes less accessible in later life.

Concurrent medical conditions or disabilities, culture, or perspectives coupled with end-of-life concerns might affect their perspectives on the importance of addressing substance misuse (Kuerbis et al. 2014). These factors also might precipitate use/misuse, be intertwined with signs and symptoms of depression, or even reflect suicidal ideation. In turn, these aspects could affect how brief interventions are introduced to older adults, their structure and content, and perhaps their effectiveness. For example, a short-term outlook on substance misuse perhaps mixed with fatalism could lead to lower motivation to change among some older adults ("Why quit now? I might as well enjoy the few years I have left"). These views will be challenging to address in brief interventions, but interventionists should be aware that some older patients may express this form of resistance to change. Focusing on the short- and intermediate-term benefits of reducing substance misuse may be an effective strategy.

Financial factors play an important role in substance use/misuse, construction of brief interventions, and engagement in needed treatment (Kuerbis et al. 2014). Older adults might be facing retirement, which could provoke specific concerns about reduced income, loss of activities, and shrinking social networks, as well as broad concerns about their life purpose. If already retired, they may be experiencing financial and other consequences of retirement that they did not anticipate. Many older adults experience housing concerns or crises, resulting from loss or reduction of income, changes in neighborhoods, or the need for assisted living or other supportive living arrangements. These unwelcome financial and social changes can precipitate or exacerbate substance misuse (Wu et al. 2011, Kuerbis et al. 2014). Financial stress could also lead to concerns about how to pay for needed treatment, with resulting continued use/misuse and avoidance of treatment. Brief interventions for older adults with substance misuse should evaluate for these issues when investigating causes of use/misuse and providing resources for assistance.

Other factors affecting the design and content and perhaps the success of substance-misuse brief interventions include demographic characteristics other than age, such as gender, race/ethnicity, education, culture, and nativity (Wu et al. 2011, St. John et al. 2010). Traditional gender roles and beliefs and perspectives regarding gender roles have changed over time, and older adults may have strong feelings about these roles, ambivalence about the changes, or harbor values and beliefs from their formative years. Women in general live longer than men, may be less likely than men of their same age group to be financially independent, and have different social supports. Older women may have a different use pattern than older men in terms of the substances they misuse (e.g., prescription pain relievers and anxiolytics), might have different views about acceptable and unacceptable use/misuse of substances, and are likely to respond to substances differently than men (e.g., increased sensitivity to the same level of use). These gender differences in later life can shape guidance on acceptable levels of use as well as symptoms, signs, and negative consequences of use/misuse (Blow et al. 2002). Race/ethnicity and concomitant culture also might affect beliefs about normative behaviors with respect to substance use vs. misuse, denial vs. openness about use/misuse, responses to interventionist and healthcare providers (e.g., acquiescence vs. mistrust), and beliefs about how to change or modify behaviors.

Demographic characteristics of the intervention recipient might have an impact on their willingness to self-report use/misuse, symptoms, and negative consequences to misuse; their responses to evaluations; and their willingness to receive feedback (St. John et al. 2010). The responses also might be affected when the demographic characteristics of interventionists and intervention recipients are dissimilar. Educational background of the recipient also might influence planned brief interventions. For example, substance-misuse interventions for those with fewer years of education might benefit from an emphasis on interventionist-directed approaches with concrete change plans, while interventions for those with more years of education might emphasize self-reflection and more active involvement in change plans. Interventionists should be sensitive to these and other demographic aspects when constructing and delivering the intervention. Given the limited knowledge on this topic, more research is needed on tailoring substance misuse interventions for older adults based on demographic characteristics.

## Brief Interventions for Prescription and Non-Prescription Drug Use/Misuse: Unique Issues for Older Adults

Prescription drug use and misuse is a growing problem in the United States, especially among older adults, and deserves special attention (Blow et al. 2012, Cooper 2012, Blazer et al. 2009). As a consequence, substance-misuse brief interventions for older adults need to be developed that are tailored to this population (Blow et al. 2012). The drugs most frequently prescribed and in turn misused by older adults are benzodiazepines and opioid analgesics (Cooper 2012, Blazer et al. 2009, Blow et al. 2012). These medications are often prescribed for "as needed" use instead of standing use. As such, they might not be mentioned in drug-use history reviews. Because of their therapeutic indications as well as their potential for problems, there are differences in opinions regarding how to characterize, define, and set diagnostic standards for misuse of prescription medications (Simoni-Wastili et al. 2006, Barrett et al. 2008). Prescription drug misuse can also present in a wide variety of ways, including use without a prescription; hoarding medications; use for its intoxicating or euphoric effects; recreational use; use for reasons other than why it was prescribed; use with alcohol or other medications to intensify their effects; use to overcome ill effects of other substances; diversion, etc. Misuse also includes sporadic or "pseudo-therapeutic" actions (e.g., taking an extra dose, taking a medication for sleep instead of for pain) (Simoni-Wastili et al. 2006). Many of these forms of misuse are not captured by traditional screening methods, may go unrecognized when reviewing medication histories, or do not meet DSM-5 or other standards for abuse or dependence. In addition, other prescription and non-prescription medications might be misused by older adults, such as medications for insomnia or pain, and these could go unrecognized through a routine screening for substance use/misuse (Blow et al. 2012, Barrett et al. 2008). Older adults, who typically have greater access to and utilization of healthcare services, have a greater likelihood of being prescribed addictive medications than do younger adults (Wu et al. 2011, Kuerbis et al. 2014). Because these drugs are prescribed, initially for medical conditions, denial of misuse is common. Beliefs that they are necessary for treatment of the medical condition and are warranted because they are approved by a clinician further entrench the denial and frustrate appeals to change behaviors. Misuse might begin with self-medicating behavior (e.g., taking extra doses for untreated pain), but could progress to psychological (e.g., marked by cravings) or physiological dependence. Use and misuse also can be secondary to misdiagnosis of underlying medical conditions, overprescribing, or multiple prescriptions from unknowing different providers (Kuerbis et al. 2014).

Even when the older patient recognizes the problems from his or her substance use, screening and evaluation efforts may be hampered by denial or minimization of misuse (Wu et al. 2011, Kuerbis et al. 2014, Kalapatapu et al. 2010). Chronic pain syndromes can further exacerbate an overreliance on opioid medications, along with resistance to use of non-narcotic pain relievers and non-medication approaches to pain relief. For older adults, it is especially important to address underlying mental health and social determinants of chronic pain syndromes, which are frequently overlooked when chronic pain becomes the presenting concern. Diversion of use for reasons other than that for which they are intended (e.g., elimination of insomnia or use for their psychoactive properties) could make misuse more difficult to address (Kuerbis et al. 2014, Kalapatapu et al. 2010, Cooper 2012). Diversion—which may include providing these medications to a spouse or other family members—might not be self-recognized (Cooper 2012), and hence should be included in a formal evaluation of all aspects of prescription drug use and misuse. Diversion also might be denied, out of concealment of engaging in a socially unacceptable or illegal behavior; caution must be taken to provide a nonjudgemental approach when investigating its existence. Use of prescription opioids or other sedative medications concurrently with alcohol, other drugs, or non-prescription medications also may result in symptoms that are misinterpreted, unrecognized, or missed by clinicians or patients themselves as anxiety, cognitive decline, infectious or other medical causes of delirium, depression, or psychosis (Kalapatapu et al. 2010).

Substance-misuse interventions for older adults need to take into account the high likelihood that prescription medications are being used. These are difficult to screen for and can be masked from the patient or interventionist out of denial, because of "as needed" use designations, shame, or fear of loss of access to these medications (Cooper et al. 2012). Diligence during screening for their use is essential. Education about their misuse vs. appropriate use, addressing "doctor shopping" behaviors or inappropriate behaviors to acquire them (e.g., feigning symptoms or lying about medical conditions), and the issue of diversion need to be included in interventions. Strategies to reduce/ eliminate prescription drug misuse, such as seeking alternatives to chronic pain relief and addressing problems that perpetuate or exacerbate their use (e.g., alcohol misuse, insomnia, mental health problems), also should be part of these interventions.

## Setting for Substance-Misuse Brief Interventions for Older Adults and Contextual Concerns

Older adults are more likely than their younger counterparts to have primary care providers and specialists, to receive care in medical settings other than primary care settings, and to be in long-term care facilities. (Blow et al. 2012; Cooper et al. 2012; Wu et al. 2011). Therefore, healthcare settings appear to be a natural setting for brief interventions for this population. However, one of the hopes for substance-misuse brief interventions is that they will be available to older adults where they might need them, at locations that are convenient, and in settings where older adults are more likely to receive other services. If such interventions are intended to be an extension of addiction services, then they might occur in medical and non-medical services. These settings include community-based organizations (e.g., community centers for older adults), medical facilities (e.g., private clinician offices, specialist offices, clinics, emergency departments, urgent care centers, acute care hospitals, long-term care facilities), psychiatric and mental health settings, religious or faith-based centers, and judicial facilities (e.g., jails, prisons, pretrial/court services, probation offices). Each setting brings a contextual element that might be included as a feature of these respective brief interventions. These features might include capitalizing on follow-up/linkage-to-care options available (e.g., inpatient hospitalization) and incorporating the reason for the visit to the setting and need for an intervention as a motivation to change behavior (e.g., "driving under the influence" charges). The setting will probably inform the experience and training of the interventionist, which in turn could affect the type of intervention delivered. The resources available at these settings also help dictate the purpose, design, and delivery of these interventions.

## Additional Considerations for Substance-Misuse Brief Interventions for Older Adults

Depending on the goals of the brief interventions, resources available to interventionists, and length of the interventions, some older adults might benefit from inclusion of caregivers, family members and medical or other providers in the interventions (Philip et al. 2010). Their roles could be to provide information about misuse history and negative consequences, particularly for older adults with cognitive deficits; offer the perspective of someone affected by the substance misuse, such as additional burdens to their care; receive the intervention, if they also are misusing substances; and encourage the person receiving the intervention by pledging their assistance and support with enacting the change plan and offering additional assistance after the intervention (Philip et al. 2010).

The optimal number of sessions for a brief intervention is not known, especially for older adults. As noted previously, some older adults might benefit from a longer, slower paced course, although this hypothesis is under-studied. The number of sessions may be determined by the setting, as well as the resources available and goals of the intervention. For example, an emergency department–initiated brief intervention might involve a single session during delivery of medical care. It might include a telephone or in-person "booster" session designed to assist with linkage-to-care after the intervention. At an extended-care facility, in contrast, intervention recipients might be offered a multi-session brief intervention. The multiple sessions could cover successive, related topics to avoid overwhelming the participant with too much material in one setting. These extended interventions might also involve skill-building or guided steps to promote insight into the substance-misuse problems and the development of care plans with feedback about their progress towards enacting treatment plans. An important additional consideration for older adults when designing multi-session brief interventions is the issue of transportation and mobility problems. Some older adults might be limited by their inability to drive or physical disabilities that restrict their involvement with in-person sessions (Kuerbis et al. 2014, Cooper 2012). Others might not have the financial or practical resources to transport themselves for these sessions. The needs of those involved and goals of the brief intervention need to be balanced against practical concerns and the potential limitations of single vs. multi-session interventions. Alternate methods of delivering additional sessions, such as by telephone or at-home visits by interventionists, may deserve consideration.

## Qualifications of Interventionists

Interventionists can come from a broad range of medical, psychological, and social service disciplines. The interventionist's role will vary depending on the setting (e.g., community outreach settings, medical or specialty clinics, social service providers, extended care facilities, emergency departments, hospital inpatient wards, etc.), as well as financial, space, and staffing resource constraints. People delivering interventions could be volunteers, community advocacy workers, public health workers, medical health care providers, mental health care providers, social workers, or substance-misuse treatment providers, or have some other professional role. Depending on the setting, they might be part of the existing infrastructure or brought in as auxiliary staff. The role of the interventionists in a given setting will in part dictate the type, format, and content of the brief intervention. For example, a brief intervention delivered by a patient's primary care doctor may be very different from one delivered by a volunteer at a community center. The goals of the interventions in certain settings also determine who provides them. For example, brief interventions in the emergency department might focus on referring older adults to treatment resources, while a community-based treatment center would probably integrate brief interventions and substance-misuse treatment. The training and skills of the interventionists in these two settings would probably be different.

Accordingly, the training and skill sets of interventionists should be commensurate with their role and the population they serve. As an example, the intervention training and skill sets required by a medical health provider who offers brief advice to older adults about alcohol abuse in a specialty care clinic are markedly less than those required by a social worker offering a series of brief interventions about prescription drug misuse to older adults at a community-based organization. Training for interventionists can be provided as part of a defined protocol towards accomplishing a specific goal in a given setting for a particular role (e.g., training of medical technicians in urgent care centers to screen and provide brief advice about smoking cessation). More intensive training would be conducted in accordance with broader goals, such as brief interventions provided by substance-abuse counselors in extended-care facilities for older adults using prescription drugs. Interventionist training might be offered at academic, health care, or community facilities, or by commercial organizations. One organization, the Motivational Interviewing Network of Trainers (MINT), offers training opportunities and certification in motivational interviewing, which is a common component of many brief interventions. This type of training could be incorporated into maintenance-of-certification training for a variety of medical and other healthcare professionals.

The ideal characteristics of an interventionist delivering brief interventions on substance misuse for older adults are not specified. The role the interventionist plays, such as providing brief advice vs. conducting a series of brief interventions, could inform who is chosen and trained for that role. Given the topic (substance misuse) and population served (older adults), ideal characteristics might include a nonjudgemental attitude towards substance misuse, experience in working with older adults, an appreciation of the unique needs of older adults with substance-misuse problems, and an ability to adapt to those needs (e.g., empathy towards concerns about shame, denial, healthcare needs), comfort with using a nonconfrontational support style, etc. (Wu et al. 2011, Kuerbis et al. 2014). Some research has suggested that older adults might respond better to members of their peer age group, given a perception of shared experiences, personal characteristics, perspectives, and cultural styles and approaches (Cooper 2012).

## Challenges of Implementing Substance-Misuse Brief Interventions for Older Adults

There are several challenges in implementing substance-misuse brief interventions for older adults. Chief among these is a lack of efficacy and effectiveness research supporting their use (both in general, and specifically for older adults), and controversy over the best methods for conducting them. Additional challenges include changing substance-misuse behaviors over time, differences in misuse patterns across age cohorts, and differences across cultures and demographic groups. Although there are general principles that unite brief intervention approaches, it is likely that a "one-size-fits-all" approach would not be equally appropriate for different substances (e.g., alcohol vs. prescription opioids), age groups (e.g., baby boomers vs. previous generations), and demographic groups (e.g., non-Hispanic black women vs. Hispanic men) (Cooper 2012). Adjusting the content, speed, number of sessions, and delivery methods of brief interventions for older adults might also affect their efficacy. Technology-enhanced interventions, such as computer-assisted feedback and information and text-messaging reminders, which might be appropriate for younger adults and aid in the effectiveness of interventions, are of unclear utility among older adults. Difficulties with access and experience with their use, as well as vision changes over time, might limit their utilization for this population.

In addition, there are several practical and resource-related challenges to be met. Implementing substance-misuse brief interventions for older adults involves training interventionists in techniques suitable to the setting, setting resources, and goals of the interventions (Babor et al. 2011, Blow et al. 2012). Implementation also involves preparing for time to deliver the interventions, which might be challenging in busy clinical settings, especially if a slower-paced, multi-session intervention is needed for older adults. Lack of, or limited, reimbursement could limit their use in some settings, especially when other, more highly reimbursed, activities are available and resources are limited. Practitioners' lack of comfort with addressing substance misuse and working with older adults, and lack of motivation and interest, perhaps related to concerns about the efficacy/effectiveness of interventions, reimbursement, and overcoming practical challenges, represent potential barriers to the implementation of such brief interventions (Babor et al. 2011, Kalapatapu et al. 2010, Blow et al. 2012). Overcoming mobility and transportation problems (Cooper 2012)—which can affect the structure, number of sessions, and delivery of brief interventions for older adults—is another practical consideration.

## Efficacy and Effectiveness of Substance-Misuse Brief Interventions for Older Adults

Research examining the efficacy or effectiveness of brief interventions for substance use in older adults is sparse in comparison to the number of studies exploring this topic among their younger counterparts. Moreover, there is more information available about the effect of brief interventions on reducing tobacco and alcohol use among older adults, as compared with prescription or illicit drugs and polysubstance use. Published studies also demonstrate conflicting results about the presence or size and duration of effect. Further complicating the interpretation of available evidence, studies vary with regard to the type of intervention, the person delivering the intervention, length of follow-up, study design, and even the characteristics of patients studied. In this final section, we will attempt to distill the available evidence on brief interventions for substance-using older adults. Table 3.1 presents a summary of studies examining the effect of in-person brief interventions on tobacco, alcohol, and drug use/misuse among older adults. Studies of telephone- or web-based interventions, or studies examining proxies for substance use (e.g., medical claims data) will be discussed, but are not included in the table.

### TOBACCO

Hill et al. (1993) was one of the first to introduce the idea of customizing treatment for older adult smokers in a study of behavioral treatment versus physical exercise, and this approach has gained ground since then. Two studies have

**Table 3.1 Summary of Studies on Brief Interventions for Substance Use in Older Adults**

| Substance | Study | Population | Sample Size (n) | Intervention | Control | Main Results | Limitations |
|---|---|---|---|---|---|---|---|
| **Tobacco** | Morgan 1996 | Outpatient clinic, Ages 50–74 | 659 | Brief intervention (BI), Nicotine Replacement Therapy (NRT), booster call | Usual care | At 6 months, quit rate = 15.4% in BI group vs. 8.2% in control ($p < 0.005$) | Details of "usual care" not provided. Study not blinded. Randomized at level of clinic, but detailed characteristics of clinics not provided. Differences in baseline characteristics of study subjects present. |
| | Kim 2005 | Outpatient (Korea) Subgroup age 50+ | 235 | BI by a nurse, booster phone calls | Advice to quit smoking | At 5 months, quit rate = 13.4% in BI group and 13% in control, risk ratio (RR) = 1.03 (0.53–1.99) | Intervention was not tailored to older smokers. |
| | Tait 2006 | Community, Age 68+ | 215 | BI and NRT, (6) telephone sessions over first 12 weeks | Continuing smokers who did not want the intervention | At 6 months, 88.5% of the intervention group had made a quit attempt and 31% had stopped smoking for at least 30 days. No one in the control group quit smoking. | Patients were self-selected for the intervention, and the comparison group was made up of patients who did not want to quit. The study is subject to recall and reporting biases. |

*(continued)*

*Table 3.1* **Continued**

| Substance | Study | Population | Sample Size (n) | Intervention | Control | Main Results | Limitations |
|---|---|---|---|---|---|---|---|
| | Doolan 2008 | Women inpatients with cardiovascular disease, Subgroup age 62+ | 277, (n = 136, age ≥ 62) | BI | Advice to quit smoking | At 6 months, the quit rate was 62% in the BI group vs. 42% in usual care group. No difference at 12 mos. Higher quit rate among older smokers than younger smokers (age < 62). | The study may have been underpowered to detect differences at 12 months. May not be generalizable to a broader population. |
| **Alcohol** | Fleming 1999 | Outpatient clinic, Age 65+ | 158 | Two 10–15 minute physician-led interventions 1 month apart | Received general health booklet | At the 3-month follow-up, the intervention group had reduced alcohol use (−34%), binge-drinking episodes (−74%), and excessive drinking (−64%) compared to controls. These effects were sustained at 12 months. | Groups were different at baseline. Alcohol use was self-reported. No difference in health outcomes was observed. |

| Study | Setting | N | Intervention | Outcome measure | Results | Limitations |
|---|---|---|---|---|---|---|
| Gordon 2003 | Outpatient clinic, Subgroup age 65+ | 45 | Randomized to: (1) BI, or (2) Motivational enhancement (more intensive BI and 2 follow-up sessions) | Alcohol assessments | All groups decreased alcohol use over time (baseline–12 months). No effect of BI. | The study had a small number of older adult participants and may have been under-powered to detect a difference. |
| Moore 2010 | Outpatient clinics, Age 55+ | 631 | Brief oral and written advice from physician, follow-up by health educator at 2, 4, and 8 weeks | Booklet on health behaviors, including alcohol use | At 3 months, the intervention group had fewer at-risk drinkers (odds ratio [OR] 4.1 [0.22–0.75]), drinking fewer drinks (−21%), and less binge drinking (OR 4.6 [0.22–0.99]). This difference was attenuated at 12 months. | Differential loss to follow-up in study groups. |

*(continued)*

Table 3.1 Continued

| Substance | Study | Population | Sample Size (n) | Intervention | Control | Main Results | Limitations |
|---|---|---|---|---|---|---|---|
| | Watson 2013 | Outpatient clinics, Age 55+ | 529 | Brief intervention with referral to treatment as needed | Brief advice (minimal intervention) | Both groups reduced alcohol use over 12 months. No difference between groups at 6 and 12 months follow-up. | Conducted in highest-risk category (AUDIT-C scores ≥ 8). |
| **Poly-substance** | Schonfeld 2010 | Community, Mean age = 75 | 1,999 | SBIRT | N/A | Reduction in alcohol use, medication misuse, and depression scores. | No control group. Medication misuse was determined by "interviewers' impressions." Selection bias— participants referred to study by a community organization. |
| | Schonfeld 2014 | Community, Age 55+ | 8,165 | SBIRT | N/A | Reduction in both alcohol (−45%) and drug use (−24%) at 6 months. | No control group. No differentiation between illicit and prescription drug misuse. |

demonstrated a benefit of a brief intervention in decreasing tobacco use at six months post-intervention compared to usual care or brief advice (Morgan et al. 1996, Doolan et al. 2008). Yet these findings conflict with a Korean study of adults over 50 years old that did not find any effect of a nurse-delivered brief intervention on smoking cessation rates at five months post-intervention (Kim et al. 2005). Notably, this latter study was not tailored to older adult smokers. Of note, the National Cancer Institute does provide smoking cessation guides tailored to those 50 years old and older (Clear Horizons) (Rimer et al. 1994).

There is still insufficient evidence to conclude whether or not positive results of brief interventions on tobacco cessation are sustained over time, since most studies have not evaluated long-term outcomes. Doolan et al. (2008) noted that at the twelve-month follow-up of their study, 58.1% of older smokers in the intervention group had quit, compared with 47.3% in the usual-care group (i.e., given advice to quit smoking); this difference was not statistically significant, but may have lacked a sufficient sample size to detect a difference between groups. Interestingly, this study also found that older smokers had higher quit rates than younger smokers, highlighting the potential benefits of brief interventions among this population.

A large study by Joyce et al. (2008) involved Medicare beneficiaries ($n = 7354$) in seven states who were enrolled voluntarily in the Medicare Stop Smoking Program. Beneficiaries were randomly assigned to one of four arms: (1) usual care (control condition), (2) reimbursement for provider counseling, (3) reimbursement for provider counseling with pharmacotherapy, or (4) telephone counseling quit-line with nicotine patch. All intervention groups had higher self-reported quit rates than the control arm, but the highest quit rates were observed in the telephone counseling plus nicotine patch arm. While this study's telephone counseling approach does not follow the typical format of a brief intervention, this finding supports that changes to health policy can have an important role in smoking cessation. These data also raise the question of whether or not brief interventions over the telephone are a viable alternative to in-person interventions. Telephone and internet-based interventions are important areas for further study. Even a mailed screening and brief intervention was found to be effective at three months in reducing at-risk drinking in individuals aged 50 and older in one study (Kuerbis et al. 2015), and this modality of intervention also deserves consideration (Table 3.1).

## ALCOHOL

Studies of brief interventions for alcohol misuse among older adults have yielded conflicting results. The largest study to date included 631 adults 55 years old and older from outpatient clinics (Moore et al. 2011). In this study, Moore et al. concluded that a brief physician-led intervention followed by three tele-phone booster sessions at two, four, and eight weeks reduced at-risk and heavy drinking at three months, but not at 12 months post-intervention. However, the self-reported quantity of drinking was reduced at three and 12 months in the intervention group. A telephone-based intervention study also revealed its short-term effectiveness of reducing at-risk drinking, but without a sustained effect at one-year follow-up (Lin et al. 2010). A study by Watson et al. (2013) found no difference between the intervention or control groups at six and 12 months. Of note, Watson's study included the highest-risk group of alcohol drinkers, those with AUDIT-C (Alcohol Use Disorders Identification Test) score of greater than 8; the recommended cutoffs to identify problem drinking are four drinks per occasion for men and three for women. This finding raises an interesting question, in that brief interventions may be more successful at lower levels of problem drinking, a topic that should be investigated in future studies. In another investigation of brief interventions, Fleming et al. (1997) enrolled patients with lower levels of alcohol use and noted a positive effect of two brief physician-led interventions. As with smoking, some research in-dicates that older adults may be more receptive than younger adults to inter-vention and treatment for problem drinking. A study on healthcare utilization among older veterans who were randomized to a brief intervention for alcohol use found that a brief intervention was associated with a short-term increase in healthcare utilization, but no long-term effects on inpatient or outpatient use were noted (Copeland et al. 2003). The heterogeneity of interventions across these studies, however, limits our ability to draw conclusions (Oslin et al. 2002).

## ILLICIT AND PRESCRIPTION DRUGS

There are no published studies of brief interventions that specifically ad-dress use of illicit drugs or misuse of prescription drugs among older adults. However, two community-based clinical trials conducted in Florida studied the impact of a brief intervention on reducing all types of substance misuse from alcohol, illicit drugs, prescription drugs, and over-the-counter medica-tions (Schonfeld et al. 2010, Schonfeld et al. 2015). These two prospective cohort studies demonstrated that, by using an SBIRT approach, substance use was decreased at one month and at six months compared to baseline use. This study is noteworthy because it was a large-scale community-based initiative as opposed to an intervention carried out in a medical setting. There were sev-eral methodological limitations to each of these two studies, but the results strongly suggest the need for more rigorous randomized controlled clinical trials to be conducted on the topic of brief interventions for drug misuse for substance-misusing older adults.

Brief interventions have been shown to decrease the use of inappropriately prescribed medications among older persons, particularly benzodiazepines (Tannenbaum et al. 2014, Salonoja et al. 2010). An example of an inappropriate medication prescribing practice would be benzodiazepines prescribed to an older person with frequent falls. However, these interventions were not targeted to patients exhibiting prescription drug misuse. Yet the results of these studies suggest that older adults on psychotropic medications can change their behaviors in response to a brief intervention.

## SUMMARY OF RESEARCH ON SUBSTANCE-MISUSE BRIEF INTERVENTIONS FOR OLDER ADULTS

Overall, we can conclude that there may be a modest benefit to brief interventions for smoking cessation in older adults, but the duration of the effect is unclear. As suggested by Doolan et al. (2008), older adult smokers may be particularly receptive to brief interventions. Overall, there is insufficient evidence to conclude whether or not a brief intervention is beneficial in reducing problematic alcohol use among older adults. It appears that there may be short-term benefit, but current evidence suggests that this benefit is not sustained. Studies are limited on drug-misuse interventions for older adults, although there is some evidence suggesting that overall substance misuse and use of inappropriately prescribed medications can be reduced through brief and related interventions.

## RESEARCH PRIORITIES FOR SUBSTANCE-MISUSE INTERVENTIONS FOR OLDER ADULTS

Preliminary work suggests that some brief interventions are effective at reducing tobacco, alcohol, and drug misuse in older adults. However, it is unclear if reductions in substance use are sustained long-term. There is still a need for more robust clinical trials of brief interventions for substance misuse in older adults, particularly with regard to illicit drugs. Furthermore, future studies should develop and test whether the presence of age-specific content increases the success of the intervention. In other words, does an intervention tailored for the older adult work better? Subsequent studies should also evaluate other health outcomes in addition to substance misuse reduction, such as social isolation, falls, hospitalizations, etc. The case for brief interventions would be considerably strengthened if reductions in substance use were also accompanied by other improvements such as tangible health or economic outcomes.

# References

American Psychiatric Association. *Diagnostic and Statistical Manual of Mental Disorders,* 5th ed. Arlington, VA: American Psychiatric Publishing; 2013.

Babor TE, McRee BG, Kassebaum PA, Grimaldi PL, Ahmed K, Bray J. Screening, brief intervention, and referral to treatment (SBIRT): toward a public health approach to the management of substance abuse. *J Lifelong Learning Psychiatry,* 2011;9(1):130–148.

Barnes AJ, Xu H, Tseng CH, et al. The effect of a patient-provider educational intervention to reduce at-risk drinking on changes in health and health-related quality of life among older adults: the Project SHARE study. *J Subst Abuse Treat,* 2016;60:14–20.

Barrett SP, Meisner JR, Stewart SH. What constitutes prescription drug misuse? Problems and pitfalls of current conceptualizations. *Curr Drug Abuse Rev,* 2008;1(3):255–262.

Blazer DG, Wu LT. Nonprescription use of pain relievers by middle-aged and elderly community-living adults: National Survey on Drug Use and Health. *J Am Geriatr Soc,* 2009;57(7):1252–1257.

Blow FC, Barry KL. Alcohol and substance misuse in older adults. *Curr Psychiatry Rep,* 2012;14(4):310–319.

Blow FC, Barry KL. Use and misuse of alcohol among older women. *Alcohol Res Health,* 2002;26(4):308–315.

Blow FC, Barry KL. Older patients with at-risk and problem drinking patterns: new developments in brief interventions. *J Geriatr Psychiatr Neurol,* 2000;13(3):115–123.

Cooper L. Combined motivational interviewing and cognitive-behavioral therapy with older adult drug and alcohol abusers. *Health Social Work,* 2012;37(3):173–179.

Copeland LA, Blow FC, Barry KL. Health care utilization by older alcohol-using veterans: effects of a brief intervention to reduce at-risk drinking. *Health Educ Behav,* 2003;30(3):305–321.

Doolan DM, Stotts NA, Benowitz NL, Covinsky KE, Froelicher ES. The Women's Initiative for Nonsmoking (WINS) XI: Age-related differences in smoking cessation responses among women with cardiovascular disease. *Am J Geriatr Cardiol,* 2008;17(1):37–47.

Fleming MF, Barry KL, Manwell LB, Johnson K, London R. Brief physician advice for problem alcohol drinkers. A randomized controlled trial in community-based primary care practices. *JAMA,* 1997;277(13):1039–1045.

Han B, Gfroerer J, Colliver J. OAS Data Review: An examination of trends in illicit drug use among adults aged 50 to 59 in the United States. *Office of Applied Studies Data Review,* Aug. 2009. Available at https://www.researchgate.net/publication/242664558_OAS_Data_Review_An_Examination_of_Trends_in_Illicit_Drug_Use_among_Adults_Aged_50_to_59_in_the_United_States. Accessed January 17, 2016.

Hill RD, Rigdon M, Johnson S. Behavioral smoking cessation treatment for older chronic smokers. *Behav Ther,* 1993;24(2):321–329.

Joyce GF, Niaura R, Maglione M, et al. The effectiveness of covering smoking cessation services for Medicare beneficiaries. *Health Serv Res,* 2008;43(6):2106–2123.

Kalapatapu RK, Sullivan MA. Prescription use disorders in older adults. *Am J Addict,* 2010;19(6):515–522.

Kim JR, Lee MS, Hwang JY, Lee JD. Efficacy of a smoking cessation intervention using the AHCPR guideline tailored for Koreans: a randomized controlled trial. *Health Promot Int,* 2005;20(1):51–59.

Kuerbis A, Sacco P, Blazer DG, Moore AA. Substance abuse among older adults. *Clin Geriatr Med,* 2014;30(3):629–654.

Kuerbis AN, Yuan SE, Borok J, et al. Testing the initial efficacy of a mailed screening and brief feedback intervention to reduce at-risk drinking in middle-aged and older adults: the Comorbidity Alcohol Risk Evaluation study. *J Am Geriatr Soc*, 2015;63(2):321–326.

Lin JC, Karno MP, Tang L, et al. Do health educator telephone calls reduce at-risk drinking among older adults in primary care? *J Gen Int Med*, 2010;25(4):334–339.

Moore AA, Blow FC, Hoffing M, et al. Primary care-based intervention to reduce at-risk drinking in older adults: a randomized controlled trial. *Addiction*, 2011;106(1):111–120.

Morgan GD, Noll EL, Orleans CT, Rimer BK, Amfoh K, Bonney G. Reaching midlife and older smokers: tailored interventions for routine medical care. *Prevent Med*, 1996;25(3):346–354.

Oslin DW, Pettinati H, Volpicelli JR. Alcoholism treatment adherence: older age predicts better adherence and drinking outcomes. *Am J Geriatr Psychiatry*, 2002;10(6):740–747.

Rimer BK, Orleans CT, Fleisher L, et al. Does tailoring matter? The impact of a tailored guide on ratings and short-term smoking-related outcomes for older smokers. *Health Educ Res*, 1994;9(1):69–84.

St. John PD, Snow WM, Tyas SL. Alcohol use among older adults. *Rev Clin Gerontol*, 2010;20(1):56–68.

Salonoja M, Salminen M, Aarnio P, Vahlberg T, Kivela SL. One-time counselling decreases the use of benzodiazepines and related drugs among community-dwelling older persons. *Age Ageing*, 2010;39(3):313–319.

Schonfeld L, Hazlett RW, Hedgecock DK, Duchene DM, Burns LV, Gum AM. Screening, brief intervention, and referral to treatment for older adults with substance misuse. *AJPH*, 2015;105(1):205–211.

Schonfeld L, King-Kallimanis BL, Duchene DM, et al. Screening and brief intervention for substance misuse among older adults: the Florida BRITE project. *AJPH*, 2010;100(1):108–114.

Simoni-Wastila L, Yang HK. Psychoactive drug abuse in older adults. *Am J Geriatr Pharmacother*, 2006;4(4):380–394.

Tannenbaum C, Martin P, Tamblyn R, Benedetti A, Ahmed S. Reduction of inappropriate benzodiazepine prescriptions among older adults through direct patient education: the EMPOWER cluster randomized trial. *JAMA: Intern Med*, 2014;174(6):890–898.

Watson JM, Crosby H, Dale VM, et al. AESOPS: A randomised controlled trial of the clinical effectiveness and cost-effectiveness of opportunistic screening and stepped care interventions for older hazardous alcohol users in primary care. *Health Technol Assess*, 2013;17(25):1–158.

Wu LT, Blazer DG. Illicit and nonmedical drug use among older adults: A review. *J Aging Health*, 2011;23(3):481–504.

CHAPTER 4

# Alcohol and Older Adults

*Anna Terajewicz LaRose and John Renner*

## Introduction

Alcohol use in older adults is an important public health concern. Alcohol is the most frequently used drug in older adults. The leading causes of death in older adults—heart disease, cancer, and stroke—can all be influenced by alcohol use (Mokdad 2004). Physiological changes associated with age make this group more susceptible to the complications of acute and long-term alcohol use. Though there is some evidence that light to moderate alcohol use may be cognitively protective in healthy adults, hazardous use can lead to negative health consequences that can affect an individual's quality of life. Historically, there has been less detection and treatment of alcohol-use disorders in older adults compared with the general adult population. This topic is especially important to address now, as the number of older adults in the general population increases. Screening for use, discussing recommendations, and treating hazardous and harmful alcohol use can lead to improvements in health and longevity for this age group.

## Prevalence

When considering the epidemiology of alcohol use in older adults, a few factors are of special importance. In 2030, estimates predict, about a quarter of the population will be over the age of 60 (U.S. Census Bureau 2008). This growth is due to increases in life expectancy and the aging of the baby-boomer generation: the individuals born between 1946 and 1964. Compared with previous generations, this cohort may have had more exposure to alcohol due to cultural shifts in attitudes about alcohol and drug use. Studies of alcohol use gathered before 2006 may underestimate actual alcohol use in this rising cohort.

Additionally, data on alcohol use in older adults have been defined in different ways across studies and countries, and some kinds of use are more harmful to health. For example, binge drinking has been associated with greater overall harm to health, and estimates of alcohol use are not always tailored to look at this and other kinds of harmful alcohol use (Esser 2014).

Alcohol use in older adults has been studied in many national and community surveys in the United States. The largest of these surveys ($n = 43,093$), the National Epidemiologic Survey on Alcohol and Related Conditions (NESARC) in 2001–2002, found that, according to the *Diagnostic and Statistical Manual of Mental Disorders, 4ᵗʰ Edition* (DSM-IV), 2.36% of males and 0.38% of females met criteria for alcohol abuse, and 0.39% of males and 0.13% of females met criteria for alcohol dependence (Grant 2004).

Another survey, the 2005–2006 National Survey on Drug Use and Health found that 43% of those over 65 reported using alcohol in the past year, 13% of men and 8% of women reported at-risk alcohol use, and more than 14% of men and 3% of women reported binge drinking (Blazer 2009). "At-risk use" was defined as two or more drinks on a usual drinking day within the past 30 days, and "binge drinking" was defined as five or more drinks on the same occasion on at least one day within the past 30 days. Furthermore, the data show that, of those over 65, 0.6% showed dependence, 0.9% showed abuse, and 12.5% showed sub-threshold dependence according to DSM-IV criteria (total = 15.4%) (Blazer 2011). At-risk drinking was found to be higher in those with more education, higher incomes, male sex, Caucasian, and tobacco use, while binge drinking was associated with being divorced, separated, or single.

The 2005–2008 National Health and Nutrition Examination Survey of the U.S. population found that 14.5% of people over 65 drink above National Institute on Alcohol Abuse and Alcoholism's (NIAAA) recommendations. These recommendations have their limits. When health status is taken into account, 53.3% of older adults who drink alcohol had hazardous or harmful alcohol use according to the Alcohol Related Problems Survey (ARPS) risk algorithm. This measure has a sensitivity and specificity of 0.93 and 0.66, respectively, to detect hazardous or harmful alcohol consumption (Wilson 2014). These data suggest that, even when formal criteria for alcohol abuse or dependence are not met, harmful alcoholic use is significant in this population if all unhealthy use is taken into account.

When considering alcohol use in older adults, there is also evidence that there are two subtypes of alcohol-dependent individuals, the early-onset older users making up two-thirds of the population of users, and the late-onset older users making up the remaining one-third of the population. There has been evidence that the first group, which begin using alcohol during their twenties or thirties, have more chronic medical problems such as cirrhosis, alcohol-related dementia, and comorbid psychiatric disorders, and are more difficult to treat. The second group generally begin using high levels of alcohol after age 40 or 50 and increase drinking during stressful life events, have fewer medical problems, and are easier to treat (Liberto 1995).

Epidemiological data show that older adults drink less alcohol than younger adults, but a significant portion of older adults who use alcohol exhibit harmful drinking behavior. The definition of "problem alcohol use" in future studies should reflect not only alcohol abuse or dependence, but also hazardous and harmful use. Finally, though the majority of those with harmful alcohol use began having problems earlier in life, up to a third develop problems later in life, and screening should be tailored to detect both subsets.

## Neurobiology of Alcohol Use and Aging

In the past, addiction to alcohol was considered to be a result of moral deficit. Thomas Trotter (U.K.) and Benjamin Rush (U.S.) were among the first to describe alcohol addiction as a disease in the early 1800s, while the term "alcoholism" was coined in 1849 by Magnus Huss. In the late 1800s, Wernicke and Korsakoff described the neurological consequences of excessive alcohol use. Alcohol addiction became considered a disease of loss of control over alcohol use with further research by Jellinek in the 1940s based on surveys of people participating in Alcoholics Anonymous (AA). The DSM identified "alcoholism" as a disorder and classified it with "sociopathic personality disturbances" in 1952. In 1966, the American Medical Association (AMA) formally began considering alcohol addiction a disease. The terms *alcohol dependence* and *alcohol abuse* were introduced formally in 1980 when the DSM-III was published. In 1997, Alan Leshner, Director of the National Institute on Drug Abuse (NIDA), discussed dependence as a neurological disease caused by neuroadaptations of the brain to alcohol (Tabakoff 2013).

The classification of alcohol addiction as a disease has been controversial. The debate hinges on the concern that when one takes personal responsibility away from people by calling alcohol use a disease, then one necessarily condones excessive alcohol use as symptomatic behavior rather than a volitional choice. The controversy partially exists as alcohol addiction manifests differently in different people across the lifespan; and up to 50–75% of people with problematic use are able to stop hazardous alcohol use on their own. This is probably a result of the complex interplay of genetic and environmental influences that lead to individual differences in the neuronal processing and adaptation of the brain to alcohol. It also may explain the increased co-occurrence of substance use in those with mental health concerns. In some individuals, the result of hazardous alcohol use is a chronic, relapsing, and progressive disorder known as "alcohol use disorder" (AUD); in others, the hazardous use never develops into an AUD. This is similar to the course of other diseases such as hypertension and type II diabetes. An individual may have genetic and environmental factors that contribute to the development of the disease, but there are also lifestyle factors that are modifiable by the individual. Some individuals with AUD have greater genetic susceptibility to this disease. Other individuals have lower genetic risk and higher environmental risk. Others may gain insight into the disease process earlier on and can find the motivation to change, halting the progression of the AUD in time.

Extensive research has been done to investigate the neurobiological underpinnings of alcohol addiction. Behaviorally, *alcohol addiction* has been described as use of alcohol that is transformed from an impulse that is positively reinforced into a compulsion that is driven by negative reinforcement. Or, as many patients like to say, "It used to be fun and made me feel good, but now I drink to just feel normal and I can't stop drinking." The neural processes that underlie the behavioral responses are complex and stem from a neuroadaptation involving the motivational, reward, stress, and arousal pathways of the brain. Once alcohol is introduced into the system, it is then reinforced by the euphoria of use. In some individuals, this can lead to alcohol abuse where alcohol continues to be positively reinforced. Alcohol abuse is followed by sensitization with repeated drug exposures, which causes a kindling process, and the cravings become stronger. At some point, the reinforcing value of alcohol changes, and addiction occurs when neuronal adaptations function to drive alcohol use through negative reinforcement; specifically, the avoidance of anxiety and dysphoria associated with cessation of alcohol use. Once adaptation occurs, withdrawal syndromes occur. Additionally, even with long-term abstinence and the extinction of the negative reinforcing value of alcohol, alcohol addiction can persist, and relapse may occur once the individual is primed again with alcohol, resulting in cycles of relapse throughout the individual's lifetime.

Various neurotransmitters and circuits have been implicated in these processes. Alcohol impacts not only $\gamma$-Aminobutyric acid (GABA), but also dopamine, opioid systems, glutamate, serotonin, neuropeptide Y (NPY), and the hypothalamic pituitary axis (HPA) through corticotrophin-releasing factor (CRF) (Gilpin 2008; Koob 2013).

The limbic system evolved to select for humans who stayed alive to reproduce by helping the individual seek things that are necessary for survival, such as food and shelter (causing positive feelings or comfort) and avoid things that are disastrous for survival, such as physical harm (causing feelings of pain and anxiety). Addiction hijacks the limbic circuitry. The specific brain regions currently identified as underlying addictions include the amygdala (fear motivation), prefrontal cortex (salience), and nucleus accumbens (reward-motivation) (Kalivas 2005).

Dopamine is the neurotransmitter that functions to control motivation in the mesolimbic circuit, which starts in the ventral tegmentum and projects to the nucleus accumbens. This circuit is partly responsible for the motivation to drink alcohol, though alcohol dependence does continue if lesions in the system exist, so this circuit is not the only player. Other players are the endogenous opioids: endorphins, enkephalins, and dynorphins. The endogenous opioids are thought to increase alcohol use by influencing the dopamine circuits and also independently by acting on the ventral tegmentum, nucleus accumbens, and central nucleus of the amygdala (Gilpin 2008).

GABA is one of the main neurotransmitters that alcohol influences. Alcohol use increases GABA release from the presynaptic neurons as well as facilitating the postsynaptic neurons. These actions of GABA occur in the nucleus accumbens, ventral palladium, stria terminalis, and amygdala. Not only do these actions occur with acute intoxication, but chronic alcohol exposure causes long-term changes in brain structure related to changes in genomic expression (Gilpin 2008).

Glutamate is another key neurotransmitter involved in the actions of alcohol. Glutamate is the main excitatory neurotransmitter in the brain and binds to the N-methyl-D-aspartate (NMDA) receptor. Alcohol inhibits glutamate in the striatum, including the nucleus accumbens, and this action may be involved with the acute reinforcing effects of alcohol. Additionally, serotonin (5-HT) may influence alcohol use, as serotonin depletion can result in impulsivity and increased alcohol-drinking in rats.

Finally, it is theorized that alcohol also affects other neuronal pathways associated with anxiety, including the hypothalamic release of CFR, which is involved in the HPA-axis stress response, as well as neuropeptide Y, which is found throughout the brain, including the amygdala.

It is important to be aware of the various factors involved in the dependence process when designing and implementing pharmacotherapy for alcohol dependence. Medications for alcohol dependence typically target the neuronal pathways responsible for relapse. For example, cravings can be attenuated by naltrexone, which blocks the opioid receptors, but also by acamprosate, which modulates glutamatergic NMDA receptors. Interestingly, different pharmacotherapies have been found to act on different parts of the relapse process. Specifically, one study modeling alcohol relapse in rats investigated whether different therapies prevented different triggers. In the study, naltrexone was able to block alcohol use related to environmental cues, while a CRF receptor antagonist was able to prevent alcohol use in response to stress (Liu 2002). This finding suggests that therapy can be tailored to patients if one can identify the specific trigger that is causing relapse, or by combination therapy that modulates multiple neuronal targets. Additionally, if pharmacotherapy were directed farther upstream in the neuronal cascade of addiction, the neuroadaptations that lead to addiction might be stopped. Finally, because alcohol dependence is multigenic, different individuals will have different susceptibilities to the neuroadaptations involved in dependence. These individuals are also likely to have different responses to various pharmacotherapies.

Alcohol addiction occurs over a spectrum. Different individuals develop unhealthy alcohol use at different ages, with different amounts of alcohol, and with different kinds of use (e.g., daily use versus binge use). This spectrum is probably related to environmental factors and genetic differences. Alcohol addiction has an approximately 60% genetic heritability in both men and women (10th Special Report, NIAAA, 2000). It is not dependent on simple Mendelian inheritance. Multigenic development of alcohol addiction is consistent with the observed broad clinical spectrum of alcohol use patterns.

The spectrum phenomenon of alcohol use has resulted in the development of different clinically observable subtypes of alcohol addiction. This observation began with Jellinek in the 1960s, who described five types of alcohol-drinking patterns, with *gamma* and *delta* types being associated with alcohol dependence. Gamma was considered to be the most common in the United States and is associated with tolerance, withdrawal, and cravings for alcohol but with the ability to abstain from use, while the delta subtype was similar, but with an inability to abstain from alcohol use. Later, in the 1980s, Cloninger suggested two subtypes, Type I, onset after age 25 with strong social influence; and Type II, onset before age 25, male, and antisocial. These subtypes have been associated with different dopamine and serotonin transporter densities in brain regions as well as genetic polymorphism in neuropeptide Y. In the 1990s, Hill expanded the Cloninger model to include a Type III subtype, those similar to Type II but without sociopathy. Following Cloninger's types, which were based on theory, Babor went on to develop subtypes based on cluster analysis. He characterized type A alcoholics as similar to Cloninger's type I, and type B alcoholics as similar to Cloninger's type II. Type A individuals have a later onset of disease and use alcohol to self-medicate, while Type B have an earlier onset, more psychopathology, and a family history of alcoholism. Other subtypes have been proposed that take into account gender differences and other subtleties. There is some limited evidence that different subtypes respond to different pharmacological and behavioral therapies. For example, sertraline has been found to be of limited benefit in Babor's Type B patients, but it has been found to benefit Type A patients. Ondansetron has been found to be helpful in those with early-onset AUD. This can explain differences in the efficacy of various pharmacotherapies across studies in different countries (Leggio 2009).

One final caveat is that genes contributing to alcohol addiction are independent from genes for the susceptibility of diseases resulting from the use of alcohol. The genes for cirrhosis and cardiomyopathy induced by alcohol are distinct from those associated with alcohol addiction. Thus some people may use more alcohol and still live to older ages, while others use less alcohol and develop alcohol-related health problems earlier on.

Though there is no specific evidence that the neurobiology of alcohol addiction is different in older adults, studies have found changes in various brain circuits related to aging that are also implicated in addiction. Dopaminergic cell bodies, dopamine levels, dopamine receptor binding, and dopamine transporter binding have been found to decrease with age; and the serotonin and glutamine systems also change with age (Dowling 2007). It is unclear how these age-related brain changes may affect the addictive process in the healthy aging adult, or those with neurological problems such as stroke, Parkinsonism, and dementias. It is possible that aging or neurological disease could lead to less prefrontal cortex inhibition and thus more impulsive behavior, including excessive alcohol use; or alternatively, that the addictive circuitry may be impaired, causing less use of alcohol, but there are no studies to date investigating either of these ideas. Additionally, it is important to note that there are likely to be neuronal differences in chronic alcoholics versus those with later onset alcohol-use disorders. Overall, the neurobiology of alcohol dependence in older adults requires more research, but it is probably affected by genetics, medical comorbidity, and especially by neurological issues and length/quantity of alcohol use over the lifetime.

## Alcohol Use Recommendations and Definitions of Unhealthy Use

When assessing drinking in older adults, it is important to be aware of what constitutes a typical drink. In the United States, one drink contains 14 grams of alcohol and is defined as one of the following (Centers for Disease Control and Prevention [CDC], 2014):

- One 12-ounce can or bottle of regular beer, ale, or wine cooler (5% alcohol by volume [ABV])
- One 8- or 9-ounce can or bottle of malt liquor (7% ABV)

- One 5-ounce glass of red or white wine (12% ABV)
- One 1.5-ounce shot glass of hard liquor; e.g., gin, vodka, whiskey (40% ABV)

The NIAAA recommends that healthy older adults (65+) drink no more than seven drinks a week and no more than three drinks on any one day, regardless of gender (Older Adults, NIAAA website 2014). The Substance Abuse and Mental Health Services Administration (SAMHSA) recommends no more than one drink per day and no more than two drinks on one occasion in older men, and lower limits in older women (Treatment Improvement Protocol [TIP[26, SAMHSA, 2008).

These recommendations were tailored toward older adult males who are in good health. Lower levels or abstinence may need to be recommended based on drug interactions, gender, and medical conditions. Additionally, not all people will have the same response to the same amount of alcohol, due to individual differences in metabolism. Defining unhealthy drinking behavior based purely on amount of alcohol consumed has limitations. To meet these limitations, different definitions of alcohol use have been described.

The DSM has been used to diagnose unhealthy alcohol use since the 1950s. The newest edition, the DSM-5, integrates the two DSM-IV disorders, alcohol abuse and dependence, into a single disorder called *alcohol use disorder* (AUD). The criteria for AUD currently include use of alcohol that leads to difficulties in at least 2 out of 11 criteria. The criteria include physiological addiction as evidenced by cravings, withdrawal, and tolerance, as well as difficulties in social or occupational functions. The severity of an AUD—mild, moderate, or severe—is based on the number of criteria met (NIAAA, AUD Comparison DSM-IV and 5, 2013) (DSM-5, 2013).

The use of the DSM-IV criteria of alcohol abuse or dependence in older adults has been criticized. A consensus panel advised that the DSM criteria are difficult to apply to older adults, lack sensitivity for older adults, and should not be the only criteria used when assessing unhealthy alcohol use (TIP 26, SAMHSA, 2008). The criteria for alcohol use in the DSM-5 are very similar to DSM-IV criteria. Whether these criteria are better able to detect unhealthy alcohol use in older adults is yet to be seen. Since the definition of AUD may not encompass all drinking behavior in older adults, alternative definitions should be considered.

A panel of the U.S. Department of Health and Human Services (DHHS) has suggested using the terms *at-risk drinkers* and *problem drinkers* when describing alcohol use in older adults. The at-risk drinker category describes those whose drinking has not yet caused problems, but may bring problems in the near future to the drinker or to others. The problem drinker category includes those who have experienced problems related to drinking, use alcohol heavily, or meet criteria for alcohol dependence or abuse (TIP 26, SAMHSA, 2008).

The World Health Organization (WHO) *International Statistical Classification of Diseases and Related Health Problems* defines harmful and hazardous use of alcohol as the following (ICD-10, 1992):

- Harmful alcohol use is defined as a pattern of use that causes damage to the physical or mental health of the individual.
- Hazardous use is defined as a pattern of use that carries a risk of harmful consequences to the user, either physical or mental.

At-risk drinking falls under the hazardous use category, while problem drinking falls under the harmful use category. The terms *harmful* and *hazardous alcohol use* may be less stigmatizing than the terms *at-risk* and *problem drinker* and may be more acceptable to patients. Stigma is an important point to consider when treating those with unhealthy alcohol use (Kelly 2015). Generally, all these terms help define use that is unhealthy and may be a better alternative to the strict AUD definition when discussing alcohol use in older adults.

"Harmful and hazardous" use depends on a number of factors. In the past, a consensus panel defined harmful and hazardous drinking in older adults as stratified by health status (Moore 1999). In general, moderate to very heavy drinking is considered hazardous, but light to very light drinking is nonhazardous in healthy older adults. Very light or light use may be hazardous in those with chronic medical conditions, medication use, smoking, and functional limitations. Older men who drink four or more drinks on an occasion and older women who drink three or more drinks on an occasion, between twice a month and three times a week, are considered hazardous drinkers (see Figure 4.1).

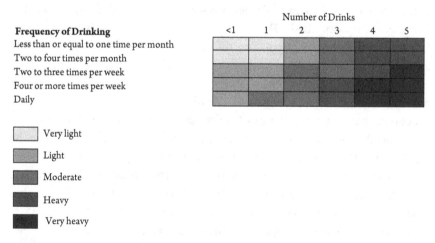

*Figure 4.1* Alcohol use classification in older adults stratified by frequency of drinking and amount used per episode. With permission. Moore AA, Morton SC, Beck JC, et al. A new paradigm for alcohol use in older persons. *Med Care* 1999; 37(2):165–179.

Alcohol-use recommendations are based on heuristics and consensus associated with health risks of use. Recommendations are lower in older adults than younger adults due to the physiological changes that occur with age. These changes include the increased ratio of body fat to body water, decreased hepatic blood flood, and reduced efficiency in the liver's ability to metabolize alcohol. Additionally, alcohol undergoes first-pass metabolism by gastric alcohol dehydrogenase, which is reduced in older adults. These changes can cause higher absolute levels of alcohol in older adults (Ferreira 2008).

Overall, the key to defining unhealthy alcohol use in older adults is to consider both the amount of alcohol consumed and the effects of the alcohol on the individual's functioning and health.

## Screening Measures

Screening for alcohol use is the first step in treating unhealthy alcohol use. The most common kinds of screens are self-reports and biomarkers. Both methods have their limitations. Generally, self-reports may not be reliable, and the specificity of biomarkers is variable. Additionally, recommendations for screening are not always implemented. The U.S. Preventive Services Task Force (USPSTF) recommends that all adults be screened for alcohol use (Moyer 2013). Primary care doctors have been found to screen only 15.7% of all adults and only 9.3% of adults 65 or older (McKnight-Eily 2014).

A range of self-report screening tools are available. These include the CAGE (Cut down, Annoyed, Guilty, Eye opener), AUDIT (AlcoholUse Disorders Identification Test), AUDIT-C (abbreviated AUDIT), MAST (Michigan Alcohol Screening Test), and single-item screens such as "Did you use alcohol in the past three months?" These screens have varying sensitivity and specificity, depending on the population studied. The CAGE is brief and is widely used. The AUDIT was developed by the World Health Organization, and the AUDIT-C is a shortened version of the test. The AUDIT performs best for hazardous or harmful drinking, and CAGE is best for alcohol dependence in general primary care populations (Berks 2008). The USPSTF currently recommends that primary care doctors screen all adults for alcohol use using the AUDIT, AUDIT-C, or a single-question screening (Moyer 2013).

The screens validated in older adults include the CAGE, MAST, MAST-G (Geriatric), SMAST-G (Short, Geriatric), AUDIT, and the ARPS (Alcohol Related Problems Survey). The studies are few and have been done in the veteran or community-dwelling setting. The CAGE has median sensitivity across studies of 66.7% (range 31–86%) and specificity of 89% (range 92–78%) (O'Connell 2004, Culberson 2006). The AUDIT has fewer data than the

CAGE, but was found to have better sensitivity and specificity, over 85% with a 5 or greater cut point for the AUDIT, or a 4 or greater cut point for the AUDIT-C (Aalto 2011). The SMAST-G has items specific to the elderly and is shorter than the 24-question MAST-G. In one trial, both had similar sensitivity and specificity when compared in patients who had suffered cerebral vascular accidents (CVA). (Johnson-Greene 2009). Interestingly, fewer than half of people screening positive on either the CAGE or the SMAST-G screened positive on both measures (Moore, Seeman 2002). The ARPS is a 10–15-minute-long questionnaire with sensitivity up to 92% and specificity of 66% and is able to identify harmful drinking, not only AUD (Moore, Beck 2002). An additional way to assess alcohol use includes asking patients to keep a log of their drinking behaviors for a week or two, but this may be limited by patient compliance and by patients' using less alcohol when monitoring themselves (Oslin 2009).

There is no single best test to detect unhealthy alcohol use in older adults. When evaluating for alcohol use, a single question can be used initially, such as "Did you use alcohol in the past three months?" followed up with a longer screening tool if this is positive, such as the AUDIT or SMAST-G if assessing for hazardous or harmful drinking, CAGE if looking for AUD, or if time allows, the ARPS for a detailed assessment. These screens should be done at initial patient encounters and reassessed annually or more frequently if patients present with nonspecific complaints such as gait disturbance, falls, confusion, weight loss, or cognitive issues. Use of family or other collaterals is useful when patients have memory disturbances.

Self-reports are the most commonly recommended screening tools for alcohol use, but they depend on valid patient recall and may take time to complete. There have been efforts to find laboratory tests to determine unhealthy drinking behaviors. In general, biomarkers are not typically used as screening measures due to their cost and low positive predictive value, but they can be of some use clinically in certain circumstances.

Physiological markers of long-term, heavy alcohol use include gamma-glutamyl transferase (GGT), the aminotransferases (AST/ALT), macrocytic volume (MCV), high density lipoprotein (HDL), and carbohydrate-deficient transferrin (CDT). The use of these markers in the general population as screening tools is not generally recommended, but they can be helpful when assessing hazardous alcohol use in certain patient populations, including those who minimize their use due to guilt, are in denial, or have cognitive deficits. The results of these tests should be interpreted cautiously. In older adults, these biomarkers have even less value due to lack of sensitivity and specificity in this population.

The kinds of biomarkers available include direct markers that detect alcohol or its metabolites, or indirect markers that look at tissue damage due to alcohol use. The traditional indirect biomarkers include gamma-glutamyl transferase (GGT), aspartate aminotransferase (AST), alanine amino-transferase (ALT), mean corpuscular volume (MCV), and carbohydrate-deficient transferrin (CDT). GGT is the most commonly used indirect biomarker. It is found in endothelial cell membranes and is detectable after heavy drinking over several weeks and returns to normal within two to six weeks after cessation of alcohol use. It can also be elevated from hepatobiliary disease, obesity, diabetes, and hypertension. The aminotransferases are enzymes that catalyze amino group transfers in hepatocytes, and elevated levels are a marker of liver damage. Typically, AST is elevated more than ALT in heavy drinkers, and the cut-off ratio for alcohol-related transaminase elevation is usually >2 AST:ALT. Like GGT, there are many other reasons for elevation of these enzymes, including physiological and viral hepatobiliary diseases. MCV may be another marker of heavy alcohol use, which can be the result of direct alcohol use or nutritional deficiencies secondary to use. In general, MCV is not very sensitive or specific and may take the longest to normalize with alcohol cessation. Transferrin is a glycoprotein metabolized by the liver. When the liver is damaged, the transferrin does not get metabolized properly, causing the accumulation of CDT in the blood. It is elevated with heavy drinking for at least two or three weeks. False positives are less likely but can be found in patients with liver diseases, kidney and pancreas transplants, or with errors of glycoprotein metabolism. CDT is more specific than other tests and is the most sensitive for detecting recent relapses (Allen 2003).

The traditional biomarkers MCV, GGT, AST, and ALT are unreliable in the elderly. CDT has higher sensitivity and specificity in younger men than in older men and women. Newer indirect biomarkers include the total amount of sialic acid in blood serum (TSA), but it is also not reliable with older adults (Kalapatapu 2009).

Direct biomarkers include ethanol and ethyl glucuronide (EtG). Ethanol can be detected readily in serum, saliva, urine, or breath with very good sensitivity and specificity. Due to its rapid elimination, it can only be used to detect recent alcohol use and does not indicate problem use unless the level is high. In the emergency setting when evaluating for altered mental status or delirium, it is important to obtain ethanol levels. Comparing ethanol level versus clinical intoxication can also be used to estimate tolerance (Kalapatapu 2009). EtG is a metabolite of alcohol that is detectible in urine for up to five days. It is very sensitive and can be found to be elevated from sources such as cough syrup and mouthwash. EtG levels may naturally increase with age. Other direct and indirect biomarkers are not readily available across laboratories, and even fewer data are available about their use in older adults.

Overall, when assessing for alcohol use in older adults, it is important to do so regularly and to use all available data. In the past, there have been barriers to identifying alcohol use in older adults. These include the myth that people with unhealthy alcohol use cannot be functioning upper-class older adults, the lack of knowledge about treatment resources for older adults, pessimism about prognosis, denial and shame, fewer social warning signs, and the fact that alcohol-related health issues can be confounded by age-related medical problems and drugs (Menninger 2002). The purpose of screening older adults should be to detect use of alcohol that is hazardous or harmful, and then to use this information to help treat the patient.

## Benefits of Alcohol Use

Over 100 population-based studies have found a J-shaped relationship between alcohol intake and mortality, with *moderate use*, one to three drinks a day, being associated with decreased relative risk of death when compared with no use or excessive use in those over the age of 50. These studies are correlational and do not take into account individual differences and should not be interpreted as clinical recommendations, especially in women and those with medical problems. The benefits of alcohol use are thought to be mediated by alcohol itself, the phytochemicals that serve as antioxidants to decrease oxidative stress generated by normal physiological processes, and by increasing social interaction and decreased stress (Ferreira 2008).

Various studies indicate that moderate use of alcohol decreases coronary heart disease, inflammation, and dementia. One recent cross-sectional study sampling over 580 multi-ethnic individuals over the age of 65 found that those who had light to moderate alcohol use were found to have larger relative brain volumes than non-drinkers. The findings were related to wine consumption and not to other types of alcohol use (Gu 2014). A recent systematic review looking at dementia in those 65 years or older found that moderate alcohol use is associated with a 38% reduced risk of dementia (Peters 2008). Other studies of brain volume and alcohol use have shown mixed results. A recent meta-analysis of ischemic heart disease and alcohol use did find decreased relative risk of ischemic heart disease that is maximized in men with around 30 grams of alcohol per day and around 15 grams of alcohol per day for women, but the studies had significant heterogeneity and large standard deviation (Roerecke 2012).

Though there have been some studies linking low-level alcohol use to increased health and longevity, a recent meta-analysis did not find a statistically significant association between low-level intake and decreased mortality, but it did confirm higher levels of mortality with use of 40 grams per day of alcohol in adult men (slightly less than three standard U.S. drinks) (Jayasekara 2014). Other studies have found alcohol use of 50–60 grams (3.5–4 standard U.S. drinks) to be toxic in older adults and in adult women. The use of alcohol above this amount was associated with an increased relative risk of mortality that continues to be directly proportionate to the amount of alcohol imbibed (Roerecke 2013).

In summary, there is some evidence correlating light-to-moderate alcohol use to improved health, but this should be interpreted cautiously. Alcohol use should not be recommended to those who do not drink alcohol. More research needs to be done on the potential health benefits of alcohol in order to clarify alcohol use recommendations.

## Risks and Medical Complications of Alcohol Use

Excessive alcohol use is toxic to every organ system. Generally, the organ damage attributable to alcohol is associated with its metabolism. The pathophysiology includes systemic accumulation of aldehyde dehydrogenase and acetaldehyde, increases in reactive oxygen species (ROS), increases of tumor necrosis factor alpha (TNFa) in brain and liver, as well as stellate cell activation in the pancreas and liver. This inflammatory response is thought to mediate apoptosis and cell death or carcinogenesis (Li 2008). There are numerous effects on various organ systems with excessive alcohol use. Older adults are at higher risk for gastritis, pancreatitis, symptomatic withdrawal, and delirium (Menninger 2002).

In the year 2000, alcohol was estimated to be the third leading preventable cause of death, attributable to 3.5% of deaths that year, following tobacco (18.1%), and poor diet and physical inactivity (16.6%) (Mokdad 2000). In working adults, alcohol-related mortality is estimated to be even higher, 9.8% (Stahre 2014). The CDC attributed 87,789 deaths to alcohol use (38,253 to chronic causes and 49,544 to acute causes) per year between 2006 and 2010. Of the chronic-illness causes of death, those attributed to at least 1,000 deaths were alcoholic liver disease, liver cirrhosis, alcohol dependence syndrome, alcohol abuse, hemorrhagic stroke, and hypertension. Medical problems related to chronic alcohol use are directly correlated to dose of alcohol and to the genetic susceptibility of the specific individual. Of the acute causes of alcohol-related deaths, those attributed to at least 1,000 deaths were motor vehicle traffic crashes, poisoning (non-alcohol), suicide, homicide, fall injuries, alcohol poisoning, and fire injuries (alcohol related disease impact (ARDI), CDC, 2013). Acute intoxication can also lead to death and disability from delirium, falls, fractures, hypertension, arrhythmias, electrolyte disturbance, decreased respiratory drive, aspiration, and insomnia. There are limited data regarding alcohol-attributable mortality in older adults. Previous epidemiological research has found that alcohol-related hospitalizations in older adults were 54.7 per 10,000 in men and 14.8 per 10,000 in women, similar to hospitalization rates for myocardial infarction (Adams, 1993). In a recent meta-analysis, the relative risk of death for men over 60 with alcohol-use disorders is 2.14, and for women over 60 it is 2.92 (Roerecke 2013).

## NERVOUS SYSTEM

The pathophysiology of neuronal damage by alcohol is complicated and not fully understood. Alcohol is thought to mediate neuronal damage directly, but also indirectly through its metabolic byproducts, nutritional deficits, electrolyte disturbance, trauma, and vascular changes. Alcohol is hypothesized to cause excitotoxicity of the NMDA receptors on glutamatergic neurons, which are found in high concentrations in the hippocampus and frontal lobes. It is also believed to cause oxidate stress and disrupt neurogenesis in the brain. Alcohol is pro-inflammatory and may cause damage by disrupting cytokines and leading to systemic and neurological inflammation. The apolipoprotein E epsilon 4 allele has been associated with increased susceptibility for neurotoxicity from alcohol (Kim 2012).

Not only does alcohol affect the brain through intoxication, blackouts, and addiction, it also can have long-term degenerative affects. Alcohol use can affect the brain by causing Wernicke-Korsakoff syndrome, Marchiafava-Bignami disease, and alcohol-related dementia. Alcohol can also cause indirect brain damage through hepatic encephalopathy and traumatic brain injury from falls resulting in subdural hematoma and cerebral contusion.

Wernicke-Korsakoff syndrome (WKS) is a spectrum of neurological disorders that are due to a deficiency in thiamine (vitamin $B_1$) and can occur in up to 12.5% of those with alcohol dependence. The classic triad of ophthalmoplegia, gait instability, and altered mental status in Wernicke encephalopathy (WE) is found in only 20% of patients; often cognitive impairment is the only symptom present. Uncorrected WE can lead to Korsakoff syndrome (KS), which is characterized by global amnesia and confabulations in addition to gait abnormalities. WE is associated with atrophy of the mammillary bodies and KS with global gray matter volume deficits. The pathophysiology of WKS is thought to include accumulation of acetaldehyde, increases in reactive oxygen species, decreased brain-derived neurotrophic factor, glutamate excitotoxicity, decreased thiamine pyrophosphate, liver dysfunction, and the synergistic effects of these processes. The brain changes associated with WKS can be corrected with thiamine supplementation and alcohol abstinence due to neuroplasticity, as evidenced by MRI studies (Zahr 2011). Marchiafava-Bignami is another neurological disease related to thiamine deficiency. It is a rare disease of chronic alcoholics in which the corpus callosum becomes progressively demyelinated, eventually leading to coma and, following recovery, seizure and dementia (Hillbom 2014).

Alcohol-related dementia (ARD) or alcohol-related brain damage (ARBD) is a clinical diagnosis describing a dementing process that is caused by brain damage due to alcohol, which results in global brain atrophy and multi-domain cognitive difficulties. Whether ARD is related to WKS is unknown, but some postulate that these degenerative brain disorders may be on a spectrum and may have related pathophysiologies (Zahr 2011). Up to 78% of those with alcohol dependence have shown brain pathology at autopsy. The brain changes related to heavy alcohol use include increases in the ventricles, especially the third ventricle; white matter loss; and atrophy of the cerebellum, and the frontal and prefrontal cortex (Ridley 2013). Heavy alcohol use has been linked not only to ARD but also to vascular dementia and mixed dementia subtypes. There is also evidence of memory and executive function impairment in those not specifically diagnosable with ARD who use alcohol excessively. The degree of deficit is related to gender, duration of use, amount used, age of onset, as well as genetic issues as alcohol-naïve subjects with family alcohol dependence have been found to have fronto-cerebellar connectivity alterations (Sinforiani 2010).

Alcohol has been controversially associated with both neuroprotection as well as cognitive decline. A recent cohort study looking at over 3,000 Australian community-dwelling men age 65 or older found that moderate use of alcohol (10–19 standard US drinks per week) was associated with reduced odds of cognitive impairment, but it was not found to be statistically significant after the analysis was adjusted for age, education, marital status, and previous cardiovascular disease. The population of heavy drinkers in the study was not large enough to detect differences (Almeida 2014).

Another study, the UK Whitehall II cohort study, looked at over 5,000 men and over 2,000 women and assessed them for cognitive changes over time, starting from a mean age of 56 years and assessing two times within 10 years after the initial assessment. The study found that men consuming at least 36 grams/day (2.5 standard U.S. drinks) had faster declines in cognitive functioning equivalent to 2.4 extra years of global cognitive decline and 5.7 years of memory decline. In women, consuming up to 9.9 grams/day of alcohol (about three-fourths of a standard American drink) was found to be protective compared to abstainers with about 5 extra years of cognitive function.

Those with at least 19 grams/day (about 1.33 standard U.S. drinks) showed a non–statistically significant association with decline in executive function of 2.4 years (Sabia 2014).

A U.S. prospective cohort study followed over 6,000 middle-aged adults in the Health and Retirement Study for up to 19 years, to assess for AUD and the risk of cognitive impairments in later life. The study found that a history of AUD was associated with a 2.21 odds of severe memory impairment and with a 1.80 odds of cognitive impairment (not statistically significant). At baseline, those with AUD were found to be younger, less educated, male, have lower socioeconomic status, have a history of cardiovascular disease, and have lower cognitive function (Kuzma 2014).

Additionally, it is important to note that alcohol-associated degenerative brain changes may lead to different outcomes in each individual. The cognitive reserve hypothesis suggests that the same amount of brain damage can have varying effects on different people. Those with greater cognitive reserve may use compensatory mechanisms to overcome brain damage (Consentino 2012). Thus the same amount of damage may not have the same clinical appearance. Taking these factors into account, as well as the fact that the studies to date do not support moderate use of alcohol, alcohol use should not be encouraged in patients as a neurocognitive aid.

Finally, other neurological problems associated with alcohol use include peripheral neuropathy ($B_{12}$ deficiency), optic neuropathy, and pellagra (dermatitis, diarrhea, and dementia) from niacin deficiency.

## GASTROINTESTINAL SYSTEM

The gastrointestinal (GI) system is affected by alcohol use. Even at low doses, alcohol can be associated with gastro-esophageal reflux disease (GERD) and mucosal inflammation, including esophagitis and gastritis. At higher doses and with longer periods of use, alcohol is associated with pancreatitis, GI bleeding, Mallory-Weiss tears (bleeding from the gastro-esophageal junction after vomiting), liver problems, and alcoholic bowel disease. Hepatic effects of alcohol occur across a spectrum, starting with fatty liver, progressing to alcoholic hepatitis, and finally cirrhosis. Women are at greater risk of developing hepatitis with fewer years of drinking and smaller amounts of alcohol. Over 90% of heavy and binge drinkers develop fatty liver, while 10–20% of them develop alcoholic hepatitis. Fewer will develop cirrhosis, but cirrhosis is highly fatal, with death rates of 60% at four years. Development of hepatitis is linked with dose, chronicity, and genetics (Mailliard 2012). Cirrhosis can lead to various complications, including portal hypertension, ascites, esophageal varices, and lower GI bleeding. Individuals with AUDs are also at higher risk for hepatitis C. Generally, these GI effects are more frequently seen in older adults who have had longstanding alcohol problems, but they can also present in older adults with more recent alcohol misuse.

Nutritionally, alcohol can interfere in absorption of nutrients, suppress appetite, and provide empty calories. This can result in malnutrition, weight loss, vitamin and mineral deficiencies including vitamins A, $B_1$ (thiamine), $B_2$ (riboflavin), $B_3$ (niacin), $B_6$ (pyridoxine), C, D, E, folate, calcium, and zinc (Chase 2005).

## CARDIOVASCULAR AND PULMONARY SYSTEMS

Alcohol can affect the entire cardiovascular system. Alcohol is known to cause cardiomyopathy, hypertension, arrhythmias such as "holiday heart" syndrome (acute arrhythmia after heavy ethanol use in a person without heart disease), stroke (ischemic and hemorrhagic), and coronary artery disease. In the pulmonary system, alcohol use is associated with snoring and worsening of sleep apnea (central and obstructive) in addition to atelectasis and aspiration pneumonia.

## MUSCULOSKELETAL SYSTEM

Acutely, alcohol use can lead to increased risk of injury from fractures and bruising due to gait instability associated with intoxication, as well as rhabdomyolysis with high levels of alcohol use and immobility. Long-term use has been associated with osteoporosis—the exact mechanism not being known but probably related to disruption of the skeletal remodeling process directly and indirectly though nutritional deficiency and hormonal regulation (10th Report, NIAAA, 2000). Alcoholic myopathy can also be observed with long-term alcohol use leading to type II fiber atrophy and decreased total muscle mass related to RNA disruption (Preedy 2001).

## HEMATOPOIETIC SYSTEM

Acute high-level alcohol use as seen in binge drinking is associated with impairment in immunity as well as an increase in inflammatory cytokines. Long-term alcohol use has been associated with anemia (folic acid deficiency), lymphocytopenia, and thrombocytopenia. These disorders have been associated with bone marrow stem cell progenitor suppression and can lead to an increased risk of infections and bleeding. Furthermore, there is evidence of alcohol-triggered autoimmunity that causes damage to other organ systems.

## CANCER

Chronic alcohol use is also known to be associated with cancers such as tongue cancer, pharyngeal cancer, pancreatic cancer, esophageal cancer, hepatocellular carcinoma, and colorectal cancer. Many studies have also implicated heavy (three or more drinks per day) alcohol use with an increased risk of breast cancer.

## PSYCHIATRIC DISORDERS

An association between alcohol and other drug use and mental disorders has been long observed in the general population. Alcohol use itself is known to precipitate depression or worsen existing depression in those who use alcohol to alleviate mood symptoms. The U.S. National Comorbidity Survey found a 2.4 odds ratio between lifetime mental disorder and alcohol and drug disorder; about half of those with AUD had at least one mental disorder, and about half of those with a mental health disorder had an AUD or drug dependence (Kessler 2004). There is some thought that the association between AUD and depression is a causal link in which AUD increases the risk for depression (Boden 2011). There is also the self-medication hypothesis, where depression is thought to lead to alcohol use. In older adults, there is also an increased risk of other mental health diagnoses, but there are limited studies on the association of AUD and mental health issues in older adults. The studies to date have shown increases in mental health issues in older adults with AUD, especially depression, anxiety, and insomnia. The association between the two realms may be causal, but there is a lack of evidence. Clinical observation suggests that it is possible in older adults that late-onset depression could be precipitated by life changes associated with aging or medical problems. Older adults may use alcohol as a way to cope with these changes. Alternatively, older adults may use alcohol more socially as they retire and be unaware of recommended levels of alcohol use, inadvertently causing depression from overuse of alcohol. This would be an important topic for further study.

# Drug Interactions

Many older adults are at risk for drug–alcohol interactions, as over 90% of older adults use prescription medications. Drug interactions with alcohol are varied and include drugs that increase blood alcohol levels (histamine H2 blockers), drugs with increased or decreased metabolism with alcohol (benzodiazepines, warfarin, propranolol), and drugs that increase hepatic toxicity (acetaminophen, isoniazid). Alcohol can also potentiate and worsen side effects of various drugs, including GI bleed with NSAIDS or aspirin; sedation when combined with benzodiazepines, narcotics, antihistamines, and antidepressants; or hypotension when combined with nitrites, alpha blockers, or antidepressants. Finally, alcohol can interact with the effectiveness of certain drugs, including those used to treat hypertension, diabetes, gout, gastritis, depression, insomnia, liver disease, and seizures (Moore 2007).

Due to the possibility of drug–alcohol interactions, it is important for clinicians to check drug interactions using websites or desk references—while recognizing that some drug-interaction websites will include alcohol as a drug in the interaction interface, but not all interactions are found. For example, warfarin, propranolol, and acetaminophen showed interactions on common websites, but other interactions, such as ranitidine and gabapentin, were not shown. Additional resources should be used when investigating drug–alcohol interactions, and potential interactions should regularly be discussed with patients when adding or adjusting medications or when discussing use of over-the-counter medications.

## Treatment

Current treatments for alcohol use consist of supportive measures for acute intoxication, management of withdrawal, brief interventions for treatment of hazardous alcohol use, and intensive treatment of long-term harmful alcohol use.

## Acute Intoxication

When older adults present to the emergency department (ED) with evidence of alcohol intoxication, the treatment should focus on supportive measures and the assessment of comorbid conditions and confounding medical and psychiatric conditions such as diabetic ketoacidosis, encephalitis, stroke, or other drug toxicity. Treatment of alcohol intoxication includes assessing the patient's alertness and orientation; stabilizing airway, breathing, and circulation; identifying injuries; checking glucose levels, and correcting electrolyte disturbances. Coma/unconsciousness usually occurs with levels exceeding 300 mg/dL, and death can occur at levels of 400mg/dL, but this depends on the patient's tolerance, and some individuals with levels as high as 600mg/dL may still be conscious. Typically, alcohol concentration decreases by 20–30 mg/dL/h, but this rate can be much faster in those with higher metabolism. Withdrawal symptoms are possible even when the blood alcohol content (BAC) is above 200 mg/dL in those who have longstanding alcohol use. An important aspect of treating acute intoxication is to assess alcohol levels and monitor vitals, then to treat withdrawal symptoms. This can be especially important in older adults with longstanding alcohol use because they are at higher risk for complicated alcohol withdrawal. Furthermore, alcohol use increases the risk of psychiatric issues as well as the danger of harm to self and others. Alcohol is involved in up to 50% of suicide attempts. Basic psychiatric screens for comorbid conditions such as depression, suicidality, and homicidality should also occur in the emergency setting when an individual presents with acute intoxication.

Another emergent problem to consider when treating intoxication in older adults is WKS. Wernicke's encephalopathy can be easily treated and is often underdiagnosed. The European Federation of Neurological Societies recommends using the criteria of two out of four of the following signs when diagnosing WKS: dietary deficiency, ocular motor abnormality, cerebellar dysfunction, and altered mental status or mild memory impairment (Zahr 2011). Treatment typically includes 100 mg of parenteral or intramuscularly administered thiamine, as oral absorption is poor in chronic alcohol users.

The emergency setting is also an important place to consider alcohol-related medical complications when older adults present with nonspecific symptoms such as altered mental status, weakness, incontinence, and frequent falls. When the patient is unable to give a thorough past medical history, involvement of family or collaterals can be very helpful.

This setting may also be used for screening and brief interventions for alcohol use, as up to 24–31% of patients in the ED have problem drinking behaviors. Numerous studies have found that interventions in the ED setting can decrease alcohol use. Lack of training, legal issues, and time constraints in the ED are among the largest obstacles to the implementation of these interventions. Alternative ways to deal with these barriers included computer-based approaches or the Project ASSERT model (Alcohol & Substance Abuse Services, Education, and Referral to Treatment). The Project ASSERT model at Boston Medical Center and Yale–New Haven Hospital uses community outreach workers or health-promotion advocates to screen, intervene, and refer patients with alcohol problems to appropriate treatment settings. This model has been found to be effective in helping patients get enrolled into treatment and is cost-effective (D'Onofrio 2004).

## Management of Alcohol Withdrawal

Acute alcohol withdrawal is a potentially life-threatening disorder that occurs with abrupt cessation of alcohol use. There is a range of symptoms associated with alcohol withdrawal, including tremor, anxiety, diaphoresis, increased pulse, hypertension, seizures, and delirium tremens (DTs). The severity of withdrawal depends on the amount used, chronicity of use, comorbid conditions, and individual factors.

In general, the onset of alcohol withdrawal can occur from a few hours to 24 hours after the last drink, depending on individual factors. Most alcohol withdrawal symptoms peak at 72 hours and will resolve within five to seven days. Alcohol withdrawal seizures and the DTs have different timelines. Withdrawal seizures usually occur 6–48 hours following cessation of alcohol intake. Typically, fewer than 10% of those with alcohol withdrawal symptoms experience withdrawal seizures. Of these, 90% develop seizures within 48 hours of cessation, while fewer than 3% of seizures occur from 5–20 days post-cessation (Trevisan, 1998). DTs usually develop three days after alcohol cessation in those with chronic alcohol use and usually last for two to three days, but can last for up to eight days. About 3–5% of those with alcohol withdrawal develop DTs, and 1–4% with DTs die as a result. Symptoms include autonomic hyperactivity, hallucinations, confusion, and disorientation. Clinical Institute Withdrawal Assessment for Alcohol (CIWA) scores above 15, elevated systolic blood pressure (>150 mm Hg), elevated pulse (>100 bpm), prior seizures, prior DTs, older age, and comorbid medial issues increase the risk of experiencing DTs (Ropper 2014).

There are few studies assessing alcohol withdrawal in older adults; those that exist are observational studies. It has long been hypothesized that advanced age is associated with increased severity of withdrawal, seizures, and delirium. Some studies have shown this to be the case, but others have not. The largest retrospective study to date found that alcohol withdrawal severity and benzodiazepine requirements do not increase with age, but that older adults are at higher risk for cognitive and functional impairments during alcohol withdrawal. This can occur in up to one-third of patients over 60 years of age (Kraemer, 1997). In addition, those with longer periods of alcohol use are at higher risk for withdrawal, though two individuals with similar chronicity and amounts of use may experience different severities of withdrawal symptoms, as withdrawal occurs across a spectrum. When assessing individuals, it is important to ask about chronicity of use, amount of use, and history of complicated withdrawal or withdrawal seizures.

There is no specific tool to use when assessing withdrawal in older adults. Assessment can be done using a standardized scale such as the Clinical Institute Withdrawal Assessment for Alcohol–Revised Version (CIWA-Ar), which assesses for autonomic and other symptoms, including nausea, tremor, the sweats, anxiety, agitation, hallucinations, and headache (Sullivan, 1989). Another tool that that was recently developed to assess for complicated alcohol withdrawal in medically ill patients is the Prediction of Alcohol Withdrawal Severity Scale (PAWSS). The PAWSS takes into account autonomic hyperactivity, blood alcohol level (BAL), and previous withdrawal or DTs (Maldonado 2014). There are no studies to date regarding the sensitivity or specificity of this test in older adults, but it may be found to be useful in older patients at risk for complicated withdrawal.

After assessment, the use of benzodiazepines has long been the standard of care for treating alcohol withdrawal in either a fixed schedule, front-loading, or symptom-triggered regimen (Kraemer, 1997). Management of withdrawal can be accomplished with a variety of different benzodiazepines, including diazepam (Valium), chlordiazepoxide (Librium), oxazepam (Serax), and lorazepam (Ativan). The benzodiazepines differ in half-life, presence of active metabolites, metabolism (hepatic and/or renal), and delivery method. The choice of using a long-acting benzodiazepine has to be weighed against the risk of delirium and over-sedation, while using a short-acting benzodiazepine may lead to breakthrough symptoms and complicated withdrawal. In older adults, especially if they have cognitive decline or a history of delirium, short-acting benzodiazepines such as lorazepam or oxazepam can be used to minimize cognitive effects. Lorazepam should be used over oxazepam in those with liver dysfunction or those who are in need of intravenous dosing. In older adults, a small study found that a symptom-triggered approach to alcohol withdrawal has been found to be superior to usual care, resulting in less-severe and shorter-duration alcohol withdrawal management (Taheri 2014). The use of other drugs for alcohol withdrawal has not been extensively studied in older adults, though anticonvulsants such as gabapentin may be found to be good alternatives to use in the future when treating older adults, given their side-effect profile. Detoxification is usually done in the inpatient setting, as outpatient detoxification is not generally recommended for older or younger adults given the medical risks associated with alcohol withdrawal.

The goals of treatment of those with complicated withdrawal, including those who develop seizures and DTs, are controlling agitation and decreasing the risk of seizure and injury. This is often done in the intensive care unit and includes treatment of withdrawal with benzodiazepines, usually intravenously. Benzodiazepine doses have been described in the literature based on uncontrolled studies but include administering loading doses to prevent seizures and autonomic dysfunction, then adding maintenance doses of 5–20 mg per hour of diazepam or 10–30 mg per hour of lorazepam as needed. Adjunctive medications to control autonomic hyperactivity or agitation include propofol, haloperidol, and dexmedetomidine (an alpha-2 agonist), but these have not been studied extensively in older adults (Schuckit 2014).

Those with longstanding AUD are at risk for general medical complications as well as alcohol-related medical complications. It is important to consider and treat these issues, which can include infectious, metabolic, traumatic, and cardiovascular issues, in those with alcohol withdrawal who do not respond to treatment. Finally, seizures in those with AUD can also occur due to head injury, metabolic disturbances, and other toxic exposure, and seizures that continue despite withdrawal treatment should be further evaluated.

## Treating Hazardous and Harmful Alcohol Use

The first step in treating hazardous or harmful alcohol use is to screen patients for alcohol use. If the individual is found to screen positively, further evaluation and brief interventions or referral for more intensive treatment should occur. If the patient has other concerning symptoms or his or her use appears to be hazardous to health, clinical evaluation (e.g. complete blood count (CBC), liver function tests (LFTs), vitamin levels) and treatment of alcohol-related conditions is recommended. Completing baseline cognitive testing using the Montreal Cognitive Assessment (MOCA) or related tools at subsequent visits may also be considered, if clinically indicated.

Brief interventions should be used for patients with hazardous and harmful drinking who do not meet the criteria for an AUD. Brief interventions can be carried out by any healthcare provider, not only by addiction specialists. Such interventions have been performed in the ED, inpatient, and primary care settings by physicians, nurses, social workers, and other healthcare providers, with good results. They involve time-limited counseling sessions that employ concepts of motivational interviewing and psychoeducation, followed by continued support at further sessions and, if necessary, medication assistance or referral to specialists.

An example of a brief intervention would be the following:

State the concern: "I am concerned that your drinking may be affecting your health; are you also concerned?"

Advise: "It would be best for your health to cut down or stop drinking. Would you like to know the recommended levels of using alcohol?"

Agree on a plan of action: "It can be difficult to make new changes. Are there any goals related to cutting down that you would like to work on that we can discuss?" or "Have you considered the positive and negatives associated with using alcohol? I would be glad to help you explore this and help you meet your goals."

These interventions should be nonjudgemental, as stigma and shame have long been known to play a part in resistance to discussing use of alcohol. Motivational interviewing was developed in the 1990s by Miller and Rollnick and is known to be an effective way to help patients talk about and make changes in a way that minimizes shame and highlights autonomy and collaboration. It includes identifying the stage of change the patient is in, then helping the patient identify the benefits the problematic behavior has had in the past, in addition to the risks the behavior poses in the present. Then specific personal goals are set to help the patient meet the difficulties it takes in making sustainable behavioral change. Most brief interventions are modeled on these techniques. Feedback, Responsibility, Advice, Menu, Empathy, Self-efficacy (FRAMES) is a useful acronym for some of the elements used in motivational interventions (Miller 2012).

In brief:

- Feedback to discuss the personal risks of substance use with the patient.
- Responsibility and the choice for change is up to the patient.
- Advice about how to cut down or stop can then be given to the patient.
- Menu or choice of treatment options is given.
- Empathy and understanding should be used when discussing these topics.
- Self-efficacy is highlighted so the patient feels able to make changes.

This model can be used when discussing substance use with individuals and has been used for a variety of diseases, including diabetes and weight loss. The model has also been adopted for use in older adults with alcohol use (Barry 2001).

The effectiveness of brief interventions has been studied in older adults. Project TrEAT (Trial for Early Alcohol Treatment) was the first study testing brief physician advice on alcohol use, and it showed decreases in alcohol use at 12 months. Another trial looked at brief interventions—Project GOAL (Guiding Older Adults Lifestyles)—in a randomized controlled trial in people 65 or older, which found decreased weekly alcohol use and binge drinking compared to the control. The intervention consisted of two 10–15-minute counseling sessions followed by two telephone calls (Fleming, 1999). Another study, Project SHARE (Senior Health and Alcohol Risk Education) used interventions that included education, diaries, advice, and telephone counseling and was found to also reduce at-risk drinking versus usual care for up to a year after the intervention (Ettner 2014). An alternative to in-office assessment of alcohol use and interventions has been proposed using newer technologies. Online and computer-based programs are already available and may be a way of providing treatment that is cost-effective and less time-intensive (Hester 2006).

Other interventions that may be helpful to some patients would include Alcoholics Anonymous, Smart Recovery, or other self-help groups. These may help some patients, but there are limits to these groups, and they should not be used exclusively for most older adults (Oslin 2005). Ultimately, the goal of treating hazardous and harmful alcohol use should focus on harm reduction. Working collaboratively and diminishing shame is an important aspect of discussing alcohol use with patients. Loneliness, loss of a partner or friends, isolation, retirement, and depression often trigger increased drinking in older adults. Involvement in hobbies, clubs, volunteering, Senior Center activities, or comparable groups may be more effective in addressing these issues than traditional self-help groups in this population. Individual or group psychotherapy may also help an individual come to terms with the stressors and life changes that led to the increased use of alcohol. In addition, it may be helpful to involve family and other providers, especially if the patient has cognitive difficulties or lacks the capacity to make informed decisions about how his/her alcohol use is impairing his/her health. Finally, the literature suggests that older adults, compared to middle-aged adults, respond better to early treatment, but that they use aftercare less (Oslin 2005; Oslin, Pettinati 2002). This finding highlights the importance of screening older adults, providing treatment, and following up with them to help decrease their alcohol use.

## Useful Websites for Screening and Brief Interventions

*Alcohol Screening and Brief Intervention* in the primary care setting and patient handouts can be found on the National Institute of Alcohol Abuse and Alcoholism (NIAAA) website: www.niaaa.nih.gov/publications

*Screening, Brief Intervention, and Referral to Treatment (SBIRT)* can be found on the Substance Abuse and Mental Health Services Administration (SAMHSA) website: www.samhsa.gov/sbirt

*The American College of Emergency Physicians* maintains a website that includes helpful resources for Alcohol Screening and Brief Intervention in the ED:

https://www.acep.org/clinical—practice-management/alcohol-screening-in-the-emergency-department/*A computer-based screening instrument* has been developed by Boston University School of Public Health based on the AUDIT, and it can be found at the following site: www. alcoholscreening.org

## Pharmacotherapy for Alcohol-Use disorders

Medication management for alcohol-use disorders is used either to decrease drinking behaviors and cravings or to treat psychiatric symptoms associated with alcohol use. Currently, there are fourmedications approved by the Food and Drug Administration (FDA) that are used to treat AUD: disulfiram, oral naltrexone, injection naltrexone, and acamprosate. Disulfiram (Antabuse), the first medication approved (in 1974), is taken daily by the patient at a dose of 250–500 mg. When an individual uses alcohol while taking the drug, it causes a disulfiram-ethanol reaction. This occurs because the inhibition of aldehyde dehydrogenase results in an increased plasma level of acetaldehyde. The reaction manifests as flushing of the skin, increased heart rate, palpitations, decreased blood pressure, nausea, shortness of breath, sweating, dizziness, blurred vision, and confusion. The disulfiram ethanol reaction can occur for up to two weeks after the last dose of the drug because it binds irreversibly to aldehyde dehydrogenase (ALDH). Its other side effects independent of alcohol ingestion include optic neuritis, peripheral neuropathy, and hepatotoxicity (Kranzler 2013). To date, there are no studies specifically focused on the use of disulfiram in older adults. Its use in older patients is not recommended due to potentially serious adverse effects.

Naltrexone was approved to treat alcohol dependence in 1995. It acts as a mu opioid receptor antagonist with possible kappa receptor partial agonist activity. Many studies have found that it decreases cravings for alcohol, resulting in lower rates of heavy drinking (Kranzler 2013). This medication is typically taken orally at a dose of 50–100 mg/day. Naltrexone is also available as a long-acting injectable formulation, VIVITROL°, which was approved by the FDA to treat alcohol dependence in 2006. It is given once a month intramuscularly at a dose of 380 mg. There are no direct comparison studies, but patient adherence appears to be better with the long-acting form of the drug. The long-term side effects include possible transaminase elevations, although this concern arose from early studies involving doses several-fold higher than those now recommended. Subsequent investigations with oral or injection naltrexone in individuals with AUD have not found evidence of hepatotoxicity (Yen 2006; Vagenas 2014). Nevertheless, it is recommended that liver function should be monitored while patients use this medication. However, those who may benefit from the long-acting form should first be started on the oral form. Oral naltrexone has been studied in older adults and was found to be more effective than placebo in a randomized controlled trial (RCT) of patients who were 50–70 years old (Cornelius, 1997). There are no studies to date of the long-term injectable naltrexone in older adults. The use of this medication may be of benefit to those with medication-compliance issues or memory deficits. This should be weighed against the risk of side effects such as wounds in the area of injection, as older adults are at increased risk of skin breakdown and ulcerations. Use of visiting nurses and family to help with dispensing medications may be also be useful to manage lower compliance rates.

The most recent FDA-approved medication for AUD is acamprosate (calcium acetylhomotaurinate). It is thought to act by weak antagonism of the NMDA receptor and inhibition of the metabotropic glutamate receptor 5, resulting in moderation of alcohol withdrawal–related anxiety, although the exact mechanism of action is not known (Kranzler 2013). It is taken orally in a split dose of 2–3 g a day. It has fewer side effects than the other medications. There have been no studies to date on the use of acamprosate in older adults. Many trials in the general adult population have shown a reduction in heavy drinking and decreased drinking days, while other studies have not been able to detect a difference compared to placebo, including the COMBINE study (Combined Pharmacotherapies and Behavioral Interventions for Alcohol Dependence), in which acamprosate was added to naltrexone. A recent systematic review and meta-analysis found no significant difference between naltrexone and acamprosate; both were associated with reductions in relapse and reduced heavy drinking days (Jonas 2014).

There are several other medications that have been studied to decrease alcohol use that have not yet been FDA-approved. Some of these medications include nalmefene, topiramate, and gabapentin. Nalmefene is an opioid antagonist similar to naltrexone, but without the possible hepatotoxic side effects. Topiramate targets GABA and glutamate and has been found in a number of studies to decrease cravings for alcohol and reduce heavy drinking days (Miller 2011). Gabapentin is a medication used for seizures and neuropathic pain that modulates GABA transmission. A recent RCT found that gabapentin was effective in decreasing alcohol use in the general adult population with AUD (Mason 2013). Given its side-effect profile, it may be found to be safe and effective in treating AUD in older adults.

Psychotropic medications may also be useful in treating other psychiatric issues associated with alcohol-use disorders, but the evidence is limited.

Protracted alcohol withdrawal symptoms can last for up to a year after alcohol-use cessation. Symptoms include insomnia, low energy, anhedonia, tremor, anxiety, depression, and increased body temperature, blood pressure and pulse. Identification and treatment of protracted withdrawal is important in order for individuals to maintain long-term abstinence from alcohol (Trevisan, 1998). Depression during protracted withdrawal should be treated, but there is not specific evidence for this in the literature. Selective serotonin reuptake inhibitors (SSRIs) or psychotherapy are the first-line treatment options for depression in older adults (Solomon 2014). The SSRIs have a more favorable side-effect profile than tricyclic antidepressants and monoamine oxidase inhibitors but still have problematic side effects in older adults, including hyponatremia, increased bleeding risk, drug–drug interactions, and hypotension. A recent meta-analysis found that these antidepressants in older adults have no advantage over placebo if the depression is of short duration (less than two years) (Nelson 2013). The potential benefits of using an antidepressant medication for a shorter-term depression related to protracted withdrawal would have to be weighed on a case-by-case basis with the side effects and compliance rates of individual patients, given the potential for relapse in this group. There are no studies to date that investigate treating insomnia and anxiety in those with prolonged withdrawal symptoms. Clinical experience suggests that non-addictive medications for depression, insomnia, and anxiety can be helpful to those in early recovery.

When considering combined treatment for dual-diagnosis older adults, the literature is sparse. A trial done in adults age 55 or older with depression and alcohol dependence found that using sertraline (Zoloft) improved depression and decreased relapse, but that the combination of sertraline and naltrexone had no added benefit (Oslin 2005). Another recent study found that, in those aged 21–75 with depression and alcohol dependence who were treated with sertraline and naltrexone, there were higher alcohol abstinence rates and lower rates of depression than in those treated with naltrexone alone, sertraline alone, or placebo (Pettinati 2010).

Overall, medication management can be helpful to some older adults with alcohol-use disorders. The FDA-approved medications that are most helpful for older adults are naltrexone (oral and long-acting injectable) and acamprosate. Other promising drugs for alcohol-use disorders in older adults include nalmefene, topiramate, and gabapentin. Medications may also be useful when treating comorbid psychiatric issues in this population, but the evidence is limited and should be done on the individual basis. In general, more research needs to be done to develop and test drugs targeted for use in older adults with AUD and those who have AUD and other psychiatric comorbidities.

## Summary

Excessive alcohol use in older adults is a growing public health concern. In the past there have been difficulties in addressing alcohol use in this population due to stigma, time constraints, and the lack of knowledge about patterns of alcohol use in older adults. The studies to date show that individuals are using alcohol above the recommended limits, and that hazardous alcohol use exists beyond the strict criteria of AUD. Additionally, these recommendations may not apply to all older adults, especially if they have medical problems or are on certain medications. Light alcohol use in healthy older adults may confer health benefits, but the evidence is weak. Excessive alcohol use is known to negatively affect health. Because of the increased risks to health in this population, screening for alcohol use should occur at primary care, emergency, and specialty clinic settings using tools tailored for older adults such as the SMAST-G. Brief interventions have been shown to be effective for hazardous use in this population, and medication management should be an option that is discussed with individuals who may benefit from it. More research needs to be done regarding evidence-based practices in recommended levels of use, identification, and treatment of hazardous and harmful alcohol use in older adult populations. Above all, assessing and tailoring treatment to the patient's individual risk factors in a nonjudgemental and collaborative way is the most important step in preventing harm from alcohol use in this population.

## References

Aalto, M., Alho, H., Halme, J. T., & Seppä, K. (2011). The Alcohol-Use Disorders Identification Test (AUDIT) and its derivatives in screening for heavy drinking among the elderly. *Int J Geriatr Psych*, 26 (9), 881–885. doi:10.1002/gps.2498

Adams WL, Yuan Z, Barboriak JJ, Rimm AA. Alcohol-related hospitalizations of elderly people. Prevalence and geographic variation in the United States. *JAMA*, 1993;270(10):1222–1225.

Allen, J, Sillanaukee, P, Strid, N, Litten, R. Biomarkers of heavy drinking. In: Allen J, Wilson V, eds. *Assessing alcohol problems: a guide for clinicians and researchers*, 2nd ed. NIH Publication No. 03-3745. U.S. Department of Health and Human Services Public Health Service, National Institutes of Health National Institute on Alcohol Abuse and Alcoholism; 2003. Available at: http://pubs.niaaa.nih.gov/publications/AssessingAlcohol/biomarkers.htm.

Almeida OP, Hankey GJ, Yeap BB, Golledge J, Flicker L. Alcohol consumption and cognitive impairment in older men: a Mendelian randomization study. *Neurology* 2014;82(12): 1038–1044.

Association AP. *Diagnostic and Statistical Manual of Mental Disorders, 5th Edition*: DSM-5. Washington, DC: American Psychiatric Publishing; 2013.

Barry KB, Blow FC. *Alcohol problems in older adults: prevention and management*, 1st ed. (Oslin D, ed.). New York: Springer Publishing Company; 2001.

Berks J, McCormick R. Screening for alcohol misuse in elderly primary care patients: a systematic literature review. *Int Psychogeriatr* 2008;20(06):1090. doi:10.1017/S1041610208007497

Blazer DG, Wu L-T. The epidemiology of alcohol-use disorders and subthreshold dependence in a middle-aged and elderly community sample. *Am J Geriatr Psych* 2011;19(8):685–694. doi:10.1097/JGP.0b013e3182006a96

Blazer D, Wu L-T. The epidemiology of at-risk and binge drinking among middle-aged and elderly community adults: National Survey on Drug Use and Health. *Am J Psych* 2009;166(10):1162–1169.

Boden JM, Fergusson DM. Alcohol and depression. *Addiction.* 2011 May;106(5):906–14. doi: 10.1111/j.1360-0443.2010.03351.x

Centers for Disease Control and Prevention. Alcohol facts. Alcohol and public health frequently asked questions, 2014. Available at: http://www.cdc.gov/alcohol/faqs.htm. Accessed August 1, 2014.

Centers for Disease Control and Prevention. Alcohol Related Disease Impact (ARDI) application, 2013. Available at http://apps.nccd.cdc.gov/DACH_ARDI/Default.aspx. Available at: http://apps.nccd.cdc.gov/DACH_ARDI/Default/Report.aspx?T=AAM&P=f6d7eda7-036e-4553-9968-9b17ffad620e&R=d7a9b303-48e9-4440-bf47-070a4827e1fd&M=AD96A9C1-285A-44D2-B76D-BA2AE037FC56&F=&D=. Accessed August 23, 2014.

Chase V, Neild R, Sadler C, Batey R. The medical complications of alcohol use: understanding mechanisms to improve management. *Drug Alcohol Rev* 2005;24(3):253–265. doi:10.1080/09595230500167510.

Consentino S, Stern Y. Chapter 2: Consideration of cognitive reserve. In: *Handbook on the neuropsychology of aging and dementia.* New York: Springer; 2012.

Cornelius JR, Salloum IM, Ehler JG, et al. Fluoxetine in depressed alcoholics. A double-blind, placebo-controlled trial. *Arch Gen Psychiatry* 1997;54(8):700–705.

Culberson JW. Alcohol use in the elderly: beyond the CAGE. Part 2: Screening instruments and treatment strategies. *Geriatrics* 2006;61(11):20–26.

D'Onofrio G, Degutis LC. Screening and brief intervention in the emergency department. *Alcohol Res Health* 2004;28(2):63.

Dowling GJ, Weiss SRB, Condon TP. Drugs of abuse and the aging brain. *Neuropsychopharmacology* 2007;33(2):209–218. doi:10.1038/sj.npp.1301412

Esser MB, Hedden SL, Kanny D, Brewer RD, Gfroerer JC, Naimi TS. Prevalence of alcohol dependence among US adult drinkers, 2009–2011. *Prev Chronic Dis* 2014;11:E206. Available at: http://www.ncbi.nlm.nih.gov/pmc/articles/PMC4241371/. Accessed February 7, 2015.

Ettner SL, Xu H, Duru OK, et al. The effect of an educational intervention on alcohol consumption, at-risk drinking, and health care utilization in older adults: the Project SHARE study. *J Stud Alcohol Drugs* 75(3):447–457.

Ferreira MP, Weems MKS. Alcohol consumption by aging adults in the United States: health benefits and detriments. *J Am Diet Assoc* 2008;108(10):1668–1676. doi:10.1016/j.jada.2008.07.011

Fleming MF, Manwell LB, Barry KL, Adams W, Stauffacher EA. Brief physician advice for alcohol problems in older adults: a randomized community-based trial. *J Fam Pract* 1999;48:378–386.

Gilpin NW, Koob GF. Neurobiology of alcohol dependence: focus on motivational mechanisms. *Alcohol Res Health* 2008;31(3):185.

Grant BF, Dawson DA, Stinson FS, Chou SP, Dufour MC, Pickering RP. The 12-month prevalence and trends in DSM-IV alcohol abuse and dependence: United States, 1991–1992 and 2001–2002. *Drug Alcohol Depend* 2004;74(3):223–234. doi:10.1016/j.drugalcdep.2004.02.004

Gu Y, Scarmeas N, Short EE, et al. Alcohol intake and brain structure in a multiethnic elderly cohort. *Clin Nutr* 2014;33(4):662–667. doi:10.1016/j.clnu.2013.08.004

Hester RK, Miller JH. Computer-based tools for diagnosis and treatment of alcohol problems. *Alcohol Res Health* 2006;29(1):36–40.

Hillbom M, Saloheimo P, Fujioka S, Wszolek ZK, Juvela S, Leone MA. Diagnosis and management of Marchiafava-Bignami disease: a review of CT/MRI confirmed cases. *J Neurol Neurosurg Psychiatry* 2014;85(2):168–173. doi:10.1136/jnnp-2013-305979

Jayasekara H, English DR, Room R, MacInnis RJ. Alcohol consumption over time and risk of death: a systematic review and meta-analysis. *Am J Epidemiol* 2014;179(9):1049–1059. doi:10.1093/aje/kwu028

Johnson-Greene D, McCaul ME, Roger P. Screening for hazardous drinking using the Michigan Alcohol Screening Test–Geriatric Version (MAST-G) in elderly persons with acute cerebrovascular accidents. *Alcohol Clin Exper Res* 2009;33(9):1555–1561. doi:10.1111/j.1530-0277.2009.00987.x

Jonas DE, Amick HR, Feltner C, et al. Pharmacotherapy for adults with alcohol-use disorders in outpatient settings: a systematic review and meta-analysis. *JAMA,* 2014;311(18):1889. doi:10.1001/jama.2014.3628

Kalapatapu RK, Chambers R. Novel objective biomarkers of alcohol use: potential diagnostic and treatment management tools in dual diagnosis care. *J Dual Diagn* 2009;5(1):57–82.

Kalivas PW, Volkow ND. The neural basis of addiction: a pathology of motivation and choice. *Am J Psychiatry* 2005;162(8):1403–1413. doi:10.1176/appi.ajp.162.8.1403

Kelly JF, Wakeman SE, Saitz R. Stop talking "dirty": clinicians, language, and quality of care for the leading cause of preventable death in the United States. *Am J Med* 2015;128(1): 8–9. doi:10.1016/j.amjmed.2014.07.043

Kessler RC. The epidemiology of dual diagnosis. *Biol Psychiatry* 2004;56(10):730–737. doi:10.1016/j.biopsych.2004.06.034

Kim JW, Lee DY, Lee BC, et al. Alcohol and cognition in the elderly: a review. *Psychiatr Invest* 2012;9(1):8. doi:10.4306/pi.2012.9.1.8

Koob GF. Theoretical frameworks and mechanistic aspects of alcohol addiction: alcohol addiction as a reward deficit disorder. *Curr Top Behav Neurosci* 2013;13:3–30. doi:10.1007/7854_2011_129

Kraemer KL, Mayo-Smith MF, Calkins DR. Impact of age on the severity, course, and complications of alcohol withdrawal. *Arch Intern Med* 1997;157:2234–2241.

Kranzler HR, Knapp CM, Ciraulo DA. Alcohol. In: *Clinical manual of addiction psychopharmacology*, 2nd ed. Washington, DC: American Psychiatric Publishing; 2013:1–69.

Kuźma E, Llewellyn DJ, Langa KM, Wallace RB, Lang IA. History of alcohol-use disorders and risk of severe cognitive impairment: a nineteen-year prospective cohort study. *Am J Geriatr Psych* 2014. doi:10.1016/j.jagp.2014.06.001

Leggio L, Kenna GA, Fenton M, Bonenfant E, Swift RM. Typologies of alcohol dependence. From Jellinek to genetics and beyond. *Neuropsychol Rev* 2009;19(1):115–129. doi:10.1007/s11065-008-9080-z

Liberto JG, Oslin DW. Early versus late onset of alcoholism in the elderly. *Int J Addict* 1995;30(13–14):1799–1818.

Li T-K. Quantifying the risk for alcohol-use and alcohol-attributable health disorders: present findings and future research needs. *J Gastroenterol Hepatol* 2008;23(s1):S2-S8. doi:10.1111/j.1440-1746.2007.05298.x

Liu X, Weiss F. Additive effect of stress and drug cues on reinstatement of ethanol seeking: exacerbation by history of dependence and role of concurrent activation of corticotropin-releasing factor and opioid mechanisms. *J Neurosci* 2002;22(18):7856–7861.

Mailliard ME, Sorrell MF. Chapter 307. Alcoholic liver disease. In: Longo DL, Fauci AS, Kasper DL, Hauser SL, Jameson J, Loscalzo J, eds. *Harrison's principles of internal medicine*, 18e. New York: McGraw-Hill; 2012. http://accessmedicine.mhmedical.com.ezproxy.bu.edu/content.aspx?bookid=331&Sectionid=40727102. Accessed February 1, 2015.

Maldonado JR, Sher Y, Ashouri JF, et al. The "Prediction of Alcohol Withdrawal Severity Scale" (PAWSS): systematic literature review and pilot study of a new scale for the prediction of complicated alcohol withdrawal syndrome. *Alcohol* 2014;48(4):375–390. doi:10.1016/j.alcohol.2014.01.004

Mason BJ, Quello S, Goodell V, Shadan F, Kyle M, Begovic A. Gabapentin treatment for alcohol dependence: a randomized clinical trial. *JAMA Intern Med* 2014;174(1):70. doi:10.1001/jamainternmed.2013.11950

McKnight-Eily LR, Liu Y, Brewer RD, et al. Vital signs: communication between health professionals and their patients about alcohol use—44 states and the District of Columbia, 2011. *MMWR Morb Mortal Wkly Rep* 2014;63(1):16–22.

Menninger JA. Assessment and treatment of alcoholism and substance-related disorders in the elderly. *Bull Menninger Clin* 2002;66(2):166–183.

Miller PM, Book SW, Stewart SH. Medical treatment of alcohol dependence: a systematic review. *Int J Psychiatry Med* 2011;42(3):227–266.

Miller WR, Rollnick S. *Motivational interviewing: helping people change*, 3rd ed. New York: Guilford Press; 2012.

Mokdad AH, Marks JS, Stroup DF, Gerberding JL. Actual causes of death in the United States, 2000. *JAMA* 2004;291(10):1238–1245.

Moore AA, Beck JC, Babor TF, Hays RD, Reuben DB. Beyond alcoholism: identifying older, at-risk drinkers in primary care. *J Stud Alcohol Drugs* 2002;63(3):316.

Moore AA, Morton SC, Beck JC, et al. A new paradigm for alcohol use in older persons. *Med Care* 1999;37(2):165–179.

Moore AA, Seeman T, Morgenstern H, Beck JC, Reuben DB. Are there differences between older persons who screen positive on the CAGE questionnaire and the Short Michigan Alcoholism Screening Test–Geriatric Version? *J Am Geriatr Soc* 2002;50(5): 858–862.

Moore AA, Whiteman EJ, Ward KT. Risks of combined alcohol/medication use in older adults. *Am J Geriatr Pharmacother* 2007;5(1):64–74. doi:10.1016/j.amjopharm.2007.03.006

Moyer VA. Screening and behavioral counseling interventions in primary care to reduce alcohol misuse: US Preventive Services Task Force recommendation statement. *Ann Intern Med* 2013;159(3):210–218.

National Institute on Alcohol Abuse and Alcoholism. AUD comparison between DSM IV and DSM 5. NIH Publication No. 13-7999; 2013.

National Institute on Alcohol Abuse and Alcoholism. Older adults. Available at: http://www.niaaa.nih.gov/alcohol-health/special-populations-co-occurring-disorders/older-adults. Accessed August 1, 2014.

Nelson JC, Delucchi KL, Schneider LS. Moderators of outcome in late-life depression: a patient-level meta-analysis. 2013. Available at: http://ajp.psychiatryonline.org/doi/10.1176/appi.ajp.2012.12070927. Accessed May 3, 2015.

O'Connell H, Chin A-V, Hamilton F, et al. A systematic review of the utility of self-report alcohol screening instruments in the elderly. *Int J Geriatr Psych,* 2004;19(11):1074–1086. doi:10.1002/gps.1214

Oslin D. Treatment of late-life depression complicated by alcohol dependence. *Am J Geriatr Psych* 2005;13:491–500.

Oslin DW, Mavandadi S. Alcohol and drug problems. In: *The American psychiatric publishing textbook of geriatric psychiatry*, 4th ed. American Psychiatric Association; 2009.

Oslin DW, Pettinati H, Volpicelli JR. Alcoholism treatment adherence: older age predicts better adherence and drinking outcomes. *Am J Geriatr Psych* 2002;10(6):740–747.

Peters R, Peters J, Warner J, Beckett N, Bulpitt C. Alcohol, dementia and cognitive decline in the elderly: a systematic review. *Age Ageing* 2008;37(5):505–512. doi:10.1093/ageing/afn095

Pettinati HM, Oslin DW, Kampman KM, et al. A double-blind, placebo-controlled trial combining sertraline and naltrexone for treating co-occurring depression and alcohol dependence. *Am J Psychiatry* 2010;167(6):668–675. doi:10.1176/appi.ajp.2009.08060852

Preedy VR, Adachi J, Ueno Y, et al. Alcoholic skeletal muscle myopathy: definitions, features, contribution of neuropathy, impact and diagnosis. *Eur J Neurol* 2001;8(6):677–687.

Ridley NJ, Draper B, Withall A. Alcohol-related dementia: an update of the evidence. *Alzheimers Res Ther* 2013;5(1):3. doi:10.1186/alzrt157

Roerecke M, Rehm J. Alcohol-use disorders and mortality: a systematic review and meta-analysis: AUD and mortality. *Addiction* 2013;108(9):1562–1578. doi:10.1111/add.12231

Roerecke M, Rehm J. The cardioprotective association of average alcohol consumption and ischaemic heart disease: a systematic review and meta-analysis. *Addiction* 2012;107(7):1246–1260. doi:10.1111/j.1360-0443.2012.03780.x

Sabia S, Elbaz A, Britton A, et al. Alcohol consumption and cognitive decline in early old age. *Neurology* 2014;82(4):332–339. doi:10.1212/WNL.0000000000000063

Schuckit MA. Recognition and management of withdrawal delirium (delirium tremens). Longo DL, ed. *N Engl J Med* 2014;371(22):2109–2113. doi:10.1056/NEJMra1407298

Sinforiani E, Zucchella C, Pasotti C, Casoni F, Bini P, Costa A. The effects of alcohol on cognition in the elderly: from protection to neurodegeneration. *Funct Neurol* 2010;26(2):103–106.

Stahre M, Roeber J, Kanny D, Brewer RD, Zhang X. Contribution of excessive alcohol consumption to deaths and years of potential life lost in the United States. *Prev Chronic Dis* 2014;11. doi:10.5888/pcd11.130293

Substance Abuse and Mental Health Services Administration. Results from the 2010 National Survey on Drug Use and Health: Summary of national findings, NSDUH Series H-41, HHS Publication No. (SMA) 11-4658. Rockville, MD: Substance Abuse and Mental Health Services Administration. 2011. Available at: http://www.samhsa.gov/data/nsduh/2k10nsduh/2k10results.htm.

Sullivan JT, Sykora K, Schneiderman J, Naranjo CA, Sellers EM. Assessment of alcohol withdrawal: the revised Clinical Institute Withdrawal Assessment for Alcohol scale (CIWA-Ar). *Br J Addict* 1989;84(11):1353–1357. doi:10.1111/j.1360-0443.1989.tb00737.x

Tabakoff B, Hoffman PL. The neurobiology of alcohol consumption and alcoholism: an integrative history. *Pharmacol Biochem Behav* 2013;113:20–37. doi:10.1016/j.pbb.2013.10.009

Taheri A, Dahri K, Chan P, Shaw M, Aulakh A, Tashakkor A. Evaluation of a symptom-triggered protocol approach to the management of alcohol withdrawal syndrome in older adults. *J Am Geriatr Soc* 2014:n/a-n/a. doi:10.1111/jgs.12932

Taylor WD. Clinical practice. Depression in the elderly. *N Engl J Med* 2014 Sep 25;371(13):1228–36. doi:10.1056/NEJMcp1402180

TIP 26: Substance Abuse Among Older Adults. HHS Publication No. (SMA) 12-3918. Rockville, MD: Substance Abuse and Mental Health Services Administration; 2008. Available at: http://store.samhsa.gov/product/TIP-26-Substance-Abuse-Among-Older-Adults/SMA12-3918. Accessed February 14, 2015.

Trevisan LA, Boutros N, Petrakis IL, Krystal JH. Complications of alcohol withdrawal: pathophysiological insights. *Alcohol Health Res World* 1998;22. Available at: http://askadeo.info/2011/61-66-isci/. Accessed July 21, 2014.

U.S. Administration on Aging. Table 12. Projections of the population by age and sex for the United States: 2010 to 2050 (NP2008-T12). Population Division, U.S. Census Bureau. 2008. Available at: http://www.aoa.gov/AoARoot/Aging_Statistics/future_growth/future_growth.aspx.

U.S. Dept. of Health and Human Services, Public Health Service, National Institutes of Health, National Institute on Alcohol Abuse and Alcoholism. 10th Special Report to the U.S. Congress on Alcohol and Health: Highlights from Current Research from the Secretary of Health and Human Services. 2000.

Wilson SR, Knowles SB, Huang Q, Fink A. The prevalence of harmful and hazardous alcohol consumption in older U.S. adults: data from the 2005–2008 National Health and Nutrition Examination Survey (NHANES). *J Gen Intern Med* 2014;29(2):312–319. doi:10.1007/s11606-013-2577-z

Vagenas P, DiPaola A, Herme M, et al. An evaluation of hepatic enzyme elevations among HIV-infected released prisoners enrolled in two randomized placebo-controlled trials of extended release naltrexone. *J Subst Abuse Treat* 2014;47(1): 35–40.

World Health Organization. Mental and behavioral disorders due to psychoactive substance use. *The ICD-10 Classification of Mental and Behavioral Disorders*. Geneva: World Health Organization; 1992. Available at: http://www.who.int/substance_abuse/terminology/ICD10ClinicalDiagnosis.pdf. Accessed February 15, 2015.

Yen MH, Ko HC, Tang FI, Lu RB, Hong JS. Study of hepatoxicity in the treatment of alcoholism. *Alcohol* 2006;38(2):117–20.

Zahr N, Kaufman K, Harper C. Clinical and pathological features of alcohol-related brain damage. *Nature Rev Neurol* 2011;7:284–294. doi:10.1038/nrneurol.2011.42

CHAPTER 5

# Abuse of Opioids and Prescription Medications

*Isis Burgos-Chapman, Louis A. Trevisan, and Kevin Sevarino*

## Introduction

The world's elderly population is growing. Along with this, the baby-boomer generation with its increased propensity to misuse or abuse drugs is entering that age group. They come on the heels of an explosion of opioid pain medication use that occurred between 1990 and 2010. The problems of opioid pain medication misuse and opioid-use disorder in the elderly are about to grow, yet, pain medication misuse and opioid-use disorder are often underdiagnosed and undertreated in the elderly. Prescription pain medication misuse and opioid-use disorders present real problems and should be on every practitioner's radar as possible reasons for problems surfacing in the elderly patient. In this discussion, we attempt to outline the magnitude of the problem and discuss ways to risk-stratify which elderly patients are at higher risk of developing problems with opioids than others. We discuss the role of opioids in chronic pain treatment in the elderly, and the pitfalls of opioid use in that population. Finally, we provide general guidelines in the treatment of the aged with pain medication misuse and/or an opioid-use disorder.

## The Growing Risk of Opioid-Use disorders in the Elderly

The number of people aged 60 years and over exceeds 700 million worldwide, the majority living in developed countries (United Nations 2009). The 2009–2013 American Community Survey five-year estimate indicates that there are 41.8 million people 65 years old or older (U.S. Census Bureau 2012). When baby boomers started turning 65 in 2011, 10,000 people were turning 65 every day. This phenomenon will continue for the next 20 years. By 2030, one in five Americans will be 65 or older (Ortman et al. 2014). Those aged 65 and older and those aged 85 and older will double and triple in number respectively by the year 2050 (Kalapatapu and Sullivan 2010). The proportion of older adults in less developed countries will rise extensively by 2050 (Wang and Andrade 2013).

"Baby boomers" are defined as those who were born following World War II, between 1946 and 1964. Currently, they are 50–69 years old. This cohort numbered about 81 million people as of July 2010 (U.S. Census Bureau 2012). It is estimated that there will be considerable change in the population aged 55 and older by the year 2020—compared to the year 2000, baby boomers older than 55 are expected to double in numbers (U.S. Census 2000 and 2014). Persons aged 65 and older will grow from 15% of the population in 2014 to 21% of the population in 2030, when the youngest baby boomer has reached 66 years (U.S. Census Bureau 2014).

In addition to these population changes, the cohort of aging baby boomers has different attitudes toward treatment than the generation that came before them (Gross 2008). In part this may be due to aging baby boomers' rates of illicit drug use. Their use of illicit drugs has historically been much higher than those of previous cohorts (Johnson and Gerstein 1998). Baby-boomers grew up during a time when generational tension due to politics and modes of authority caused dramatic social and cultural change that, along with music and mainstream experimentation with substances, influenced their identity. This group will have a more lenient attitude and greater need for treatment for substance use than previous generations (Gross 2008). By 2011, those aged 50–59 accounted for 83% of all substance-abuse treatment admissions for everyone age 50 and older (Wu and Blazer 2011). Consistent with this observation, drug use is increasing among people in their fifties. Furthermore, addiction specialists and organizations for the elderly anticipate that a large number of baby boomers will need help with fighting prescription pain medication misuse. Baby boomers as a cohort are rapidly moving into the treatment realm of the practicing primary care physicians, as well as general, geriatric, and addiction psychiatrists (Offsay 2007).

## Prevalence of Opioid-Use Disorders and Opioid Misuse in the Elderly

When looking at prevalence of opioid misuse in the older patient, the definition of what constitutes "older" or "elderly" must be specified. Unfortunately, without a standard definition, studies vary widely in applying this term, with some considering people 55 and older as elderly, others 60 and older, and others 65 and older. The definition of who is "old" has come under increased scrutiny as America's population ages. The US Social Security Administration (SSA) recently increased the age for eligibility requirements for full Social Security from 65 to 66.5 years old, and this will again increase in the future. Typically in the geriatric literature, the age of 65 is considered *young-old*, above 75 is considered *old*, and over 85 is considered *old-old*. These definitions are still actively being debated. An added complexity is that many patients with substance abuse or opioid-use disorders may be biologically older than age-matched controls without substance abuse (Patterson and Jeste 1999). Aging substance-abusing patients carry a much higher disease burden than the non–substance-abusing population, including those who also receive opioid treatment for chronic pain (Patterson and Jeste 1999, Parikh and Chung 1995). Thus, chronological age in this population may not accurately reflect biological age. This definitional ambiguity is important to acknowledge, because this chapter is meant to be all-inclusive. Therefore, in the present discussion, people over the age of 50 with lifetime or recent onset opioid-use disorder may be considered as "elderly" or "older" patients.

Also to be considered in the elderly is the definition of *addiction*, or in DSM-5 parlance, an *opioid-use disorder*. Of course, those with a prior history of an opioid-use disorder who continue this behavior into their older years, diagnostic clarity is not in question. However, for many without such a prior history, interference in their occupational functioning may not be a factor in the retiree. Social withdrawal is difficult to define in the nursing home patient with restricted independence, or one living at home with dementia. As discussed, overstating one's pain to obtain additional opioids, if driven by a desire to use the substances for non-prescribed reasons (e.g., helping with sleep or anxiety), would meet a DSM criterion. Add a family member or spouse being upset by the elderly person remaining on opioids, and one meets two DSM-5 criteria, consistent with at least a mild opioid-use disorder. The elderly patient may be at risk for physically hazardous use that would not affect a younger patient, including falls, cognitive clouding, and delirium. Thus, while difficulties with opioids in the elderly are often classified as "misuse," to be clear, these consequences allow one to diagnose either an Opioid-Use Disorder or an Unspecified Opioid-Related Disorder (American Psychiatric Association 2013). Misuse or non-medical use may be distinguished from persistent abuse or dependence typical of as an opioid-use disorder (Culbertson et al. 2008, Blow 1998). For example, use of the opioid to help with sleep or anxiety is misuse. Compared to abuse of illicit drugs, misuse of prescription pain medications and non-medical use of prescription pain medications is an important and emerging issue in the elderly (Wang and Andrade 2013).

Currently, older adults account for 13% of the U.S. population but use one-third of all medications prescribed in the United States (National Institute on Drug Abuse (NIDA) 2014). Nationally, 2.8 million adults over age 50 abused prescription medications in the last year, second only to cannabinoids. This number is expected to reach over 4.4 million by the year 2020, as predicted by Substance Abuse and Mental Health Services Administration (SAMHSA). Opioids represent the largest class of medications abused non-medically—about 75% of the total non-medical use of prescription drugs (NMUPDs). Opioids (33%), then benzodiazepines (21%), were the two most-cited drugs for NMUPDs in emergency department (ED) visits by those over 55, often in combination with alcohol (SAMHSA 2009). And 7.2 million older Americans receive at least one opioid prescription annually. This is three times more than the general population. On average, older persons take 4.5 medications per day (National Survey on Drug Use and Health (NSDUH) 2013, Simoni-Wasila and Yang 2006). Up to 11% of older women misuse and abuse prescription drugs (Simoni-Wasila and Yang 2006, Culbertson and Ziska 2008). Lifetime prevalence of NMUPDs is 4.7% for opiates, 4.1% for sedatives, 3.4% for tranquilizers, and 4.7% for stimulants (Culbertson and Ziska 2008). The RADARS (Researched Abuse, Diversion and Addiction-Related Surveillance) System indicated that rates of reported elderly opioid abuse in those 60 and older peaked in late 2012, at a rate of 15% of the rate for those 20–59 (West et al. 2015). Reported rates of misuse peaked in mid-2011, at a rate about 45% of that of the younger cohort, and three times that for overt abuse. Yet Americans, while constituting only 4.6% of the world's population, consume 80% of the global opioid supply, 99% of the global hydrocodone supply, and two-thirds of the world's illegal drugs (Han et al. 2009). Despite recent RADARS data, it is a logical conclusion that drug use among the aging baby boomers will increase at an alarming rate (Patterson and Jeste 1999).

Relative to younger cohorts, illicit opioid-use disorders have a much lower prevalence in the elderly (e.g., Ives et al. 2006, Edlund et al. 2007, Denisco et al. 2008). NSDUH (2013) figures indicate that in those 50 and older, 1.9% had prior lifetime heroin use, compared to 1.0% of that age cohort in 2002. Reflective of recent use, under 0.1% (the lowest reported level) had used in the prior year in 2012, vs. 0.1% in 2002. The vast majority had initiated the opioid use prior to age 30, and risk factors for continued use in the 50–59 age group included being male, unmarried, and of low education and income status (Wang and Andrade 2013). Methadone-maintained elderly are not well studied, so there are inconsistencies in the literature. Some studies indicated that males in particular suffered poorer physical health than younger cohorts, and women suffered higher risk for comorbid mental health diagnoses (Wu and

Blazer 2011). Unfortunately, continued illicit opioid use is not uncommon in former illicit opioid users living into their fifties and beyond (Hser et al. 2007).

Per NSDUH (2013) for pain relievers, 8.0% of respondents had ever used, compared to 5.8% in 2002, and 0.8%, the highest percentage, had used 26–100, or over 100, days in the prior year, compared to 0.6% in 2002. For those 50 and older, in the years 2005–2006, non-medical use of prescription pain medications was 1.4%, much higher than for tranquilizers (0.46%) and other classes of prescription medications (Blazer and Wu 2009). Risk factors included being male, American Indian/Alaskan Native, having depression in the prior year, and being an alcohol or cannabis user. Surprisingly, 21% reported their first non-medical use of opioids occurred at age 50 or later. This does not mean those that all who had used opioid pain relievers met criteria for an opioid-use disorder or were misusing a drug, but it marks a clear trend that exposure to these substances and frequency of use are rising relative to heroin itself. In earlier studies, older age was associated with lower likelihood of abuse and misuse of opioids (Ives et al. 2006, Reid et al. 2002). However, the landscape is changing. Exposure to opioids rapidly rose since those studies, and the baby boom cohort represents an ever-increasing percentage of those over 55. Thus, relative to opioid-use disorders, opioid misuse is likely to rise in the future with increased age and pain conditions (Becker et al. 2008).

The distinction between intentional misuse of opioids, which is generally accepted to be a marker of addiction, and unsafe use of opioids, is often not easy. Estimates are that, of those who misused opioid pain medications in the prior year, 9–10% developed an opioid-use disorder (Blazer and Wu 2009, Wu and Blazer 2011). Edlund et al. (2007) found American veterans aged 60 and older taking opioids for chronic non-cancer pain (CNCP) had a rate of diagnosed opioid abuse or dependence of 1%, compared to 4% for those younger than 60. This ratio is far higher than the rate of opioid-use disorders in general in the elderly, compared to their younger counterparts. Kolodny et al. (2014) argue that non-medical use of pain medications should not be viewed as significantly different from that of opioid addiction in general. Over 75% of opioid poisoning deaths occur in those with a preceding history or a history suggestive of an opioid-use disorder, though these data do not specifically address the elderly (Johnson et al. 2013, Hall et al. 2008).

Retail sales of commonly used opioid medications increased from a total of 50.7 million grams in 1997 to 126.5 million grams in 2007. This was an overall increase of 149%, with increases ranging from 222% for morphine, 280% for hydrocodone, 319% for hydromorphone, 525% for fentanyl base, 866% for oxycodone, to 1293% for methadone. Average *per capita* sales of opioid medication increased from 74 milligrams in 1997 to 369 milligrams in 2007, a 402% increase (Manchikanti and Laxmaiah 2007). As early as 1999, nearly

15% of community-dwelling elderly received more than one opioid analgesic (Simoni-Wastila et al. 2005). Parallel to this was a dramatic increase in the number of new non-medical users of therapeutics. In those 50 years and older, the NMUPD rate was 2.1%, second only to cannabinoids/marijuana 2.8%, but for those over 65, NMUPD had the highest rate, at 0.8% (NSDUH 2008). Pain relievers are the group of medications that are by far the most misused, nearly doubling the amount of the next most frequently misused medication, tranquilizers. The non-medical use of opioid prescription medications is endemic and, as discussed, particularly problematic in the older patient.

The Treatment Data Sets (TEDS) project that older adults in need of substance-abuse treatment will increase to 4.4 million in 2020 from 1.7 million in 2000/2001. It is estimated that there will be an increase of 50% in the number of older adults, and an increase of 70% in the number of older adults needing treatment (Gfroerer et al. 2003). Lofwall et al. (2008) reported that, in 2005, 10% of substance-abuse treatment admissions were for those 50 and above. Per TEDS (SAMHSA 2014a)( (accessed at http://www.samhsa. gov/data/sites/default/files/2012_Web_Tables_as_of_2014_Q4/TEDS_ 2012_Substance_Abuse_Treatment_Admissions_Tables.html#US12, April 18, 2016), in 2012, heroin was the principal abused substance for substance-abuse treatment admissions in 0.4% of those over 65 vs. 11.1% of those 51+, for other opioids, 0.3% for 65+ vs. 6.3% for 51+. The number of those citing heroin as a problem has grown steadily between 1998 and 2008 (Arndt et al. 2011). Comparing 2012 to 2002, in those 55 and older, heroin was the principal substance of abuse for those admitted, at 14.8% vs. 13.0%, but for non-heroin opioids and methadone, the rates were 4.8% vs. 2.1% (SAMHSA 2015). Non-heroin opioid use is growing at a significantly higher rate than heroin use. Per SAMHSA (2014), the admission rates for opiates other than heroin were between 120% and 419% higher in 2012 than in 2002 in all nine U.S. Census divisions. Admission rates for opiates other than heroin were higher in 2012 than in 2002 in the lower 48 states, though this decreased marginally for New Mexico (SAMHSA 2014). For those aged 65 or older, between 1995 and 2005, the proportion of treatment admissions for heroin/opioids grew from 6.6–10.5% (SAMHSA 2007).

Between 1999 and 2002, the number of opioid analgesic poisonings on death certificates rose 91.2%. During this time period, poisoning from opioid analgesics surpassed both cocaine and heroin poisoning as the most frequent type of drug poisoning found on death certificates in the United States (Paulozzi et al. 2006). The age-adjusted rate for opioid-analgesic poisoning deaths nearly quadrupled, from 1.4 per 10,000 in 1999 to 5.4 per 100,000 in 2011, though the rate has slowed since 2006 (Chen et al. 2014). The significance of substance abuse in older adults is highlighted by mortality data from the Drug

Abuse Warning Network (DAWN) that indicate that the rate of drug-related deaths among adults age 55 and over increased from 5.0 per 100,000 population in 2003 (DAWN 2003) to 17.0 per 100,000 population in 2007* and 26.6 per 100,000 in 2014*. Exacerbating this death rate is the concurrent prescribing of benzodiazepines in the elderly (Jones et al. 2012). Benzodiazepine use increases steadily with age, exceeding 8% in those 65–80 (Olfson et al. 2015.) Used principally for insomnia and/or anxiety, benzodiazepines' rates of use are much higher for women than for men: at age 80, approximately 12% of women compared to about 6% of men received a benzodiazepine prescription in 2008. Combined use of benzodiazepines with opioid pain relievers (or alcohol) significantly increases the risk of serious emergency department outcome (inpatient admission or death). Per 2005–2011 DAWN data, in those over 65, this outcome was 39% for benzodiazepines alone, 59% for the combination with opioids, and 70% when alcohol was also present (SAMHSA 2014).

In the elderly with opioid-use disorders, there is higher all-cause mortality than in their younger counterparts as a combination of drug-related events along with non–drug-related causes, the latter of which rise naturally with age while the former remains relatively stable (Larney et al. 2015, Beynon et al. 2010). The elderly with opioid-use disorders suffer a greater burden of medical comorbidity. Older (50+) compared to younger veterans with opioid-use disorders have higher rates of hepatitis C, human immunodeficiency virus (HIV), chronic pain, neuropathy, mood disorders, and post-traumatic stress disorder (Larney et al. 2015). Between veterans with opioid-use disorders and those without, those older than 50 showed elevated deaths due to HIV and liver-related causes (Larney et al. 2015). In a large cohort of opioid users in England, similar findings have been reported. Higher comorbidity of illness continued into the elder years, and some causes of death worsened, including infectious disease, cancer, and liver disease. With aging, gender differences between drug-related deaths declined from a relative risk of 1.9 below age 35, to 1.2 from 45–65 (Pierce et al. 2015).

## Sources of Opioid Medications

Equally important in the epidemiology of elderly opioid misuse and opioid-use disorders is identifying the source of the misused prescription opioid medications. The idea that most people in this group are getting their prescription medications from illicit sources including the internet and dealers on the street

---

* Calculated at http://wonder.cdc.gov/ using death codes X40- 45, and summing ratesfor all age groups 55 and older; accessed 4/18/16.

does not capture the true picture. According to the NSDUH (2013), the major source of pain relievers for the most recent non-medical use among past-year users aged 12 and older was a single friend who received the medications from a single doctor for a treatable condition (53%). Other methods of obtaining pain medications for non-medical use were: prescription from one doctor (21.2%), bought or taken from a friend (14.6%), doctor shopping (2.6%), and obtained from a drug dealer (4.3%). Of people receiving prescription pain medications from a friend or relative, the source of that medication was one doctor 83.8% of the time (NSDUH 2013). One-third of the prescription drugs sold in the United States are used by the elderly, mainly for chronic pain, insomnia, and anxiety. For the elderly as for most people, the method of obtaining prescription pain medications is most likely from one doctor, either through a friend or a family member, or directly prescribed (Gfroerer et al. 2003, Han et al. 2009). Indeed, it is probable that the elderly are more likely than younger folk to seek legitimate sources for their opioids. Cicero et al.2012 reported the odds ratio in those older than 45 is much higher than in the general population for using a legitimate prescriber for their opioid, perhaps because it becomes easier to get one as one ages (Cicero et al. 2008, Cicero et al. 2012). Inciardi et al. (2009a) found in a study of opioid misusers that a significant percentage of the elderly admitted to overstating their chronic pain to obtain opioids, and in turn they were able to divert these medications in part for economic gain.

## Risk Factors

Risk factors for prescription pain medication misuse and/or opioid-use disorders in the elderly include being female, having a personal or family history of substance abuse, having comorbid psychiatric disorders such as Cluster B personality disorders, having multiple medical problems, and having chronic pain (American Geriatric Society 2009). The risk factors of overt opioid-use disorders in the general population and those with chronic pain are similar (Simoni-Wasili and Yang 2006, Brown et al. 1996). For misuse, the risk factors may be less clear. In some, but not all, studies, high levels of pain are associated with greater risk of pain medication misuse (Park and Lavin 2010). Of note, this study did not support gender as a risk factor for opioid medication misuse. Typical warning signs that a patient may be misusing prescription pain medications include: over-reporting symptoms, refusal of generic equivalents, arguments about pharmacology, or insistence on getting a controlled-substance prescription on the first visit. Other warning signs include: frequent requests to move appointments up, keeping a pain appointment but skipping or missing other doctor appointments, appearing grossly disheveled or cognitively impaired, reporting lost or stolen prescriptions, frequent unauthorized dose escalations, and positive urine toxicology tests for illicit drugs (Simoni-Wasili and Yang 2006).

Levi-Minzi et al. (2013) have specifically examined characteristics of opioid pain medication misusers in a predominantly male South Florida population aged 60 years and older. Though a small sample was studied ($n = 88$), and the population was somewhat atypical, with nearly a fifth reporting they were military veterans and about a quarter having been homeless in the prior 90 days, this is one of the few examinations of those not in treatment who reported opioid misuse. Mean age of the group was 63.3 years, and 86.4% reported severe pain issues; 80.7% reported misuse of their *prescribed* opioid for pain control. Just over half of these obtained their opioid from their primary care physician (PCP). It was notable that those in severe pain were over 12 times as likely to obtain the opioid from their PCP, and had a much lower odds ratio of using a dealer (odds ratio [OR] = 0.20). This is not to say that this misusing population was solely a chronic pain group without prior substance-use history. A significant portion endorsed recent use of cocaine or crack (35.2%), heroin (14.8%), and cannabis (30.7%). Just over 10% reported selling their prescription medication in the prior month, and 26% indicated they obtained their opioid from a dealer. About half had had prior formal substance-abuse treatment. A high percentage reported past-90-days benzodiazepine use (48.9%). Sixty-four percent reported severe depression or anxiety in the prior year. Interestingly, alcohol, cannabis, and benzodiazepine users all had over four times the odds ratio of using a dealer relative to those who did not report use of these substances. Importantly, this study strongly supports the risk factors of prior substance-abuse history and concurrent psychiatric comorbidity as predictive of opioid misuse or use disorder.

## Managing Risks of Opioid Abuse/Misuse

Recently, medical providers have begun to hesitate more to initiate treatment with opioids, given the abuse potential with this class of medication (Culberson and Ziska 2008). "Opiophobia," as coined by Barkin et al. (2005), can then lead to underuse of opiates in moderate to severe pain management. To aid prescribers in their decision making, several risk assessment tools have been developed to help evaluate risk of opioid misuse (Table 5.1). In the elderly, risk assessment scales are available for those with mild-to-moderate, as well as severe, cognitive impairment (Abdulla et al., 2013; Closs et al. 2004). The Opioid Risk Tool (ORT) and Opioid Assessment for Patients with Pain–Revised (SOAPP-R) are helpful questionnaires to assess initial risk. These

*Table 5.1* **Risk Assessment Tools**

| | |
|---|---|
| Universal Precautions in Pain Medicine | 10-step guide to aid in assessment and chronic treatment of pain (Gourlay et al., 2005) |
| Opioid Risk Tool (ORT) | Brief validated questionnaire; assigns sex-specific score for future aberrant opioid-related behavior |
| Screener & Opioid Assessment for Patients with Pain (SOAPP-R) | Used to identify which chronic pain patients may be at risk for problems with long-term opioid medication |
| Current Opioid Misuse Measure (COMM) | 17-question self-assessment for patients already on opioids, designed to identify ongoing patient misuse of opioid medication |

*Source*: American Geriatrics Society, 2009.

scales stratify individuals into having low, medium, or high risk of aberrant opioid use (Webster & Webster, 2013). The Current Opioid Misuse Measure (COMM) is helpful in assessing risk in individuals who are already being pre-scribed opioids (Butler et al. 2007, Butler et al. 2008). The Pain Medication Questionnaire also appears useful for screening community-dwelling elderly for pain medication misuse (Park et al. 2010).

It is advised that every pain assessment consist of a detailed patient inter-view, including personal and family history of substance abuse (Chang and Compton 2013). A detailed physical exam with random toxicology screens should be used as means of assessing medication adherence and to monitor for other potential problematic drug use. Tools such as the Universal Precautions in Pain Management (Gourlay 2005) have been developed to aid clinicians in making pain assessments and stratifying risk vs. benefits of opioid use. Additional resources can be found through the Physicians for Responsible Opioid Prescribing (http://www.supportprop.org/).

# Pain

It is beyond the scope of the current review to fully examine pain management in the elderly, and the reader is referred to earlier reviews (Makris et al. 2014, Tracy and Morrison 2013, Stewart et al. 2013, Camacho-Soto et al. 2011, Fine 2009). As regards opioid-use disorders and opioid misuse in the elderly, the role of opi-oids in pain management must be examined in regard to (1) how prescribed opi-oids contribute directly to opioid-use disorders, and (2) how opioid misuse, both by end users and prescribers, contributes to opioid-use disorder in the elderly.

Chronic pain and addiction are closely linked. This is true for the elderly prescription pain medication abuser as well as the younger adult. Chronic pain and addiction share several common features, including loss of function, loss of control over one's life, and a loss of sense of self. As discussed later, chronic pain is very common in the elderly. Chronic pain is seen in 25–50% of community-dwelling older persons and 40–80% of the nursing home population (Chai and Horton 2010).

## The Role of Opioids in Pain Management in the Elderly

There are, of course, several types of pain that can be broadly grouped: pain secondary to cancers; and in palliative care, acute pain secondary to injury, infection, etc.; chronic non-cancer pain (CNCP); and the distinction between neuropathic vs. nociceptive pain. In the main, we will review the literature regarding CNCP, with notation where there is information regarding cancer pain. Acute pain management will not be addressed, although there will be instances where an acute injury results in a prescribed opioid that in turn may trigger relapse to an opioid-use disorder. There is no definite understanding of whether short-term prescribing of an opioid in a patient without a prior opioid-use disorder results in development of an opioid-use disorder in the geriatric population, though it is suspected this would be exceedingly rare.

The management of pain in the elderly has been extensively reviewed (Malec and Shega 2015, National Opioid Use and Guideline Group 2010, American Geriatric Society 2009, Pergolozzi et al. 2008). About one in four elderly receive opioids for chronic pain (Solomon et al. 2006). In the 15 years following 1995, the use of opioids increased nine-fold in the elderly (Olfson et al. 2013). Fairly large studies indicate opioids relative to other pain medications confer substantial risks when used to treat CNCP in the elderly, including all-cause mortality (Solomon et al. 2010a, Simoni-Wasili et al. 2006, Hajjar 2003). Two opioids that differ substantially in potency, codeine and oxycodone, have the highest risk of elevated overall cause mortality (Solomon et al. 2010b). One cannot escape the controversies surrounding opioid use in the management of CNCP in all ages: Do they work, are they necessary, do their benefits outweigh the risks, should there be more definitive guidance on dosing and monitoring post-prescribing etc.? The inability to clearly demonstrate their efficacy is more complicated in the elderly, as there are precious few data about functional outcomes in this population. Furthermore, cognitive and communication deficits, stoicism, and reluctance to try an opioid medication contribute to reduced use of opioids in the elderly (Spitz et al. 2011, Upshur et al. 2006). As a result, many argue pain is relatively under-treated in this population (Monroe et al. 2014, Levi-Minzi et al. 2013, McLachlan et al. 2011, Reynolds et al. 2008, Auret and Schug 2005, Landi et al. 2001). Even in cancer-related pain, a surprising proportion of the elderly are not prescribed an opioid; e.g., one-third of those with severe pain (Barbera et al. 2012). Rates of opioid prescribing decline in those over age 85, as well as in those with low cognitive performance (Mercandante and Arcuri 2007a). However, a Danish study, perhaps reflecting the effects of increased opioid use since the 1990s, shows an increase in opioid prescribing with age, and higher prescribing in nursing home residents than in community-dwelling elderly (Jensen-Dahm et al. 2015). Several studies provide suggestive, though not direct, evidence that under-treatment of pain in the elderly contributes to the rise of pain medication misuse (Levi-Minzi et al. 2013). Furthermore, under-treatment of pain can result in lower quality of life, behavioral and mood disturbances, and impairments in working memory (see Jensen-Dahm 2014). Complicating matters, opioids themselves may have a small but real negative effect on mental health functioning (Papaleontiou et al. 2010).

Interestingly, geriatricians report less concern than internists about addiction in the elderly, and more concern about the under-treatment of pain (Lin et al. 2007). In rank order, fear of causing harm (77%), subjectivity of pain (62%), lack of training in pain management (31%), fear of causing addiction (19%), fear of regulatory oversight (12%), and concern about family/caregiver abuse (12%) were cited as provider barriers to using opioids in elderly with CNCP (Spitz et al. 2011). Compared to similar surveys related to younger cohorts, the fear of contributing to addiction or drug diversion was much less of a concern, even though the elderly, along with their family and friends, represent a significant source of diverted opioids (Inciardi et al. 2009b).

Pain is a common occurrence among elderly adults, affecting this group more than any other (Weiner 2007). Approximately 25–50% of community-dwelling elderly, and 40–80% of nursing home elderly residents, experience pain of sufficient severity or duration to be considered chronic (Chai and Horton 2010). In the elderly, women are generally more likely to report persistent pain than men are (Tsang et al. 2008, Campbell et al. 2010). Treatment of pain in the elderly requires a delicate balance between adequately controlling pain and simultaneously monitoring for potentially adverse effects. Some argue that opiates should not be used at all for long-term treatment of chronic pain, given their side-effect profile and possible abuse potential. Currently, there is a lack of conclusive data regarding the effectiveness and safety of long-term opioid use in many populations, including the elderly (Papaleontiou et al. 2010). Given limited alternatives for pain management, however, opiates remain a mainstay treatment option and continue to be widely used. Therefore, it is important to be aware of possible risks associated with opiate use in this population.

Older people differ from their younger counterparts in several critical ways regarding pain and its management. First, most studies indicate the elderly suffer more chronic pain, as would be expected because of the accumulation of wear and tear injuries and diagnoses, especially osteoarthritis, degenerative spine and other joints, claudication, and peripheral vascular disease and cancers (Rosen et al. 2011, Donald and Foy 2004, Helme and Gibson 2001). Over half of all cancer patients are 65 years or older (Marcandante and Arcuri 2007). The prevalence of neuropathic pain also rises with age (Fine 2009). Estimates of chronic pain in those 65 and older range from 45–85%, though the definitions of the pain frequency and duration vary widely (Krueger and Stone 2008, Sjogren et al. 2009). As noted, women are at greater risk for developing chronic pain conditions (Hurley and Adams 2008). In the elderly, pain management issues become more central to care.

Second, the detection of pain in the elderly is complicated by cognitive decline, receptive and expressive communication difficulties, and sometimes by a tendency of the elderly to under-report their pain for various reasons, including stoicism and cultural factors (Molton and Terrill 2014, Dowling et al. 2008, Etzioni et al. 2007, Mercandante and Arcuri 2007a, Yong 2006). Reduced reporting of pain by the elderly runs counter to some neurobiological data indicating that reduced central pain modulating systems causes increased sensitivity to noxious stimuli, as well as the overall increase in chronic pain in the elderly (Cole et al. 2010). Pain under-reporting leads to the under-treatment of pain in the elderly (Landi et al. 2001, Chodosh et al. 2001). Provider attitudes can also compromise treatment of pain in the elderly (Malex and Shega 2015, Spitz et al. 2011, Bruckenthal et al. 2009, American Geriatric Society 2009). Under-detection and under-treatment of pain appears to be a particular problem for nursing-home residents, those with cognitive impairment, and in ethnic minorities (Sawyer et al. 2006, Won et al. 2004, American Geriatrics Society 2002). Specialized screening tools have been developed to overcome challenges in assessment of pain in the elderly (Fine 2009, Schofield 2012).

Third, despite the fact that the elderly's access to medications is more restricted due to transportation and financial issues, they are at much higher risk for polypharmacy (Molton and Terrill 2014, Nobili et al. 2011). The risk of drug interactions complicates the increased risk of adverse effects in the elderly, necessitating careful dose titration and close monitoring (Rastogi and Meek 2013, American Geriatric Society 2009). Polypharmacy reduces patient compliance, as does cognitive impairment, worsening the tendency of the elderly to be less adherent to pain medication recommendations than the younger population (Markotic et al. 2013, DiMatteo et al. 2007, Sale et al.

2006). In a random screening of 20% of Medicare beneficiaries who filled at least one scrip for an opioid, hospital admissions rose proportionally with the number of opioid prescribers (Jena et al. 2014). The Updated Beers Criteria (American Geriatrics Society 2012) for potentially inappropriate medications for the elderly focus much more on psychotropics such as benzodiazepines, antipsychotics, and antidepressants than on opioids, and include only meperidine and pentazocine on the "to avoid" list.

Fourth, pain guidelines for the treatment of chronic pain must be modified for the elderly, given their added susceptibility to renal, cardiovascular, and gastrointestinal adverse effects from NSAIDs, and intolerance to side effects of agents such as the tricyclic antidepressants (see American Geriatrics Society 2009). This makes the choice of opioids more frequent in pain management paradigms.

The rates of opioid use for pain have been rising in the elderly as they have for other age groups, essentially doubling between 1997 and 2005. From 1997 to 2005, the CONSORT Study demonstrated that rate of increase in men 65 and older was slower than for younger men (Campbell et al. 2010). For women age 65 and older, the rate of increase paralleled that of other cohorts. However, the rate of opioid prescribing for elderly women was about five-fold higher than for men of the same age group in two large health plans in California and Washington (Campbell et al. 2010). Long-term opioid use in elderly women reached 8–9%. Between 1993 and 2012, by far the largest increase in hospitalization for opioid-related causes occurred in the age groups 65–84 and in those 85 and older (Owens et al. 2014).

## Physiological Changes Associated with Aging

There are normal physiological changes in gastrointestinal, renal, and hepatic functions that occur as people age that can place elders at a higher risk for experiencing side effects from opioids (Fine 2009, American Geriatric Society 2009). Aging is associated with an increase in body fat, decrease in lean body mass, and decrease in total body water, which can have an effect on drug distribution (Chau et al. 2008). As a result, lipophilic medications can take longer to be eliminated from the body. Age-related decline in hepatic and renal function can have an impact on onset of action, rate of elimination, and half-life of opiates (Tracy and Morrison 2013, Pergolizzi et al. 2008). As a practical matter, despite significant changes in gastrointestinal and hepatic functions, oral bioavailability of opioids is not markedly changed with aging, but 25–50% dose reductions are advised because of reduced first-pass metabolism and increased sensitivity to side effects such as sedation (Malec and Shega 2015). Especially in the presence of liver disease, such as cirrhosis, hepatitis B or C, and cancers, starting doses of opioids should be reduced by about 50%, and dosing intervals doubled (Verbeeck 2008). Codeine efficacy is predicted to be decreased in the presence of hepatic failure because of reduced conversion to morphine (Mercadante and Arcuri 2007a).

Reductions in renal clearance with aging more markedly affect opioid clearance, because opioids, with the exception of methadone and buprenorphine, are largely cleared by the kidneys. Elimination of the morphine metabolites morphine-3-glucuronide (M3G) and morphine-6-glucuronide (M6G) is markedly slowed in those with renal failure. These metabolites are active, but M3G is also neurotoxic, lowering the seizure threshold. M6G can accumulate in the presence of dehydration (Pergolizzi et al. 2008, Faura et al. 1998). Hydromorphone suffers similar risks to morphine (Mercandante and Arcuri 2007b), but oxycodone and hydromorphone can be used with caution in renal failure. Codeine is partly metabolized to morphine, and so can induce some of the same neurotoxicity. Below a creatinine clearance of 30 mL/min, codeine should not be used because of substantial toxicity. The same creatinine clearance warning is also true for meperidine and propoxyphene (Hanlon et al. 2009). With the exception of buprenorphine and methadone, the half-life of all opioids and their respective metabolites is increased in older adults who may be experiencing renal dysfunction. It is important to monitor creatinine clearance in these individuals and make slow changes to dosages (Dean 2004).

The "start low, go slow" mantra for the elderly is partly based on the universal reduction in renal function with aging. Fentanyl catabolism appears significantly slowed in those over 75 versus those younger than 60, yet dosage reductions are not usually made (Pesonen et al. 2009, Smith 2009). Tramadol elimination half-life roughly doubles with liver or renal failure (Mercadante and Arcuri 2004), yet recommendations are to reduce doses by only 20%. Oxycodone, methadone, and buprenorphine appear least affected by renal impairment, and fentanyl by liver impairment (Mercadante and Arcuri 2007a, Tracy and Morrison 2013, British Geriatrics Society 2013). As a practical matter, pharmacodynamic alterations affect dosing paradigms for the elderly much more than pharmacokinetic changes (Malec and Shega 2015, Gupta and Avram 2012). The American Geriatrics Society 2002 and 2009 guidelines recommend that pain medications be started one at a time and at a low dose. Doses should be started about 25–50% lower than doses given to young adults (Chau et al. 2008). Excellent reviews of drug–drug interactions and metabolic changes caused by renal and hepatic decline in the elderly for specific opioids are found in Huang and Mallet, 2013; Gloth, 2011; and Pergolizzi et al., 2008.

The elderly are more sensitive to acute sedation and analgesia with opioids (Gupta and Avram 2012, Pesonen et al. 2009). The effective analgesic dose in an 80-year-old is predicted to be about half that of a 40-year-old, due to an increase in intrinsic potency and not cerebral opioid uptake (Gupta and Avram 2012). However, multiple other factors in the elderly can make predicting what is both a safe and effective starting dose of opioids problematic. Erring on the side of safety may often lead to inadequate analgesia, at least in the first several days of treatment. Being older does not mean one should be deprived of pain treatment. Wilder-Smith and Oliver (2005) argue it is important to take into account an older adult's state of fitness in addition to considering chronological age.

## Adverse Opioid Side Effects

Relatively few studies have explored the link between age and opioid-related adverse events (Barber and Gibson 2009). A post-hoc analysis of a randomized controlled trial found that older participants (> 65 years old) had a higher rate of constipation (27.5 vs. 16.8), fatigue (8.6 vs. 4.3), pruritus (10.4 vs. 6.9), and anorexia (5.9 vs. 2.6) than their younger subjects (Vorsanger et al. 2007). Two other studies reported up to three times the rate of somnolence in older versus younger adults (Rosenthal et al. 2004, Roth et al. 2000). Another retrospective cohort study within a primary care practice in New York City found that the most common side effects associated with opiate use were constipation (22% of sample), mental status change (16%), nausea (10%), lethargy (9%), and urinary retention (2%). Four participants (3%) met criteria for abuse/misuse behaviors, but no formal screening tools were used. Forty-eight percent of the participants in this study dropped out due to side effects and lack of analgesic efficacy (Reid et al. 2010). A large meta-analysis by Papalentiou et al. (2010) found rates of 30% for constipation, 28% for nausea, and 22% for dizziness, resulting in a discontinuation rate of 25%.

Table 5.2 lists a compilation of commonly reported adverse effects from opioids. A detailed discussion of the more serious adverse effects follows.

### RESPIRATORY DEPRESSION AND INCREASED RISK OF OVERDOSE DEATH

Respiratory depression is often the most concerning side effect associated with opiates (American Geriatrics Society 2009). All opioids come with a black-box warning for respiratory depression, along with the risk of abuse and diversion. Respiratory depression is mediated via dose-dependent agonist activity of opioids at the μ-opiate receptor. Respiratory depression can result from rapid dose escalation, drug–drug interactions with other

*Table 5.2* **Commonly Reported Opioid-Related Adverse Effects**

| | |
|---|---|
| Cognitive Impairment | Opioid Induced Hyperalgesia |
| Constipation | Pruritus |
| Hormonal Changes | QT Prolongation |
| Immunological Effects | Respiratory Depression |
| Myoclonus | Sedation |
| Nausea | Urinary Retention |

sedating medications/drugs (e.g., benzodiazepines, alcohol), and drug concentration accumulation that could occur with liver and/or renal dysfunction (American Geriatrics Society 2009, Pergolizzi et al. 2008). Chronic diseases in the elderly, including chronic obstructive pulmonary disease (COPD) and congestive heart failure, and the general loss of physiological reserves, compound the risk. For hospitalized patients, the risk of respiratory depression steadily climbs from the seventh to ninth decades of life, going from 2.8 to 8.7 times the risk in younger patients (Cepeda et al. 2003). Accumulation of the morphine metabolites M3G and M6G is especially problematic in renal failure, contributing to prolongation of respiratory depression. Another important consideration is that certain opioids such as methadone have a variable pharmacokinetic profile that can lead to accidental overdoses (Fishman et al. 2002, Santiago et al. 1985).

High doses of opioids and/or combination with other central nervous system depressants can lead to apnea. This side effect can be minimized if opiates are started at a low dose and increased slowly. Most opioids, including morphine, oxycodone, hydromorphone, fentanyl, and methadone, cause dose-dependent decreases in respiration (Pergolizzi et al. 2008). Buprenorphine is the only opioid found to have a ceiling effect for respiratory depression, and respiratory rate with this medication rarely falls below 10 breaths per minute (Pergolizzi et al. 2008).

Not all overdoses are accidental, and it is well known the elderly, especially white males, display increased suicide rates (Parks et al. 2014). The increased incidence of multiple losses and medical illness with aging probably account for some of this increased risk (Juurlink et al. 2004). Suicide rates have increased somewhat over the first decade of the twenty-first century, with the highest rate among those over 75 (Rockett et al. 2012). In 2012 and 2013, the rates of death from opioid overdose, based on analysis of the RADARS Poison center program, for those 60 and older exceeded those for ages 20–59. Rates for 2013 suicidal *intent* in this system were 0.869 per 100,000, compared to 2.429 per 100,000 in the younger cohort, implying *accidental* overdose occurred to a significant degree (West et al. 2015). Of concern, the rate of elderly suicidal intent with opioids continued to climb as of 2013, while it had peaked in the younger cohort in 2011. In a U.S. veteran cohort aged 50 and above between 2000 and 2011, those with opioid-use disorder versus those without were at elevated risk of accidental drug-related death (risk ratio 9.5) vs. suicide (risk ratio 2.1) or violent death (risk ratio 2.0) (Larney et al. 2015). However, these rates did *not* differ between older and younger veterans with active opioid-use disorders. In the large English cohort of opioid users in drug treatment or the criminal justice system, studied by Pierce et al. (2015), relative to age- and gender-matched controls, elevated rates of opioid overdose deaths persisted from younger to older cohorts, and in fact progressively increased in both genders in age groups 18–34, 35–44, and 45–64. From 1999 to 2011 in the United States, the age group 55–64 experienced the greatest (over six-fold) increase in opioid-analgesic poisoning deaths compared to all younger age groups, though the 2011 rate of 6.3/100,000 was still under the per 100,000 rates for those 45–54 (11.2), 35–44 (9.3), and 35–34 (8.5), but higher than that for 15–24 year olds (3.6) (Chen et al. 2014). White women aged 55–64 have experienced the largest increase in accidental opioid overdose death in the past 10 years (Centers for Disease Control and Prevention [CDC] 2013).

## CONSTIPATION AND NAUSEA

Gastric pH tends to increase as people age. Other age-related changes include reduced gastric and intestinal motility, along with decreased enzyme activity and absorption. These changes can make constipation more frequent (about one-third) in older adults (Pergolizzi et al. 2008, Papaleontiou et al. 2010). As a result, it is often advised that prophylactic treatment for constipation be initiated as soon as opioid treatment is started. However, even elderly in long-term care treated with opioids are not consistently treated with laxatives (Max et al. 2007). Constipation tends to be long-lasting, unlike other opioid-related side effects (Benyamin et al. 2008). Buprenorphine and transdermal fentanyl may confer less risk of reduced colonic motility (Pergolizzi et al. 2008). The elderly may be at somewhat reduced risk of nausea related to others, but this side effect is still common (see Tracy and Morrison 2013 for review). Gastrointestinal side effects represent a major cause of treatment failure for this class of agent in the elderly (Reid et al. 2010).

## ANTICHOLINERGIC EFFECTS AND DELIRIUM

The elderly tend to have a higher sensitivity to anticholinergic medications. It has been noted that certain opioids tend to have anticholinergic side effects that can lead to urinary retention, increased sedation, and mental status change. Frail and dehydrated elderly individuals are at most risk for developing opioid neurotoxicity when given high doses for long periods of time (Pergolizzi et al. 2008). All opioids, though buprenorphine less so, have been associated with central nervous system effects, though more data are needed to prove the safety of buprenorphine. Tolerance to these side effects usually develops but requires a slow titration schedule to minimize likelihood of anticholinergic side effects and non-adherence.

The elderly are at increased risk of several factors associated with development of delirium, including renal insufficiency, baseline cognitive impairment, and polypharmacy (McNicol et al. 2003). However, it should be noted that untreated severe pain, a danger when the older person has communication deficits, can also contribute to delirium. In the elderly hospitalized for hip fracture, careful use of opioids can reduce the incidence of delirium (Morrison et al. 2003).

## SEDATION AND COGNITIVE SUPPRESSION

Especially in those with pre-existing cognitive decline, opioids in the elderly are associated with excess sedation and cognitive slowing (Papaleontiou et al. 2010, Manfredi et al. 2003). The combination of opioids with other sedating medications, such as benzodiazepines, antidepressants, and antipsychotics, further increases risk of sedation and falls. Consequently, it is important in this patient population to consider the risk of polypharmacy and monitor carefully when prescribing opioids.

## DEPRESSION

There appears to be a bidirectional and complex relationship between opioid use and depression (Scherrer et al. 2015). One might expect improvements in mood with improved pain management, and conversely, more depression with worsening pain (Roth et al. 1998, Lindsay and Wyckoff 1981). There is disagreement as to whether opioid use in CNCP is associated with elevated rates of depression (Papaleontiou et al. 2010). A large meta-analysis concluded there was a small but significant negative association between mental health and opioid use for CNCP in the elderly (Papaleontiou et al. 2010). Recently, an association of morphine-equivalent doses (MED) of 50 mg or higher was associated with an odds ratio of 2.65 for depression. Dose increase of 10.1 MEDs also predicted development of depression, and conversely, the presence of depression predicted higher MEDs (Scherrer et al. 2015). Park and Lavin (2010) reported depression as a risk factor for opioid medication misuse in community-dwelling elderly. Grattan et al. (2012) found, for all adults, including a cohort over 65 without a prior history of a substance-use disorder, moderate to severe depression was associated with misuse of opioids for relief of stress or insomnia, and overuse of prescribed opioids.

## CARDIAC EFFECTS AND INCREASED RISK OF MYOCARDIAL INFARCTION

Elevated risk of cardiovascular events, including myocardial infarction, has been found with opioid use in the elderly relative to those prescribed NSAIDs (Solomon et al. 2010a) and in general (Khodniva et al. 2014). The Khodniva abstract reported an 18% risk of events, and 33% increased risk of cardiovascular-related death, in a study of nearly 30,000 individuals. Though unexplained, codeine appears to confer higher risk of cardiovascular events than other opioids (Solomon et al. 2010b). Opioid-related cardiac side effects are uncommon. There has been an association between morphine and histamine release that can lead to vasodilation and hypotension (Benyamin 2008). Notably, methadone has been found to be associated with QT prolongation and *torsade de pointes* in those taking doses as low as 30 mg daily (Benyamin 2008). When prescribing methadone, it is recommended to monitor cardiac function through EKGs when initiating treatment, making dose changes, or when adding medications that are Cytochrome P450 (CYP)3A4 inhibitors.

## INCREASED RISK OF FALLS

Falls are a leading cause of traumatic injury in the elderly (Stevens 2006). Given that both pain and opioids are implicated in fall risk, the relationship of opioid prescribing to falls is controversial (Malec and Shega 2015). In those 60 years and older, Saunders et al. (2010) found fractures occurred at a rate of 10.0/100 person-years in those prescribed opioids for chronic pain, versus 3.8/100 for nonusers, with older women being at particular risk. Many other studies have supported an elevated risk of falls in the elderly with opioid use (Rolita et al. 2013, O'Neil et al. 2012, Miller et al. 2011, Solomon et al. 2010a, Buckeridge et al. 2010, Vestergaard et al. 2006). The risk increases during periods of initiation, and at higher doses (Miller et al. 2011). Tramadol and propxyphene appear to incur less fall risk than other opioids (Solomon et al. 2010b). Given that psychotropic and benzodiazepine drug use are the most consistently associated with falls in the elderly, and these are at increased use in older age, the addition of opioids further adds risk (Huang et al. 2012). However, an extensive review of fall risk in those with cancer did not support an increased risk with opioid use (Wildes et al. 2014, Stone et al. 2012). Factors such as prior history of falls, use of benzo-diazepines, lack of independence for activities of daily living (ADLs), and presence of depression or use of an antidepressant were all significantly as-sociated with falls in community-dwelling elderly with cancer, while opioid use was not.

## HEPATIC FUNCTION AND MYOCLONUS

In the baby-boomer generation, elevated rates of hepatitis B and C will cer-tainly contribute to impairments in liver function as this cohort ages (Nave 2013). Reduced first-pass metabolism may necessitate dosage reductions of opioids, and reduced metabolism by the liver would render codeine less able to metabolize to morphine, and thus attenuate its analgesic effect (Brecher and West 2014, Tegeder et al. 1999). Both fentanyl and buprenorphine may be preferred agents in those with marked hepatic impairment (Tegeder et al. 1999, Pergolizzi et al. 2008). Myoclonus has been cited as a dose-dependent central nervous system side effect on those receiving chronic opioid treat-ment. This side effect has been especially noted with oral morphine, and it has been suggested to be the result of metabolites produced by the liver (Chau et al. 2008).

## OPIOID-INDUCED HYPERALGESIA

Opioid-induced hyperalgesia (OIH) is an increased sensitivity to both painful and non-painful stimuli despite taking high doses of opiates. In part, this is believed to be accumulation of toxic metabolites of opioids such as M3G and the activation of N-methyl-D-aspartate (NMDA) receptors associated with the long-term use of high doses of opiates (Benyamin et al. 2008). In addi-tion, downregulation of central inhibitory pain pathways and/or central sensi-tization of pro-nociceptive pathways are also believed to play a role (Lee et al. 2011). However, there is controversy regarding the differentiation of OIH from tolerance and disease progression. Using the cold-water task, sensitivity to pain appears to be elevated by current as well as prior (up to weeks) opioid maintenance (Wachholtz and Gonzalez 2015). The ability to tolerate the pain improved more quickly with cessation of opioids, though it did not reach the baseline of the opioid-naïve after weeks. OIH can play a critical role in the fail-ure of chronic opioid therapy to relieve pain and/or improve function, but it is unclear whether the elderly are at increased or decreased risk to develop OIH relative to younger patients.

## IMMUNOSUPPRESSION

Aging is associated with a decreased function and responsiveness of the immune system known as *immunosenescence* (Rinder et al. 1997). Therefore, the body is more susceptible to infectious disease and cancer. Pain can be both a psychological and a physiological stressor that can affect one's immune system as well. While it is very important to provide pain relief to decrease suffering and the stress response, it is worth noting that certain opioids have immunosuppressive properties. These immunosuppressive properties have been implicated in heroin addicts' increased susceptibility to HIV (Benyamin et al. 2008). Morphine has been found to be the most immunosuppressive opioid, while buprenorphine, hydromorphone and oxycodone have been found to be less so (Martucci et al. 2004, Sacerdote et al. 1997). Currently, there are no available data to determine the precise long-term effects of these immunological effects. Per an international expert panel consensus statement, opioids with minimal immunosuppressive properties should be preferentially used in the elderly (Pergolizzi et al. 2008). Specifically, this panel advised against use of fentanyl and morphine because of their immunosuppressive effects, as well as recommending the avoidance of higher doses of opioids where possible.

## HORMONAL CHANGES

Opioids act on the endocrine system via the hypothalamic-pituitary-adrenal (HPA) axis and the hypothalamic-pituitary-gonadal axis. This leads to decreases in serum luteinizing hormone (LH) and cortisol levels, and increases in prolactin (Chau 2008). Furthermore, suppression of estradiol and androgen production might provide a mechanism for the reduced bone density and increased risk of fracture discussed previously (Katz and Mazer 2009). Heroin use has also been associated with acute suppression of LH followed by decrease in testosterone levels. Men using prescribed or illicit opioids have been found to experience sexual dysfunction, depression, and decreased energy levels as a result. Women have also been found to have reduction of estrogen levels and experienced depression, sexual dysfunction, and possibly decreased bone mineral density. Women on methadone maintenance were noted to have decreased estrogen levels (Daniell 2008). The clinical significance of the link between chronic opioid use and osteoporosis and fractures remains controversial.

# Treatment

Age-specific treatment approaches for substance-use disorders result in better adherence and fewer relapses (Oslin 2005). Treatment guidelines from SAMHSA (Blow 1998) indicate that treatment should include age-appropriate group therapy, address loss early in treatment, and teach skills to rebuild social support networks. It is recommended that staff be experienced in working with the elderly, proceed at a slower pace, and employ age-appropriate content. A culture of respect with an atmosphere of support and change rather than confrontation should be created within the therapeutic setting (Schonfeld and Dupree 1998 and 1997).

While there have not been studies looking specifically at the treatment of opioid-use disorders in the elderly, there have been several studies looking at the effectiveness of treatment in elder-specific alcohol-use disorders. These can be used to illustrate effective approaches to engage and treat substance-use disorders in elderly patients in general. Kashner et al. (1992) assessed participants in the Older Alcoholics Rehabilitation Program of the Veterans Administration who were randomly assigned to reminiscence therapy versus traditional care programs. They found that developing patient self-esteem and peer relationships was superior to confrontational approaches typical of traditional care programs. Several studies have shown that brief interventions and motivational techniques work well in the elderly population for alcohol-misuse problems. The Guiding Older Adult Lifestyles (GOAL) project used brief physician advice for 156 at-risk drinkers, who showed reduced alcohol consumption in 35–40% of the participants at 12 months follow-up (Fleming et al. 1999). Results of the Health Profile Project ($n = 454$) demonstrated that a motivational enhancement session reduced at-risk drinking at 12 months (Blow et al. 2000). The Staying Healthy Project undertaken by the American Society on Aging noted that about 6% of the older adults sampled reported at-risk drinking, and that a brief intervention resulted in about 40% reduced consumption of alcohol (Barry et al. 2006). The Gerontology Alcohol Project targeted adults with late-life-onset alcohol abuse. Using day treatment and a group format (cognitive-behavioral therapy), 75% of the participants maintained drinking goals, and no one returned to steady drinking (Dupree et al. 1984). The Computerized Alcohol-Related Problems Survey demonstrated that a brief intervention that provided feedback and psycho-education to at-risk drinkers was effective in primary care settings (Nguyen et al. 2001). The Primary Care Research in Substance Abuse and Mental Health (PRISM) trial randomized 414 older at-risk alcohol users to integrated primary care intervention or to referral to a specialist provider, such as a substance-abuse clinic. The trial showed that elder alcohol users who received the integrated intervention were twice as likely to stay in treatment (Oslin et al. 1997).

In some cases of elderly pain medication misuse, brief interventions can work. Where they fail, a more comprehensive evaluation is recommended, including a thorough drug and alcohol use history. If there is a diagnosis of opioid-use disorder or opioid misuse, then the clinician's focus should turn to comprehensive treatment, including issues of detoxification, rehabilitation, aftercare or continuing care, treatment of co-occurring illnesses, and adequate pain management. Treatment should be holistic and include integrated teamwork between patient, physician, therapists, case managers, family, and friends. Clinicians should be aware of the physical, behavioral and spiritual well-being of the older individual. While medications are an important part of a multidisciplinary plan, they are only one part of the multimodal approach often needed in treatment of either chronic pain of an opioid-use disorder.

Medications for treatment of opioid pain medication misuse or opioid-use disorder in the elderly include possible treatment with methadone, buprenorphine/naloxone (Suboxone), and naltrexone (Office of National Drug Control Policy [ONDCP] 2012). Methadone is a synthetic opioid with a long half-life that has been researched extensively for addiction and pain use. When this medication is used in relation to opioid-use disorder, it should be prescribed and dispensed from a federally licensed methadone clinic. Methadone is safe to use in the elderly when the individual is closely monitored and followed medically. Buprenorphine is a partial opioid agonist having many desirable properties compared to methadone, including lower abuse potential, lower level of physical dependence, relative non-lethality if ingested in overdose quantities, less difficulty in dosing, less euphoria, and possibly less OIH induction. It has a prolonged therapeutic effect, so it can be taken daily or up to every three days. It appears to be as effective as methadone for people with moderate levels of opioid-use disorders. Lastly, naltrexone is used in the patients who must abstain from opioids due to legal or other considerations. It is not recommended for use in the elderly for prescription pain medication abuse, as naltrexone can often block the effect of other appropriately used opioid pain medications and can have several unpleasant side effects.

In general, when using medications in the elderly, the rule is "start with a low dose and increase the dose slowly, but keep going." This dictum of geriatric medicine holds true for opioid-use disorder pharmacological intervention as well. Monitoring elderly patients closely is key, as the elderly may metabolize medications more slowly, are often on multiple medications increasing the likelihood of drug–drug interactions, have a reduced volume of distribution necessitating lower doses of medications for the same effect, and may have increased pharmacodynamic sensitivity to medications. While not specifically studied in the elderly, as previously described, supported non-pharmacological modalities include CBT (cognitive behavioral therapy), relapse prevention, and age-specific 12-Step programs (Alcoholics Anonymous or Narcotics Anonymous [AA or NA]) and Rational Recovery (RR). Counseling and case management are often needed by the elderly, as well as brief interventions with the physician or clinician. Motivational interviewing and motivational enhancement have not been studied in the elderly. The most effective approach to any group intervention with the elderly is to have age group–appropriate cohorts in treatment. The elderly prefer to be in treatment with other patients their own age. Simoni-Wastila and Yang (2006) provide useful general approaches to improve the treatment of prescription drug abuse in older adults.

## Summary

The problem of opioid-use disorders and prescription pain medication misuse in the elderly is an escalating challenge, as it is in the general population. Two facts—the expansion of the elderly population, and the increased representation of baby-boomers in that population—make the problem likely to expand. Yet, there is little direct examination of these problems in the elderly. Chronic pain needs in the elderly deserve to be adequately addressed. Along with this, risk-stratification for opioid use in the elderly should become standard practice, as should routine screening for opioid misuse and opioid-use disorders in the elderly. Once identified, there are established treatments available, including medications and psychotherapies that can be tailored to the meet the specific needs of the older patient. Brief treatment and interventions appear to work well with the elderly and should be tried in cases of pain medication misuse. When the older patient has a well-defined opioid-use disorder, then referral to specialty substance-abuse treatment is recommended. Along with appropriate medication-assisted therapies, issues such as loss, cohort issues, medical problems, psychiatric comorbidities, and social isolation should be the focus of supportive approaches that avoid confrontation. The benefits of using a multidisciplinary approach are well recognized for the chronic pain patient, and this strategy needs to become just as recognized for the elderly patient with either pain medication misuse or an overt opioid-use disorder.

## References

Abdulla A, Adams N, Bone M, Elliott AM, et al. Guidance on the management of pain in older people. *Age Ageing* 2013;42(Suppl 1):i1–57.

Alliance of Aging Network. 2006. Available at http://agingresearch.org/content/article/detail/826.

American Geriatric Society Panel on the Pharmacological Management of Persistent Pain in Older Persons. Pharmacological management of persistent pain in older persons. *J Am Geriatr Soc* 2009;57:1331–1346.

American Geriatrics Society Panel on Persistent Pain in Older Persons. The management of persistent pain in older persons. American Geriatrics Society. *J Am Geriatr Soc* 2002;50:S205–S224.

American Geriatrics Society, Beers Criteria Update Expert Panel. American Geriatrics Society updated Beers criteria for potentially inappropriate medication use in older adults. *JAGS* 2012;60:616–631.

American Psychiatric Association. *Diagnostic and Statistical Manual of Mental Disorders, Fifth Edition,* Washington, DC: American Psychiatric Publishing Washington DC; 2013.

Arndt S, Clayton R, Schultz SK. Trends in substance abuse treatment 1998–2008: Increasing older adult first time admissions for illicit drugs. *Am J Geriatr Psych* 2011;19:704–711.

Auret K, Schug SA. Underutilization of opioids in elderly patients with chronic pain: Approaches to correcting the problem. *Drugs Aging* 2005;22:641–654.

Ballantyne JC. (2012). "Safe and effective when used as directed": The case of chronic use of opioid analgesics. *J Med Toxicol* 2012;8:417–423.

Barber JB, Gibson SJ. Treatment of chronic non-malignant pain in the elderly: Safety considerations. *Drug Saf* 2009;32:457–474.

Barbera L, Seow H, Husain A, Howell D, et al. Opioid prescription after pain assessment: A population-based cohort of elderly patients with cancer. *J Clin Oncol* 2012;30:1095–1099.

Barkin RL, Barkin SJ, Barkin DS. Perception, assessment, treatment, and management of pain in the elderly. *Clin Geriatr Med* 2005;21:465–490.

Barry K, et al. The effectiveness of implementing a brief alcohol intervention with older adults in community settings: Staying Healthy Project (SHP). American Society on Aging; 2006.

Becker WC, O'Connor PG. The safety of opioid analgesics in the elderly. *Arch Intern Med* 2010;170:1986–1988.

Becker WC, Sullivan LE, Tetrault JM, et al. Non-medical use, abuse and dependence on prescription opioids among U.S. adults: Psychiatric, medical and substance use correlates. *Drug Alcohol Depend* 2008:94:38–47.

Benyamin R, Trescot AM, Datta S, et al. Opioid complications and side effects. *Pain Physician* 2008;11, S105–S120.

Beynon C, McVeigh J, Hurst A, Marr A. Older and sicker: Changing mortality of drug users in treatment in North West of England. *Int J Drug Policy* 2010;21:429–431.

Blazer DG, Wu LT. Nonprescription use of pain relievers by middle-aged and elderly community-dwelling adults: National Survey on Drug Use and Health. *J Am Geriatr Soc* 2009;57:1252–1257.

Blow FC. Substance abuse among older adults. Treatment Improvement Protocol (TIP) #26. DHHS Pub. No. (SMA) 98–3179, Rockville, MD, SAMSHA, 1998.

Blow FC, Barry K. Older patients with at-risk and problem drinking patterns: New developments in brief interventions. *J Geriatr Psychiatry Neurol* 2000;13:115–123.

Brecher DB, West TL. Pain management in a patient with renal and hepatic dysfunction. *J Palliat Med* 2014;17:249–52.

British Geriatrics Society/British Pain Society. Guidance on the management of pain in older people. *Age Aging* 2013;42, I1–I57.

Brown RL, Patterson JJ, Rounds LA, Papasouliotis O. Substance abuse among patients with chronic back pain. *J Fam Pract* 1996;43:152–160.

Bruckenthal P, Reid MC, Reisner L. Special issues in the management of pain in older adults. *Pain Med* 2009;10:S67–S78.

Buckeridge D, Huang A, Hanley J, et al. Risk of injury associated with opioid use in older adults. *J Am Geriatr Soc* 2010;58(9):1664–1670.

Butler SF, Budman SH, Fernandez KC, et al. Development and validation of the Current Opioid Misuse Measure. *Pain* 2007;130:144–1456.

Butler SF, Fernandez K, Benoit C, et al. Validation of the revised Screener and Opioid Assessment for Patients with Pain (SOAPP-R). *J Pain* 2008;9:360–372.

Camacho-Soto A, Sowa G, Weiner DK. (2011). Geriatric pain. In HT Benzon, SN Raja, SS Liu, SM Fishman, & SP Cohen, Eds., *Essentials of Pain Medicine*, 3rd ed. Philadelphia, PA: Elsevier Saunders; 2011:409–421.

Campbell CI, Weisner C, LeResche L, et al. Age and gender trends in long-term opioid analgesic use for non-cancer pain. *Am J Pub Health* 2010;100:2541–2547.

Centers for Disease Control and Prevention (CDC). Vital signs: Overdoses of prescription opioid pain relievers and other drugs among women—United States, 1999–2010. *MMWR* 2003;66:537–542.

Cepeda MS, Farrar JT, Baumgarten M, et al. Side effects of opioid during short-term administration: Effects of age, gender and race. *Clin Pharmacol Ther* 2003;74:102–112.

Chang Y-P, Compton P. Management of chronic pain with chronic opioid therapy in patients with substance use disorders. *Addict Sci Clin Pract* 2013;8:21–32.

Chau DL, Walker V, Pai L, Cho L. Opiates and elderly: Use and side effects. *Clin Interv Aging* 2008;3:273–278.

Chen LH, Hedegaard H, Warner M. Drug poisoning deaths involving opioid analgesics: United States, 1999–2011. NCHS Data Brief No. 166, Hyattsville, MD, National Center for Health Statistics, pp. 1–9, 2014.

Chodosh J, Ferrell BA, Shekelle PG, Wenger NS. Quality indicators for pain management in vulnerable elders. *Ann Intern Med* 2001;135:731–735.

Cicero TJ, Lynskey M, Todorov A, et al. Co-morbid pain and psychopathology in males and females admitted to treatment for opioid analgesic abuse. *Pain* 2008;139:127–135.

Cicero TJ, Surratt HL, Kurtz SP, et al. Patterns of prescription opioid abuse and comorbidity in an aging treatment population. *J Subst Abuse Treat* 2012;42:87–94.

Closs J, Barr B, Briggs M, et al. The clinical utility of five pain assessment scales for nursing home residents with varying degrees of cognitive impairment. *J Pain Sympt Manag* 2004;27:196–205.

Cole LJ, Farrell MJ, Gibson SJ, et al. Age-related differences in pain sensitivity and regional brain activity evoked by noxious pressure. *Neurorbiol Aging* 2010;31:494–503.

Culberson JW, Ziska M. Prescription drug misuse/abuse in the elderly. *Geriatrics* 2008;63:22–31.

Daniell HW. Opioid endocrinopathy in women consuming prescribed sustained-action opioids for control of nonmalignant pain. *J Pain* 2008;9:28–36.

Dean, M. Opioids in renal failure and dialysis patients. *J Pain Sympt Manag* 2004;28:497–504.

Denisco RA, Chandler RK, Compton WM. Addressing the intersecting problems of opioid misuse and chronic pain treatment. *Exp Clin Psychopharmacol* 2008;16(5), 417–428.

DiMatteo MR, Haskard KB, Williams SL. Health beliefs, disease severity, and patient adherence: A meta-analysis. *Med Care* 2007;45:521–528.

Donald IP, Foy C. A longitudinal study of joint pain in older people. *Rheumatology (Oxford)*, 2004;43:1256–1260.

Dowling GJ, Weiss SR, Condon TP. Drugs of abuse and the aging brain. *Neuropsychopharmacology*. 2008;33:209–218.

Drug Abuse Warning Network. Area profiles of drug-related mortality. 2003. At http://archive.samhsa.gov/data/dawn/files/ME2003/ME03FullReport.pdf (accessed 4/18/2016).

Dupree LW, Broskowski H, Schonfeld L. The Gerontology Alcohol Project: A behavioral treatment program for elderly alcohol abusers. *Gerontologist* 1984;24:510–516.

Edlund MJ, Steffick D, Hudson T, et al. Risk factors for clinically recognized opioid abuse and dependence among veterans using opioids for chronic non-cancer pain *Pain* 2007;129:355–362.

Etzioni, S, Chodosh J, Ferrell BA, & MacLean CH. Quality indicators for pain management in vulnerable elders. *J Am Geriatr Soc* 2007;55(Suppl 2), S403–S408.

Faura CC, Collins SL, Moore RA, et al. Systematic review of factors affecting the ratios of morphine and its major metabolites *Pain* 1998;74:43–53.

Fine P. Chronic pain management in older adults: Special considerations. *J Pain Sympt Manag* 2009;38:S4–S14.

Fishman SM, Wilsey B, Mahajan G, et al. Methadone reincarnated: Novel clinical applications with related concerns. *Pain Med* 2002;3:339–348.

Fleming MF, Manwell LB, Barry KL, et al. Brief physician advice for alcohol problems in older adults: A randomized community-based trial. *J Fam Pract* 1999;48:378–384.

Gfroerer JC, Penne MA, Pemberton MR, Folsom RE. Substance abuse treatment need among older adults in 2020: The impact of the aging baby-boom cohort. *Drug Alcohol Depend* 2003;69:127–135.

Gloth FM.III. Pharmacological management of persistent pain in older persons: Focus on opioids and non-opioids. *J Pain* 2011;12:S14–S20.

Gourlay DL, Heit HA, Almahrezi A. Universal precautions in pain medicine: A rational approach to the treatment of chronic pain. *Pain Med* 2005;6:107–112.

Grattan A, Sullivan MD, Saunders KW, et al. Depression and prescription opioid misuse among chronic opioid therapy recipients with no history of substance abuse. *Ann Fam Med* 2012;10:304–311.

Gross J. New generation gap as older addicts seek help. *The New York Times*. March 6, 2008. Available at http://www.nytimes.com/2008/03/06/us/06abuse.html.

Gupta DK, Avram MJ. Rational opioid dosing in the elderly: Dose and dosing interval when initiating opioid therapy. *Clin Pharmacol Ther* 2012;91:339–343.

Hajjar ER. Adverse drug reaction risk factors in older adults. *Am J Geriatr Pharmacother* 2003;1:82–89.

Hall AJ, Logan JE, Toblin RL, et al. Patterns of abuse among unintentional pharmaceutical overdose fatalities. *JAMA* 2008;300:2613–2620.

Han B, Gfroerer JC, Colliver JD, Penne MA. Substance use disorder among older adults in the United States in 2020. *Addiction* 2009;104:88–96.

Hanlon JT, Aspinall SL, Semla TP, et al. Consensus guidelines for oral dosing of primarily renally cleared medications in older adults. *J Am Geriatr Soc* 2009;57:335–340.

Helme RD, Gibson SJ. The epidemiology of pain in elderly people. *Clin Geriatr Med* 2001;17:417–431.

Hser Y-I, Hung D, Chou CP, Anglin MD. Trajectories of heroin addiction: Growth mixture modelling results based on a 33-year follow up study. *Eval Rev* 2007;31:548–563.

Huang AR, Mallet L, Rochefort CM, et al. Medication-related falls in the elderly: Causative factors and preventive strategies. *Drugs Aging* 2012;29:359–376.

Huang AR, Mallet L. Prescribing opioids in older people. *Maturitas* 2013;74:123–129.

Hurley RW, Adams MC Sex, gender and pain: An overview of a complex field. *Anesth Analg* 2008;107:309–317.

Inciardi JA, Surratt HL, Cicero TJ, Beard RA. Prescription opioid abuse and diversion in an urban community: The results of an ultra-rapid assessment. *Pain Med* 2009a;10:537–548.

Inciardi JA, Surratt HL, Cicero TJ, et al. The "black-box" of prescription drug diversion. *J Addict Disord* 2009b;28:332–347.

Ives TJ, Chelminski PR, Hammett-Stabler CA, et al. Predictors of opioid misuse in patients with chronic pain: A prospective cohort study. *BMC Health Serv Res* 2006;6:46–56.

Jena AB, Goldman D, Weaver L, & Karaca-Mandic, P. Opioid prescribing by multiple providers in Medicare: Retrospective observational study of insurance claims. *BMJ* 2014;348:g1393. Published online Feb. 19, 2014. doi:10.1136/bmj.g1393

Jensen-Dahm C, Gasse C, Astrup A, et al. Frequent use of opioids in patients with dementia and nursing home residents—a study of the entire elderly population in Denmark. *Alzheimer Dementia* 2014;11:691–699.

Johnson EM, Lanier WA, Merrill RM, et al. Unintentional prescription opioid-related overdose deaths: Description of decedents by next of kin or best contacts, Utah, 2008–2009. *J Gen Intern Med* 2013;28:522–529.

Johnson RA, Gerstein DR. Initiation of use of alcohol, cigarettes, marijuana, cocaine, and other substances in US birth cohorts since 1919. *Am J Public Health* 1998;88:27–33.

Jones, JD, Mogali S, Comer SD. Polydrug abuse: A review of opioid and benzodiazepine combination use. *Drug Alcohol Depend* 2012;125:8–18.

Juurlink DN, Herrmann N, Szailai JP, Kopp A, Redelmeier DA. Medical illness and the risk of suicide in the elderly. *Arch Intern Med* 2004;164:1179–1184.

Kalapatapu RK, Sullivan MA. Prescription use disorders in older adults, *Am J Addict* 2010;19:515–522.

Kashner TM, Rodell DE, Ogden SR, et al. Outcomes and costs of two VA inpatient treatment programs for older alcoholic patients. *Hosp Commun Psychiatry* 1992;43:985–989.

Katz N, Mazer NA. The impact of opioids on the endocrine system. *Clin J Pain* 2009;25: 170–175.

Khodniva Y, Muntner P, Kertesz S, Safford MM. Prescription opioid use and risk of cardiovascular disease among older adults from a community sample. *Drug Alcohol Depend* 2014;140:e103.

Kolodny A Courtwright DT, Hwang CS, et al. The prescription opioid and heroin crisis: A public health approach to an epidemic of addiction. *Ann Rev Public Health* 2014;36:1–25.

Krueger AB, Stone AA. Assessment of pain: A community-based diary survey in the USA. *Lancet* 2008;371:1519–1525.

Landi F, Onder G, Cesari M, et al. Pain management in frail, community-living elderly patients. *Arch Intern Med* 2001;161:2721–2724.

Larney S, Bohnert ASB, Ganoczy D, et al. Mortality among older adults with opioid use disorders in the Veteran's Health Administration, 2015;2000–2011. *Drug Alcohol Depend* 147:32–37.

Lee M, Silverman SM, Hansen H, et al. A comprehensive review of opioid-induced hyperalgesia. *Pain Physician* 2011;14:145–161.

Levi-Minzi MA, Surratt HL, Kurtz SP, Buttram ME. Under treatment of pain: A prescription for opioid misuse among the elderly? *Pain Med* 2015;14:1719–1729.

Lin JJ, Alfandre D, Moore, C. Physician attitudes towards opioid prescribing for patients with persistent non-cancer pain. *Clin J Pain* 2007;23:799–803.

Lindsay PG, Wycoff M. The depression-pain syndrome and its response to antidepressants *Psychosomatics* 1981;22:571–573.

Lofwall MR, Schuster A, Strain EC. Changing profile of abused substances by older persons entering treatment. *J Nerv Ment Disord* 2006;196:898–905.

Makris UE, Abrams RC, Gurland B, Reid MC. Management of persistent pain in the older patient: A clinical review. *JAMA* 2014;312:825–836.

Malec M, Shega JW. Pain management in the elderly. *Med Clin North Am* 2015;99, 337–350.

Manchikanti L. National Drug Control Policy and Prescription Drug Abuse: Facts and fallacies. *Pain Physician* 2007;10:399–424.

Manfredi P, Breuer B, Wallenstein S, et al. Opioid treatment for agitation in patients with advanced dementia. *Int J Geriatr Psych* 2003;18:700–705.

Markotic F, Cerni Obrdalj E, Zalihic A, et al. Adherence to pharmacological treatment of chronic nonmalignant pain in individuals aged 65 and older. *Pain Med* 2013;14: 247–256.

Martucci C, Panerai AE, Sacerdote P. Chronic fentanyl or buprenorphine infusion in the mouse: Similar analgesic profile but different effects on immune responses *Pain* 2004;110:385–392.

Max EK, Hernandez JJ, Sturpe DA, Zuckerman IH. Prophylaxis for opioid-induced constipation in elderly long-term care residents: A cross-sectional study of Medicare beneficiaries. *Am J Geriatr Pharmacother* 2007;5:129–136.

McLachlan AJ, Bath S, Naganathan V, et al. Clinical pharmacology of analgesic medicines in older people: Impact of frailty and cognitive impairment. *Brit J Clin Pharmacol* 2011;71:351–364.

McNicol E, Horowicz-Mehler N, Fisk RA, et al. Management of opioid-related side effects in cancer-related and chronic noncancer pain: A systematic review. *J Pain* 2003;4:231–256.

Mercandante S, Arcuri E. Pharmacological management of cancer pain in the elderly. *Drugs Aging* 2007a;24:761–776.

Mercandante S, Arcuri E. Opioids and renal function. *J Pain* 2007b;5:2–19.

Miller M, Sturmer T, Azrael D, et al. Opioid analgesics and the risk of fractures in older adults with arthritis. *JAGS* 2011;59:430–438.

Molton IR, Terrill AL. Overview of persistent pain in older adults. *Am Psychologist* 2014;67: 197–207.

Monroe TB, Misra SK, Habermann RC, et al. Pain reports and pain medication treatment in nursing home residents with and without dementia. *Geriatr Gerontol Int* 2014;14:541–548.

Morrison R, Magaziner, J, Gilbert M, et al. Relationship between pain and opioid analgesics on the development of delirium following hip fracture. *J Gerontol* 2003;58:76–81.

National Institute of Drug Abuse (NIDA) (2014). Research Report Series: Prescription Drug Abuse; NIH Pub. No. 15-4881, Dept. of Health and Human Services, accessed at: http://www.drugabuse.gov/publications/prescription-drugs-abuse-addiction/preventing-recognizing-prescription-drug-abuse.

National Opioid Use and Guideline Group. 2010. Canadian guideline for safe and effective use of opioids for chronic non-cancer pain, version 4.5; http://nationlapaincentre.mcmaster.ca/opioid/.

Nave RL. Baby boomers and the hepatitis C boom. *Ann Emerg Med* 2013;62:19A–21A.

Nguyen K, Fink A, Beck JC, Higa J. Feasibility of using an alcohol-screening and health education system with older primary care patients. *J Am Board Fam Pract* 2001;14:7–15.

Nobili A, Garattini S, Mannucci PM. Multiple diseases and polypharmacy in the elderly: Challenges for the internist of the third millennium. *J Comorbidity* 2011;1:28–44.

O'Neil CK, Hanlon JT, Markum ZA. Adverse effects of analgesics commonly used by older adults with osteoarthritis. *Am J Geriatr Pharmacother* 2012;10:331–342.

Office of National Drug Control Policy (ONDCP). 2012. Healthcare Brief: Medication-Assisted Treatment for Opioid Addiction, Executive Office of the President. Accessed at https://www.whitehouse.gov/sites/default/files/ondcp/recovery/medication_assisted_treatment_9-21-20121.pdf.

Offsay JJ. Treatment of alcohol-related problems in the elderly. *Ann Long Term Care* 2007;15:39–44.

Olfson M, King M, Schoenbaum M. Benzodiazepine use in the United States. *JAMA Psychiatry* 2015;72:136–142.

Olfson M, Wang S, Iza M, Crystal S, Blanco C. National trends in the office-based prescription of Schedule II opioids. *J Clin Psychiatry* 2013;74:932–939.

Ortman JM, Velkoff VA, Hogan H. (May 2014). U.S. Census Bureau: An aging nation: The older population in the United States. Current population reports. Available at http://www.census.gov/prod/2014pubs/p25-1140.pdf. Accessed on May 10, 2016.

Oslin DW. Treatment of late-life depression complicated by alcohol dependence. *Am J Geriatr Psych* 2005;13:491–500.

Oslin D, Liberto JG, O'Brien J, Krois S. Tolerability of naltrexone in treating older, alcohol-dependent patients. *Am J Addict* 1997;6:266–270.

Owens PL, Barrett ML, Weiss AJ, Washington RE, Kronick R. 2014. Hospital inpatient utilization related to opioid overuse among adults. Healthcare Cost and Utilization Project (HCUP) Statistical Briefs [Internet]. Rockville (MD): Agency for Health Care Policy and Research (US); 2006–2014 Aug. Available at: http://www.ncbi.nlm.nih.gov/books/NBK246983/. Accessed on April 21, 2016.

Papaleontiou M, Henderson CRJr, Turner BJ, et al. Outcomes associated with opioid use in the treatment of chronic noncancer pain in older adults: A systematic review and meta-analysis. *J Am Geriatr Soc* 2010;58:1353–1369.

Parikh SS, Chung F. Postoperative delirium in the elderly. *Anesth Analg* 1995;80:1223–1232.

Park J, Lavin R. Risk factors associated with opioid medication misuse in community-dwelling older adults with chronic pain. *Clin J Pain* 2010;26:647–655.

Park J, Clement R, Lavin R. Factor structure of pain medication questionnaire in community-dwelling older adults with chronic pain. *Pain Pract* 2010;11:314–324.

Patterson TL, Jeste DV. The potential impact of the baby-boom generation on substance abuse among elderly persons. *Psychiatr Serv* 1999;50:1184–1188.

Paulozzi LJ, Budnitz DS, Xi Y. Increasing deaths from opioid analgesics in the United States. *Pharmacoepidemiol Drug Saf* 2006;15:613–617.

Pergolizzi J, Boger RH, Bidd K, et al. Consensus statement: Opioids and the management of chronic severe pain in the elderly: Consensus statement of an international expert panel with focus on the six clinically most often used World Health Organization step III opioids (buprenorphine, fentanyl, hydromorphone, methadone, morphine, oxycodone). *Pain Pract* 2008;8:287–313.

Pesonen A, Suojaranta-Ylinen R, Hammaren E, et al. Comparison of effects and plasma concentrations of opioids between elderly and middle-aged patients after cardiac surgery. *Acta Anesthesiol Scand* 2009;53:101–108.

Pierce M, Bird SM, Hickman M, Millar T. National record linkage study of mortality for a large cohort of opioid users ascertained by drug treatment or criminal justice sources in England, 2015;2005–2009. *Drug Alcohol Depend* 146:17–23.

Rastogi R, Meek BD. Management of chronic pain in elderly, frail patients: Finding a suitable, personalized method of control. *Clin Intervent Aging* 2013;8:37–46.

Reid MC, Engles-Horton LL, Weber MB, et al. Use of opioid medications for chronic non-cancer pain syndromes in primary care. *J Gen Intern Med* 2002;17:173–179.

Reid MC, Henderson CRJr, Papaleontiou M, et al. Characteristics of older adults receiving opioids in primary care: Treatment duration and outcomes. *Pain Med* 2010;11:1063–1071.

Reynolds KS, Hanson LC, DeVellis RF, et al. (2008). Disparities in pain management between cognitively intact and cognitively impaired nursing home residents. *J Pain Sympt Manag* 35:388–396.

Rinder CS, Mathew JP, Rinder HM, et al. Lymphocyte and monocyte subset changes during cardiopulmonary bypass: Effects of aging and gender. *J Lab Clin Med* 1997;129:592–602.

Rockett IR, Regier MD, Kpausta MD, et al. Leading causes of unintentional and intentional injury mortality: United States 2000–2009. *Am J Public Health* 2012;102:e84–e92.

Rolita L, Spegman A, Tang X, Crostein BN. Greater number of narcotic analgesic prescriptions for osteoarthritis is associated with falls and fractures in elderly adults. *J Am Geriatr Soc* 2013;61:335–340.

Rosen D, Hunsaker A, Albert SM, Cornelius JR, Reynolds CF. Characteristics and consequences of heroin use among older adults in the United States: A review of the literature, treatment implications, and recommendations for further research. *Addict Behav* 2011;36:279–285.

Rosenthal NR, Silverfield JC, Wu SC, et al. Tramadol/acetaminophen combination tablets for the treatment of pain associated with osteoarthritis flare in an elderly patient population. *J Am Geriatr Soc* 2004;52:374–380.

Roth SH. Efficacy and safety of tramadol HCl in breakthrough musculoskeletal pain attributed to osteoarthritis. *J Rheumatol* 1998;25:1358–1363.

Roth SH, Fleischmann RM, Burch FX, et al. Around-the-clock, controlled-release oxycodone therapy for osteoarthritis-related pain: Placebo-controlled trial and long-term evaluation. *Arch Intern Med* 2000;160:853–860.

Sacerdote P, Manfredi B, Mantegazza P, Panerai AE. Antinociceptive and immunosuppressive effects of opiate drugs: A structure-related activity study. *Br J Pharmacol* 1997;121:834–840.

Sale JE, Gignac M, Hawker G. How "bad" does the pain have to be? A qualitative study examining adherence to pain medication in older adults with osteoarthritis. *Arthritis Rheum* 2006;55:272–278.

Santiago TV, Edelman NH. Opioids and breathing. *J Applied Physiol* 1985;59:1675–1685.

Saunders KW, Dunn KM, Merrill JO, et al. Relationship of opioid use and dosage levels to fractures in older chronic pain patients. *J Gen Intern Med* 2010;25:310–315.

Sawyer P, Bodner EV, Ritchie CS, et al. Pain and pain medication use in community-dwelling older adults. *Am J Geriatr Pharmacother* 2006;4:316–324.

Scherrer JF, Salas J, Lustman PJ, Burge S, Schneider FD. Change in opioid dose and change in depression in a longitudinal primary care patient cohort. *Pain* 2015;156: 348–355.

Schonfeld L, Dupree L. Treatment alternatives for older alcohol abusers. In *Older Adults' Misuse of Alcohol, Medicines, and Other Drugs*. New York: Springer Publishing; 1997:113–131.

Schonfeld L, Dupree L. Relapse prevention approaches with the older problem drinker. *Southwest J Aging* 1998;14:43–50.

Simoni-Wastila L, Yang HK. Psychoactive drug abuse in older adults. *Am J Geriatr Pharmacother* 2006;4:22–31.

Simoni-Wastila L, Zuckerman IH, Singhal PK, et al. National estimates of exposure to prescription drugs with addiction potential in the community-dwelling elders. *Subst Abuse* 2005;26:33–42.

Sjogren P, Ekholm O, Peuckmann V, Gronbaek M. Epidemiology of chronic pain in Denmark: An update. *Eur J Pain* 2009;13:287–292.

Smith HS. Opioid metabolism. *Mayo Clin Proc* 2009;84:613–624.

Solomon DH, Avorn J, Wang PH, et al. Prescription opioid use among older adults with arthritis or low back pain. *Arch Rheum* 2006;55:35–41.

Solomon DH, Rassen JA, Glynn RJ, et al. The comparative safety of analgesics in older adults with arthritis. *Arch Intern Med* 2010a;170:1968–1978.

Solomon DH, Rassen JA, Glynn RJ, et al. The comparative safety of opioids for nonmalignant pain in older adults. *Arch Intern Med* 2010b;170:1979–1986.

Spitz A, Moore AA, Papaleontiou M, et al. Primary care providers' perspective on prescribing opioids to older adults with chronic non-cancer pain: A qualitative study. *BMC Geriatr* 2011;11:35–44.

Stevens JA. Fatalities and injuries from falls among older adults—United States, 1993–2003 and 2001–2005. *MMWR* 2006;55:1222–1224.

Stewart C, Schofield P, Gooberman-Hill R, et al. Geriatric pain management. In H Benzon, JP Rathmell, CL Wu, DC Turk, CE Argoff, RW Hurley, Eds., *Raj's Practical Management of Pain*, 5th ed. Philadelphia, PA: Elsevier Mosby; 2013:467–473.

Stone CA, Lawlor PG, Savva GM, et al. Prospective study of falls and risk factors for falls in adults with advanced cancer. *J Clin Oncol* 2012;30:2128–2133.

Substance Abuse and Mental Health Services Administration (SAMSHA). 2014a. Center for Behavioral Health Statistics and Quality. Treatment Episode Data Set (TEDS): 2002–2012. State Admissions to Substance Abuse Treatment Services. BHSIS Series S-72, HHS Publication No. (SMA) 14-4889. Rockville, MD: SAMHSA.

Substance Abuse and Mental Health Services Administration (SAMSHA). 2014b. Center for Behavioral Health Statistics and Quality. (December 18, 2014). The DAWN Report: Benzodiazepines in Combination with Opioid Pain Relievers or Alcohol: Greater Risk of More Serious ED Visit Outcomes. Rockville, MD.

Substance Abuse and Mental Health Services Administration (SAMSHA). 2009. Emergency Department Visits Involving Nonmedical Use of Selected Pharmaceuticals. Rockville, MD: SAMHSA.

Substance Abuse and Mental Health Services Administration (SAMSHA). 2007. The DASIS Report: Adults Aged 65 or Older in Substance Abuse Treatment. Rockville, MD: SAMHSA.

Tegeder I, Lotsch J, Geisslinger G. Pharmacokinetics of opioids in liver disease. *Clin Pharm* 1999; 37:17–40.

The Substance Abuse and Mental Health Data Archive (SAMHDA). 2015. Center for Behavioral Health Statistics and Quality (CBHSQ), Substance Abuse and Mental Health Services Administration (SAMHSA), U.S. Department of Health and Human Services (HHS). Available at http://www.icpsr.umich.edu/icpsrweb/content/SAMHDA/index.html. Accessed on April 18, 2016.

Tracy B, Sean Morrison R. Pain management in older adults. *Clin Ther* 2013;35:1659–1668.

Tsang A, Von Korff M, Lee S, et al. Common persistent pain conditions in developed and developing countries: Gender and age differences and co-morbidity with depression-anxiety disorders. *J Pain* 2008;9:883–891.

U.S. Census Bureau. 2000. National Population Projections: Summary Tables, 2006–2010; available at http://www.census.gov/population/projections/data/national/natsum.html.

U.S. Census Bureau. 2012. American Community Survey 5 Year Estimates: 2009–2013; available at http://.wwwcensus.gov/popest/national/

U.S. Census Bureau. 2014. National Population Projections: Summary Table 3; available at http://www.census.gov/population/projections/data/national/natsum.html

U.S. Department of Health and Human Services, SAMHSA. 2013. National Survey on Drug Use and Health: Summary of National Findings.

United Nations Department of Economic and Social Affairs. 2009. World Population Ageing 2009. New York: United Nations; 2009. Accessed from http://www.un.org/esa/population/publications/WPA2009/WPA2009_WorkingPaper.pdf. on April 18, 2016.

Upshur CC, Luckmann RS, Savageau JA. Primary care provider concerns about management of chronic pain in community clinic populations. *J Gen Intern Med* 2006;21:652–655.

Verbeeck RK. Pharmacokinetics and dose adjustments in patietns with hepatic dysfunction. *Eur J Clin Pharmacol* 2008;64:1147–1161.

Vestergaard P, Rejnmark L, Mosekilde L. Fracture risk associated with the use of morphine and opiates. *J Intern Med* 2006;260:76–87.

Vorsanger G, Xiang J, Jordan D, et al. Post hoc analysis of a randomized, double-blind, placebo-controlled efficacy and tolerability study of tramadol extended release for the treatment of osteoarthritis pain in geriatric patients. *Clin Ther* 2007;29:2520–2535.

Wachholtz A, Gonzalez G. Pain sensitivity and tolerance among individuals on opioid maintenance: Long term effects. *Drug Alcohol Depend* 2015;146, e14.

Wang Y-P, & Andrade H. Epidemiology of alcohol and drug use in the elderly. *Curr Opin Psychiatry* 2013;26:343–349.

Webster LR, Webster RM. Predicting aberrant behaviors in opioid-treated patients: Preliminary validation of the Opioid Risk Tool. *Pain Med* 2013;6:432–442.

Weiner DK. Office management of chronic pain in the elderly. *Am J Med* 2007;120:306–315.

West NA, Severtson SG, Green JL, Dart RC. Trends in abuse and misuse of prescription opioids among older adults. *Drug Alcohol Depend* 2015;149:117–121.

Wilder-Smith, Oliver HG. Opioid use in the elderly. *Eur J Pain* 2005;9:137–40.

Wildes TM, Dua P, Fowler SA, et al. Systematic review of falls in older adults with cancer. *J Geriatr Oncol* 2015;6(1):70–83.

Won AB, Lapane KL, Vallow S, et al. Persistent nonmalignant pain and analgesic prescribing patterns in elderly nursing home residents. *J Am Geriatr Soc* 2004;52:867–874.

Wu L-T, Blazer D. Illicit and nonmedical drug use among older adults: A review. *J Aging Health* 2011;23:481–504.

Yong HH. Can attitudes of stoicism and cautiousness explain observed age-related variation in levels of self-rated pain, mood disturbance and functional interference in chronic pain patients? *Eur J Pain* 2006;10:399–407.

# CHAPTER 6

# Cannabis, Nicotine, and Stimulant Abuse in Older Adults

*Christina A. Brezing and Frances R. Levin*

## Introduction

This chapter presents the current literature on cannabis, nicotine, and stimulant use in older adults. Notably, there is a dearth of evidence-based research on these substances in an older adult population. This paucity is the result of many factors, including exclusion of older adults based on age and co-occurring medical disorders from clinical research studies on substance-use disorders, as well as misconceptions about substance use in this population. As a result, there is a limited understanding of individuals who develop a substance-use disorder later in life or who persistently use substances throughout their lives; this knowledge gap points to under-explored areas of research, such as the epidemiology, identification, and age-appropriate treatment interventions for older populations. As the general population continues to age, understanding how to address the unique concerns of older adults with cannabis, nicotine, and stimulant-use disorders will become an increasingly important matter.

## Epidemiology

### GENERAL CONSIDERATIONS

Compared to rates of substance use in youth, younger, and middle-aged adults, rates in older adults are lower, but still substantial. Because of the misconceptions that older adults abstain from substance use and that younger adults with substance-use disorders "recover" by the time they are older adults, this has historically been an under-investigated area of identification and characterization. As a result, our epidemiological data on cannabis, tobacco, and cocaine use are limited to mainly large national surveys, with few studies available that more thoroughly characterize subpopulations in terms of social factors, pertinent clinical history, coping styles, co-occurring medical and psychiatric disorders, and more specific demographic information. In conjunction with evidence that older adults under-report substance use as obtained by current methods (Rockett et al. 2006), there is a significant opportunity to improve this deficit in knowledge.

## EPIDEMIOLOGY OF CANNABIS IN OLDER ADULTS

Cannabis is the most widely used illicit drug of abuse in the United States (NSDUH 2013). Recently, much of the popular media and clinical research focus has been directed towards adolescent cannabis use, due to noted rising rates of use, decreasing perceptions of harm, and the known negative health consequences for young brains as a result of earlier use. However, despite receiving less attention, cannabis is also the most commonly used illicit drug in older adults, and there is evidence that the number of older adults using cannabis is increasing (Dinitto et al. 2011). The 2008 National Surveys on Drug Use and Health (NSDUH) showed that 2.8% of older adults (age 50–65+) were past-year marijuana users (Dinitto et al. 2011). This is 2.5 times the percentage of past-year older adult marijuana users from the 1999–2001 national survey results (1.1% past-year older adult marijuana users) (Colliver et al. 2006) and reflects a faster rate of growth than what was previously projected in this population Colliver et al. (2006. projected that 2.9% of older adults would be marijuana users by 2020, taking into account only patterns of use in aging baby boomers, born from 1946 to 1964. This generation is historically more likely than previous generations to have been exposed to marijuana in their youth, and consequentially a greater percentage of them will be lifetime users. Given that the percentage of older adult marijuana users reached projected rates 12 years sooner than expected, there are probably other factors not considered in these initial calculations that are contributing to increasing marijuana use by older adults. Data from the 2012 NSDUH showed that 4.6 million adults aged 50 years or older reported past-year marijuana use, while less than one million reported use of cocaine, inhalants, hallucinogens, methamphetamine, or heroin combined (NSDUH 2013, Blazer et al. 2009). Notably, these rates collected from the national surveys on cannabis use in older adults precede or coincide with the large-scale political and social movements that have led to medicalization of marijuana in nearly half of all states in the United States, and its legalization following closely behind in Washington, Colorado, and more recently in Oregon, Alaska, and Washington, D.C.

While much debate still exists regarding the medical benefits of marijuana, the acceptance of its therapeutic potential as reflected by state law and the booming economic business driven by consumer demand make it likely that the use of this drug will continue to increase across the entire population. Older adults may be particularly susceptible to increasing rates of use, as they may be attracted to marijuana to ease pain or other symptoms of medical conditions that worsen with age. Medical marijuana state laws generally allow its recommendation in the treatment of neurological conditions like multiple sclerosis and Parkinson's disease, in addition to other conditions such as chronic pain, nausea and fatigue associated with chemotherapy, glaucoma, and cardiovascular conditions. Older adults are the primary population suffering from these conditions and may be drawn to marijuana as a potential treatment for medical disorders and symptoms. The message of marijuana as "medicine" is likely to be having an impact on the largest consumers of medications—the aging and older adult population. Additionally, as social views about marijuana change to reflect its greater acceptance, recreational use by older adults may also increase. Similar to the pattern with adolescents, as the perception of harm by this population wanes, the use of marijuana is likely to increase. Older adults also have more free time for recreational activities as they decrease the time they spend working, or retire, leaving less structured time and increased opportunity for substance use. For these reasons, it is likely that there will continue to be increasing rates of older adults using marijuana as the longer-term consequences of these policy changes come into effect (see Box 6.1).

---

*Box 6.1* **Summary of Epidemiological Trends and Characteristics of Older Adult Cannabis Users**

- Cannabis is the most widely used illicit drug by older adults.
- Aging baby boomers are more likely than previous generations to use cannabis.
- Older adults may be more susceptible to using medical marijuana for conditions where a recommendation exists.
- Older adults, particularly those who are retired, may have more free time to engage in recreational cannabis use.
- Older cannabis users are likely to be chronic, lifetime users with co-occurring psychiatric and other substance-use disorders.

Interestingly, of the 2.8% of older adults recently using marijuana in the 2008 NSDUH data, 23% of these individuals used on at least half of the days of the year, suggesting regular use that is a routine part of their lifestyle (Dinitto et al. 2013). Those who are recent cannabis users are also more likely than non-recent users to have first used marijuana at less than 18 years of age or from 19–29 years of age, further suggesting that older adults smoking marijuana are chronic, long-term users. Compared to "non-recent" and "never" marijuana users, they are more likely to be "younger" older adults (50–64 years old), not those over 65 years old. Recent older-adult users are also more likely to be men, black, unmarried, have less than a high school education, endorse higher psychological distress scores, have major depression, smoke cigarettes, binge drink, endorse current or past use of other illicit drugs (including cocaine, heroin, or hallucinogens), and have undergone past substance-abuse treatment (Dinitto et al. 2013, Blazer et al. 2009). Taking all of this into account, older adult marijuana users may represent a clinically more severe and impaired population whose use does not remit as a result of changes across the lifecycle, suggesting they are in some ways refractory to factors that promote change in marijuana use. This may be a particularly vulnerable population whose pattern of use may be more consistent with a cannabis use disorder, suggesting that they would probably benefit from more targeted and intensive treatment. (See Box 6.1 for a summary of epidemiological trends and characteristics of older adult cannabis users.)

## EPIDEMIOLOGY OF NICOTINE IN OLDER ADULTS

Smoking rates tend to be lower in adults aged 65+ years than in the general population. Unfortunately, this is thought to be due to premature deaths from smoking-related causes. Tobacco, while used with lower frequency than by adults of younger age, is still a substance commonly used by older adults. Approximately 14% of adults aged 65 years and older report using tobacco in the last 12 months (Moore et al. 2009), and more than 6% used both tobacco and alcohol together in the last 12 months, a combination that puts these adults at risk for severe health consequences, including head and neck and gastrointestinal malignancies. Tobacco and alcohol are known to be common co-occurring substances in older adults. Smoking tobacco increases the likelihood of being an at-risk drinker in this population (Moore et al. 2009). Like older adult cannabis users, older adults who use tobacco are observed in smoking cessation clinical trials to be long-term, heavy smokers who are physiologically dependent on nicotine products (Hall et al. 2009). This subpopulation of tobacco smokers is most at risk of developing serious medical consequences from chronic inhalation of tobacco products.

## EPIDEMIOLOGY OF STIMULANTS IN OLDER ADULTS

There is limited epidemiological evidence, in comparison to alcohol, marijuana, and tobacco, of stimulant use in older adults. For the purpose of this chapter, the focus will be on cocaine and prescription stimulants, such as methylphenidate and dextroamphetamine, as limited evidence is available for use of other stimulants, such as crystal methamphetamine, in this population. Cocaine is the second most common (cannabis being the first) illicit drug of abuse used by older adults. Data pooled from the 2005–2006 NSDUH reveal that adults aged 50–64 years were more likely than those aged 65+ years to have used cocaine in the past year (0.7% vs. 0.04%), and that the combined rates of past-year use of inhalants, hallucinogens, methamphetamine, and heroin were very low in comparison (<0.2%) (Blazer et al. 2009). In this same pooled sample, younger age (50–64 years), male gender, being Native American or black, unemployed, being separated/divorced/widowed, never-married, and having past-year major depression increased the odds of cocaine use (Blazer et al. 2009). Of these past-year cocaine users, 43.9% met criteria for a cocaine-use disorder (Blazer et al. 2009). Notably, data from this large survey sample only account for non-institutionalized adults, and rates of cocaine use might be higher if institutionalized adults were also included. In this same pooled sample, 0.16% of older adults had past-year non-medical use of prescribed stimulants (Blazer et al. 2009).

Looking outside the large national surveys, a study to assess the mental health and substance abuse needs of older prison inmates found that older inmates aged 55+ years were more likely to use cocaine as their primary illicit drug use than were younger inmates, who were more likely to report marijuana or methamphetamine as their primary illicit drugs of use. More than a third of these older inmates with substance-use problems had never received treatment (Arndt et al. 2002).

Despite prevailing misconceptions about the "rarity" or "unusualness" of substance-use disorders in older adults, epidemiological evidence suggests that millions of older adults use marijuana and cocaine, in addition to tobacco. Future research should attempt to better characterize this large population, in addition to looking at older adults with cannabis, cocaine, and tobacco use in smaller subpopulation studies.

# Impact on Health of Cannabis, Nicotine, and Stimulants in the Older Adult

## GENERAL CONSIDERATIONS

As individuals age, there are significant changes that result in reductions in lean body mass, decreases in total body water, decreased ability of the liver and kidneys to process and excrete substances, increased permeability of the blood–brain barrier (BBB), and fluctuations in neuronal receptor sensitivity, which increase older adults' vulnerability to drug effects and drug interactions. This becomes especially important when considering the effects of substances of abuse like cannabis, nicotine, and stimulants, particularly in terms of acute intoxication effects, withdrawal, tolerance, and metabolism in the context of either prescribed medications or abuse of other substances. In an older adult, even small amounts or less frequent use of marijuana or stimulants may have more significant negative consequences for health. It is also critical to consider potential drug–drug interactions, both illicit and prescribed, in older adults who are frequently on multiple medications. For example, nicotine consumed as a result of regular tobacco use affects the metabolism of a number of medications, which leads to changes in drug levels. Additionally, marijuana is known to increase the sedative effects of drugs such as barbiturates, benzodiazepines, and opiates (Kuerbis et al. 2014). In combination with alcohol, sedation can be even more substantial.

## IMPACT OF CANNABIS ON HEALTH

The data concerning the impact of cannabis on health are limited and need further exploration before definitive conclusions can be drawn. As it stands, there is mixed evidence regarding the health effects of marijuana in older adults. Past-year older adult marijuana users who responded to the NSDUH in 2008 rated their health as "good" to "very good," with no significant difference between non-recent users and never-users (Dinitto et al. 2011, Joy et al. 1999). However, they also endorsed higher levels of self-reported psychological distress, depression, and use of other substances. So while subjectively they reported no difference in health, other factors associated with poorer mental and physical health were greater in recent marijuana users. Notably, though, they did not associate their psychological distress with their marijuana use, reporting no problems from marijuana, including emotional problems, and few endorsed any desire to cut back or abstain from marijuana. One possible explanation for this finding is that marijuana use in older adults is a marker for other problems, but is not a problem in and of itself. In this case, older adults may be using marijuana to cope with psychological distress or as self-medication, and they perceive the drug as having calming and beneficial effects.

In 1999, the Institute of Medicine (IOM) report on marijuana for medical purposes concluded that cannabinoids, mainly THC (tetrahydrocannabinol), had potential therapeutic value in the treatment of pain, nausea, vomiting, and appetite stimulation. This same report also noted that smoked marijuana was a "crude THC delivery system that also delivers harmful substances (p. 4)." (Joy et al. 1999) Studies since the IOM report have found additional evidence for the potential of cannabinoids in the treatment of multiple sclerosis spasticity, HIV- and non-HIV-related neuropathic pain, amyotrophic lateral sclerosis, Parkinson's disease, Huntington's disease, epilepsy, cancer, and inflammatory bowel disease. However, the use of cannabinoids for additional medical indications is an area that does not have definitive evidence, and more rigorous research is needed.

In addition to the health effects and potential of marijuana found in the 1999 IOM report, some preclinical data have suggested that cannabidiol, one of many cannabinoids in marijuana, is neuroprotective in its ability to reduce neuroinflammation and mitigate neurodegeneration. As a result, there has been interest and theories that cannabinoids may serve a role in the prevention or treatment of dementia due to Alzheimer's disease or other causes, although this is a nascent area of study (Krishnan et al. 2009).

There are recognized negative health effects of cannabis as well. Acute intoxication with cannabis is known to cause impairment in short-term memory, poor judgement, increased heart rate, increased respiratory rate, elevated blood pressure, anxiety, panic attacks, paranoid thoughts, hallucinations, and more overt cannabis psychosis. Older adults, who have less physical reserve in terms of both cognitive and cardiorespiratory systems, may be at greater risk for health compromise. Additionally, due to the predominant route of administration by smoking plant-form marijuana, respiratory compromise including chronic bronchitis has been demonstrated in heavy, chronic cannabis smokers (Kalant 2004). It is common for cannabis smokers to utilize components of tobacco products in their joints, "blunts," and bowls, which over time has the same negative health consequences as smoking tobacco products alone. Cannabis also has a withdrawal syndrome that is characterized by other unpleasant symptoms, including anger, aggression, anxiety, depressed mood, irritability, restlessness, sleep disturbances, strange dreams, decreased appetite, and weight loss upon abrupt discontinuation of cannabis in chronic users (Haney 2005).

## IMPACT OF NICOTINE ON HEALTH

Approximately 50% of smokers die of tobacco-caused disease, and in comparison to non-smokers, individuals who smoke even as few as 1–4 cigarettes per day have a significantly higher premature mortality risk (Bjartveit et al. 2009), with cardiovascular (hypertension, cardiovascular accidents, peripheral vascular disease, strokes, myocardial infarctions), pulmonary (chronic obstructive pulmonary disease, bronchitis, emphysema), and oncological diseases (lung, head and neck, bladder, and gastrointestinal malignancies) being the leading causes of death. Smoking tobacco is also associated with decreased exercise capacity, cataracts, premature aging of skin, gum disease, tooth decay and loss, postoperative infections, development of osteoporosis, risk of hip fractures, loss of mobility, and overall poor physical functioning and decreased quality of life (LaCroix et al. 1992). Smoking tobacco also impairs or inhibits effective treatments for these conditions (Kuerbis et al. 2014).

Given that many older adults are on at least one medication and many have polypharmacy regimens to manage chronic disorders associated with aging, it is very important to consider any pharmacokinetic and pharmacodynamic interactions of these medications with nicotine and other components of smoked tobacco products. Polycyclic aromatic hydrocarbons (PAH) in tobacco smoke are not only significant carcinogens, but are also potent inducers of hepatic cytochrome P450 (CYP) enzymes 1A1, 1A2, and 2E1 (Zevin et al. 1999). CYP1A2 notably is responsible for the metabolism of many medications, and in conjunction with tobacco smoking, patients may require higher doses of these medications metabolized by this isoenzyme to maintain effective levels in the body. As a correlate, if older patients quit smoking and maintain their current medication dosing, they may be at risk to toxicity from increasing levels of medication. Nicotine itself also has important drug interactions. The most clinically consequential effects are on theophylline, caffeine, tacrine, imipramine, haloperidol, petazocone, propanolol, flecainide, and estradiol (Zevin et al. 1999). Nicotine also appears to have pharmacodynamic effects as a result of its stimulant properties that lead to a decreased impact of beta blockers on heart rate and blood pressure, decreased sedating effects of benzodiazepines, and decreased analgesic effects of some opioids. Nicotine appears to increase clearance of heparin and decrease absorption through vasoconstriction of subcutaneous insulin (Zevin et al. 1999). Given these many potential PAH–drug or nicotine–drug interactions, healthcare providers should check for these interactions in an older adult tobacco smoker.

## IMPACT OF STIMULANTS ON HEALTH

Stimulants are associated with a number of serious medical problems. Stimulants increase the monoamines dopamine and norepinephrine in both the brain and the body. As a result, they increase blood pressure and heart rate, constrict blood vessels, and increase glucose. In older adults, who are more susceptible to the systemic effects of stimulants in conjunction with baseline co-occurring medical and psychiatric problems, abuse of stimulants can lead to serious negative health consequences. These include unintentional weight loss due to decreased appetite, insomnia, severe hypertension, arrhythmias, myocardial infarctions, stroke, hyperthermia, cardiovascular failure, or seizures. Stimulants can also have negative psychiatric effects, including precipitation of anxiety and panic attacks, irritability, hostility, paranoia, and psychosis. With older adults who use stimulants, it is important to discuss the risks of taking over-the-counter cold medications that contain other "hidden" stimulants, such as pseudoephedrine, which in combination can exacerbate and compound the effects of any of these stimulants alone. Withdrawal from stimulants, as a result of an abrupt discontinuation in use, is marked by fatigue, depression, and sleep disturbances and should be considered on the differential diagnosis when older adults present with these symptoms.

## Screening and Identification of Cannabis, Tobacco, and Stimulant-Use Disorders in Older Adults

### GENERAL CONSIDERATIONS

Given that millions of older adults in the United States are utilizing cannabis, nicotine, and stimulants, these substances have negative health consequences, and the older population that is affected may have greater comorbidity and refractory substance-use disorders, it is critical that physicians and other healthcare providers screen for and identify use of these substances as well as possible cannabis, nicotine, and stimulant use disorders so that appropriate interventions and referrals can be made. Older adults tend to see their primary healthcare providers more regularly than younger adults for other medical concerns, providing a key opportunity for screening for substance use. However, physicians are unlikely to screen for or even consider substance-use disorders in older adults. In one study, hundreds of primary medical doctors were presented with a hypothetical presentation of an older patient displaying symptoms related to problematic substance use. Only 1% of these physicians considered a substance-use disorder on the differential diagnosis (SAMHSA 1998).

Many factors contribute to challenges in appropriately identifying these disorders in an older adult population. To start with, older adults typically have more medical problems. In the current healthcare environment, physicians face time constraints and limited resources that may result in giving greater attention to more "obvious" medical complaints, while screening and consideration of substance-use disorders are overlooked. Additionally, it is important to remember that cannabis- and stimulant-use disorders, in particular, may present differently in older adults than younger adults due to the confounding effects of other medical and mental health problems on an older patient's presentation in a healthcare setting, complicating the clinical picture. An older adult with a substance-use disorder may present with confusion, falls, and/or cognitive changes, all of which have a broad differential diagnosis and consequentially large medical work-up. It is essential to consider drugs of abuse like cannabis and stimulants in these non-specific presentations. Finally, the criteria for characterizing one of these substance-use disorders in older adults are skewed towards under-diagnosis in the older population. These criteria for substance-use disorders are outlined by the *Diagnostic and Statistical Manual of Mental Disorders, 5th Edition* (APA 2013). Impairment in social responsibilities and role obligations, particularly around occupation, household activities, and social engagements, may be less pertinent and harder to identify in an older adult who is retired, no longer responsible for taking care of children, and more socially isolated due to the loss of a spouse and peers to death, or due to personal struggles with their own physical limitations or medical problems. Physiological criteria may also be less applicable to older adults. Age-associated changes in metabolism of and intoxication from substances that increase the psychoactive effects of these drugs can lead to a decrease in tolerance and differences in withdrawal presentations, interfering with identification of these key physiological use-disorder criteria. Cognitive impairment in older adults as a result of substance use or other causes can limit their ability to accurately self-monitor and report other criteria such as loss of control, amount of substance used, and time spent obtaining it. Furthermore, because smaller amounts of substance can have significant effects, less time may be needed to obtain or use the substance. For these reasons, DSM-5 criteria are deemphasized in characterizing substance-use disorders in the elderly, and those within the field performing research consider using a two-tier system that stratifies older adults who use these substances as at-risk or problem users of substances (SAMHSA 1998). At-risk use of prescription drugs like dronabinol or amphetamines is defined as intentional or unintentional off-label use of prescription or over-the-counter medications, or taking medication, even occasionally, that is not prescribed directly. At-risk use of illicit substances is defined as any use of same. Problem use is characterized as substance use that results in social, medical, or psychological consequences regardless of quantity or frequency of use (Kuerbis et al. 2014),and individuals do not need to meet DSM-5 substance-use disorder criteria.

In addition to the methods utilized to identify and screen substance abuse in older adults, further consideration needs to be given to healthcare providers' style of interactions when screening for cannabis, nicotine, and stimulant use. Stigma, on the part of both the provider and the patient, can lead to discomfort in assessing and being assessed for drug use, resulting in an additional barrier for older adult patients to honestly and openly discuss their substance use. Healthcare providers should approach screening and providing intervention for identified substance-use disorders as engaging in a collaborative partner-ship with the older adult patient. Being compassionate, empathetic, nonjudge-mental, and non-confrontational is preferred to assertive or oppositional styles of assessment and intervention. Screening and a thorough assessment with the older adult around their use of cannabis, nicotine, and stimulants, in addition to other substances, should focus on the patients' own goals for health and the obstacles that using these substances pose in achieving these goals, in addition to information about the quantity, frequency, route of administration, and duration of use. In conjunction with screening for current use, assessment of past use of substances is critical in the older adult, as long-term negative health sequelae may present years after last use, particularly in the case of tobacco.

Unfortunately, screening assessments for cannabis, nicotine, and stimulants have not been specifically validated in the older adult population (Culberon et al. 2008). Utilization of screening tools that have been validated in other age groups is helpful, although problems with applicability of screening criteria, as with the DSM-5 criteria, must be considered when such instruments are adapted to this age group. The SBIRT model (Screening, Brief Intervention, and Referral for Treatment) may be particularly effective in older adults. Data from the Florida Brief Intervention and Treatment for Elders (BRITE) proj-ect showed that this intervention increased the number of substance users screened, and identified, and treated, and improved substance-use outcomes in the population (Schonfeld et al. 2010).

Finally, technology may have an important role in streamlining and seizing opportunities to screen older adults for substance use when they visit their pri-mary care physicians. The Drug and Alcohol Problem Assessment for Primary Care (DAPA-PC) is a self-administered, internet-based screening instrument for substance use that identified alcohol and drug abuse in adults aged 55+ years as confirmed with in-person visits (Nemes et al. 2004). Notably, it picked up rates of substance use in older adults that were similar to those in younger adults, with one difference: older adults saw their use as less problematic as compared to younger adults. (See Table 6.1 for a summary of general and substance-specific considerations in screening older adults.)

## SPECIFIC CONSIDERATIONS IN SCREENING FOR CANNABIS USE

It is thought that the measured rates of cannabis use in older adults are underes-timates, due to factors that influence self-report of substance use by older adults using generalized screening tools, i.e., not specific to this population. Previous studies have found that adults aged 65 and older are more likely to under-report substance use that was identified by urine toxicology in the emergency

**Table 6.1  Considerations for Screening, Characterization, and Treatment of Cannabis, Nicotine, and Stimulant Use and Use Disorders in Older Adults**

| Substance | Screening and Identification | Treatment |
|---|---|---|
| Across substances (general considerations) | • Be aware of biases about older adults' substance use.<br>• Protect time in an initial visit to screen for substance use.<br>• Consider substance use on the differential diagnosis of chief complaints.<br>• Don't depend on the DSM criteria—it's skewed to underdiagnose.<br>• Adopt a collaborative, empathic, and nonjudgemental style of interaction.<br>• Identify prior as well as current use. | • Treatment admissions for older adults are increasing.<br>• Be aware of resources specific to the older adult in the community (tailored AA meetings, geriatric substance-abuse units, clinical experts, etc.).<br>• Consider barriers and solutions for older adults in treatment plans.<br>• Comprehensive treatment must take into account co-occurring medical and psychiatric disorders, which includes medication interactions.<br>• Case management may be particularly helpful.<br>• Motivations for treatment may be more aligned with improving health and maintaining independence. |
| Cannabis | • Older adults are more likely to under-report their cannabis use.<br>• Consider prescribed forms of THC (dronabinol and nabilone) and newer formulations of illicit THC (waxes, oils, vaping). | • Make use of evidence-based treatments found to be effective in other adult populations.<br>• SBIRT is effective with older adults. |
| Nicotine | • Utilize the five A's.<br>• Identify former smokers who are at risk for relapse and long-term health consequences. | • Smoking cessation has health benefits for adults of all ages, including older adults.<br>• Evidence-based treatments for smoking cessation are effective in older adults and should include nicotine replacement therapy (NRT), other medications, brief interventions, and psychosocial therapy. |
| Stimulants | • In addition to detailed history-taking, consider use of Modified CAGE screening tool.<br>• Ask about abuse or misuse of prescribed stimulants. | • Cocaine admissions make up a disproportionate percentage of older adult substance abuse treatment admissions.<br>• Utilize evidence-based treatments effective in other adult populations. |

*Source*: Blazer DG, Wu LT. The epidemiology of substance use and disorders among middle aged and elderly community adults: National survey on drug use and health. *Am J Geriatr Psych* 2009;17(3):237–245.

department compared to younger adults (Rockett et al. 2006), and marijuana may be more likely than other illicit drugs not to be self-reported by older adults (Glintborg et al. 2008). Less obvious forms of THC, the psychoactive component of marijuana, should be screened for and considered in older adults as well. In addition to traditional forms of using cannabis through smoking marijuana in joints, blunts, pipes, and water pipes, the rapid expansion of the marijuana industry in the United States as a result of medicalization and legalization has led to forms of extracted THC and other cannabinoids in oils and waxes, smoked through water-vaporizing devices (hookahs), and consumed in edible products or forms. Additionally, abuse of prescription THC, such as dronabinol (plant-derived) or nabilone (synthetic), should also be considered in older adults prescribed these medications if clinical presentation suggests overuse.

## SPECIFIC CONSIDERATIONS IN SCREENING FOR TOBACCO AND NICOTINE USE

It is recommended that all healthcare providers utilize the "five A's" outlined by the US Preventative Health Services Task Force when screening and assessing for tobacco use. First, *ask* all patients if they smoke, and characterize their smoking behaviors (number of cigarettes/day, past quit attempts, etc.). Second, *advise* them to quit if they do. Third, *assess* the patient's motivation to make a change and quit. Fourth, the healthcare provider should *assist* the patient by offering evidence-based medication and counseling in addition to free resources, coaching, and other available applications to aid in their smoking cessation efforts. Fifth and finally, providers should *arrange* for follow-up or refer the person for additional specialized treatment. While the five A's have not been specifically validated in older adults, it is still an effective framework to use when working with this population.

Another important consideration is recognition of former smokers in the older adult population. This group is uniquely at risk for relapse to using tobacco products when entering treatment for other mental health or substance-use disorders. As important as identifying current smokers, former smokers are part of a group that continues to be at risk for the health consequences of past repeated exposure to tobacco products.

## SPECIFIC CONSIDERATIONS IN SCREENING FOR STIMULANTS

As with cannabis and other substance use screening, the Modified CAGE screening tool for both alcohol and drug abuse has been shown to be an effective instrument in identifying stimulant use in older adults. In addition to illicit stimulants, more and more older adults are prescribed prescription stimulants for off-label uses targeting motivational and attentional deficit symptoms, including depression, apathy, fatigue and adult attention-deficit hyperactivity disorder (ADHD). Abuse of prescription stimulants should also be screened for in older adults taking these medications. Of note, being female is associated with greater likelihood of prescription drug abuse in older adults and should be considered, if appropriate, in older adult women patients (Simoni-Wastila et al. 2006).

## Treatment Considerations

Even if we do identify older adults using these substances, a clear gap still exists in appropriate evidence-based interventions and treatments targeted to this population. This is concerning, as treatment-seeking older adults are rising in number. Looking at data from the Treatment Episode Data Set (TEDS), admissions for older adults (aged 50+ years) made up 10% of the 1.8 million treatment admissions for substance abuse reported to the Substance Abuse and Mental Health Services Administration (SAMHSA) (Blazer et al. 2009). A national survey of substance-abuse treatment programs identified only 18% of the sample as taking into account specific needs of the older adults. Access to age-appropriate services may be limited even when it is available, and evidence suggests that mental health utilization by older adults is lower than that of any other age group. Many barriers exist for older adults in accessing specialized substance-abuse treatment care. Regular travel to mutual-help or treatment groups, physician, and therapy appointments may be restricted, given transportation limitations. (Does the individual drive? Can he/she navigate public transportation?) Moreover, groups that have a predominantly younger population in attendance might be intimidating or uncomfortable for an older patient, while it might be difficult to find older-age groups that create a community with similar experiences and perspectives.

Older adults' motivations for changing their substance use are likely to be more aligned with avoiding negative health consequences and prolonging their ability to engage in regular activities and independence, compared to motivating factors in a younger population. All interventions should be aligned with the patient's own values and goals in order to be most effective, keeping in mind the different needs and vulnerabilities of an older person.

Finally, more comprehensive treatment may be appropriate to address the complex medical, psychiatric, and social needs common in the older adult population. Utilization of case management to connect older adults with needed community resources such as low-cost food, visiting nurses, assistance with remembering and keeping appointments, and assistance with medication and treatment adherence can be essential in facilitating better communication with healthcare providers and coordination of resources.

Generally, there are no specific recommendations for medication-assisted and psychotherapeutic treatments for older adults as distinct from adults of younger age in terms of managing cannabis, tobacco, and stimulant-use disorders. However, when treating patients in this age group, it becomes even more important to check for drug–drug interactions, consider the increased vulnerability of older adults to side effects and potential cognitive limitations that may interfere with psychotherapeutic interventions. As with all subpopulations, considering individual needs is critical. Given that many older adults face loneliness and isolation due to loss of peers, spouses, and physical independence, peer support through mutual-help groups should be considered to expand their community. If mutual-help group and peer support is appropriate for the patient, clinicians should attempt to find groups with peers of a similar age so that the focus and discussions of the group can be relevant to their shared experiences. See Table 6.1 for a summary of treatment recommendations for older adults.

## CANNABIS TREATMENT

From 2001 to 2005, SAMSHA reported that the numbers of older adults in substance abuse treatment increased by 25%. Similar to projected rates of older adult marijuana users, projected numbers of older adults in treatment for substance abuse by 2020 are predicted to be threefold the number of older adults in treatment for substance abuse in 2000 (Gfroerer et al. 2003). With increasing rates of marijuana use across all age groups, including older adults, it is estimated that there will be a 60% increase in the need for treatment related to marijuana use in older adults by 2020. Given these rising rates of both older adults using marijuana and the subset of these folks requiring targeted substance-abuse treatment, healthcare providers will need to appropriately screen for and identify at-risk populations to provide appropriate interventions and referrals for more specialized treatment as needed. While most healthcare providers are attuned to screening for alcohol and tobacco use in the older adult population, some evidence suggests that there is bias in practitioners towards thinking older adults do not use illicit drugs, should be allowed to do whatever they choose at their age, or that, even if identified, they would not be good candidates for substance-abuse treatment (Blow et al. 2000). These biased attitudes impede healthcare providers' standard procedures for recognizing and assessing substance use. In conjunction with evidence that older adults under-report their marijuana use, it may be difficult to identify marijuana use and provide appropriate interventions. For this reason, healthcare providers should refer to SAMSHA's recommendations on Screening, Brief Intervention, and Referral for Treatment (SBIRT) for all substance-use disorders, particularly when working with older adults, when their bias may be most likely to interfere with their standard procedures. Any identified marijuana use is a positive screen, and requires further follow-up questioning to better characterize the patterns of use, provide education concerning the potential negative health outcomes of using marijuana, and treatment options, including more regular visits, to assist in decreasing marijuana use or abstinence or referral to substance-abuse specialist providers.

Currently, there are no FDA-approved medications for the treatment of cannabis-use disorder. Further research is needed in this area, and side effect profiles of medication that may make the older adult more vulnerable to adverse health consequences should be considered. Psychosocial treatments, such as behavioral therapies targeting relapse prevention and motivational interventions, have not been specifically developed for the treatment of older adults. However, they would probably provide similar benefits and should be considered as part of any treatment plan until more tailored interventions for older adults are developed.

## NICOTINE TREATMENT

Smoking cessation leads to reduction in the risk of premature death, improvement in cardiac and respiratory symptoms within days to weeks, improved quality of life, and increased ability to perform activities of daily living. It is essential to aid older adults in smoking cessation to improve their health and prevent future negative health consequences.

Data from a study looking at adults aged 50+ years who utilized emergency services showed that, of the substance users who presented, 50% were current cigarette smokers and had a higher rate of cardiovascular and pulmonary diseases than non-cigarette-smoking substance users (Blazer et al. 2009). The combination of older drug users who also smoke cigarettes suggests profound negative health consequences.

Brief interventions are effective for tobacco-use problems. Normative feedback in which education is provided about the hazards of chronic tobacco use, options for treatment, enhancement of motivation for change, and referral to resources in the environment are all aspects of a brief intervention for tobacco use. Older adults should be offered nicotine replacement therapy and evidence-based medications for smoking cessation, including bupropion and varenicline, although neither medication has been studied specifically in older adults for this indication. Motivational interviewing for smoking cessation in older adults has evidence for effectiveness when combined with case management in more formal treatment (Conigliaro et al. 2000, Kennedy 1999).

## STIMULANTS TREATMENT

Cocaine, along with alcohol and opioids, is associated with treatment use in older adults more than any other substance. Cocaine admissions for treatment account for 10–13% of all substance-abuse admissions for adults aged 50–59 years (Blazer et al. 2009). The proportion of admissions to treatment for cocaine use doubled from 1995 to 2005, from 2.1–4.4% for adults age 65+ years. Additionally, in a study looking at emergency service utilization in older adults using substances, the most commonly used illicit drug identified was cocaine (63% of older adult substance-abuse presentations to the emergency room) (Blazer et al. 2009).

Similarly to the treatment status for marijuana, there are currently no FDA-approved medications for the treatment of cocaine-use disorder and no specific psychosocial treatments for cocaine-use disorder in the older adult. Much like with treatment of cannabis-use disorders in the older adult, making use of the principles of SBIRT is probably the optimal model to operate under until further research provides clarifications on best practices in older patients. In addition, practitioners may utilize current evidence-based treatments for cocaine-use disorder that have demonstrated effectiveness in general adult populations.

## Conclusion

The small but expanding literature on cannabis, nicotine, and stimulant abuse in older adults makes a strong case that this is a large and growing problem, and this population probably has unique needs, differing from those of adults of younger age. Clinicians will greater serve their older patients by familiarizing themselves with common presentations of substance use in an older person, educational materials and information regarding the consequences of use of these substances, screening tools to identify problematic use, age-appropriate interventions and counseling, and referral resources in the community when more specialized addiction treatment is warranted. Little investigation has been done into age-specific factors contributing to use of these substances or treatments targeting them. Until further research is completed in this area, utilizing current evidence-based therapies and medications effective for cannabis, tobacco, and stimulant-use disorders in younger adults is recommended.

# References

APA. *Diagnostic and Statistical Manual of Mental Disorders, 5th ed.* Arlington, VA: American Psychiatric Publishing; 2013.

Arndt S, Turvey CL, Flaum M. Older offenders, substance abuse, and treatment. *Am J Geriatr Psych* 2002;10:733–739.

Bjartveit K, Tverdal A. Health consequences of sustained smoking cessation. *Tobacco Control* 2009;6;18(3):197–205.

Blazer DG, Wu LT. The epidemiology of substance use and disorders among middle aged and elderly community adults: National survey on drug use and health. *Am J Geriatr Psych* 2009;17(3):237–245.

Blow FC, Walton MA, Chermack ST, Mudd SA, Brower KJ. Older adult treatment outcome following elder-specific inpatient alcoholism treatment. *J Subst Abuse Treat* 2000;19(1):67–75.

Colliver JD, Compton WM, Gfroerer JC, Condon T. Projecting drug use among aging baby boomers in 2020. *Ann Epidemiol* 2006;16(4):257–265.

Conigliaro J, Kraemer K, McNeil, M. Screening and identification of older adults with alcohol problems in primary care. *J Geriatr Psych Neurol* 2000;13(3):106–114.

Culberson JW, Ziska M. Prescription drug misuse/abuse in the elderly. *Geriatrics* 2008;63(9):22–31.

Dinitto DM, Choi NG. Marijuana use among older adults in the U.S.A.: User characteristics, patterns of use, and implications for intervention. *Int Psychogeriatr IPA,* 2011;23(5):732–741.

Gfroerer J, Penne M, Pemberton M, Folsom R. Substance abuse treatment need among older adults in 2020: The impact of the aging baby-boom cohort. *Drug Alcohol Depend* 2003;69(2):127–135.

Glintborg B, Olsen L, Poulsen H, Linnet K, Dalhoff K. Reliability of self-reported use of amphetamine, barbiturates, benzodiazepines, cannabinoids, cocaine, methadone, and opiates among acutely hospitalized elderly medical patients. *Clin Toxicol (Phila)* 2008;46(3):239–242.

Hall SM, Humfleet GL, Munoz RF, Reus VI, Robbins JA, Prochaska JJ. Extended treatment of older cigarette smokers. *Addiction,* 2009;104(6):1043–1052.

Haney M. The marijuana withdrawal syndrome: Diagnosis and treatment. *Curr Psychiatr Rep* 2005;7(5):360–366.

Joy JE, Watson SJ, Benson JA. *Marijuana and medicine: Assessing the science base.* Washington, DC: Institute of Medicine; 1999.

Kalant, H. Adverse effects of cannabis on health: An update of the literature since 1996. *Prog Neuro-Psychopharmacol Biol Psych* 2004;28(5):849–863.

Kennedy M. Tobacco and alcohol: Still masters of addiction. *Wisc Med J* 1999;98(1):30–34.

Krishnan S, Cairns R, Howard R. Cannabinoids for the treatment of dementia. *Cochrane Database Syst Rev* 2009; (2), CD007204.

Kuerbis A, Sacco P, Blazer DG, Moore AA. Substance abuse among older adults. *Clin Geriatr Med* 2014;30(3):629–654.

LaCroix AZ, Omenn GS. Older adults and smoking. *Clin Geriatr Med* 1992;8(1):69–87.

Moore AA, Karno MP, Grella CE, et al. Alcohol, tobacco, and nonmedical drug use in older U.S. adults: Data from the 2001/02 national epidemiologic survey of alcohol and related conditions. *J Am Geriatr Soc* 2009;57(12):2275–2281.

Nemes S, Rao PA, Zeiler C, Munly K, Holtz KD, Hoffman J. Computerized screening of substance abuse problems in a primary care setting: Older vs. younger adults. *Am J Drug Alcohol Abuse,* 2004;30(3):627–642.

NSDUH. Results from the 2012 National Survey on Drug Use and Health: Summary of national findings. 2013;Accessed HHS Publication No. SMA (13–4795).

Rockett IR, Putnam SL, Jia H, Smith GS. (2006). Declared and undeclared substance use among emergency department patients: A population-based study. *Addiction,* |101(5):706–712.

SAMHSA. Substance Abuse Among Older Adults in Primary Care: Treatment Improvement Protocol (TIP) Series 26. 1998. Rockville, MD: Substance Abuse and Mental Health Services Administration.

Schonfeld L, King-Kallimanis BL, Duchene DM, et al. Screening and brief intervention for substance misuse among older adults: The Florida BRITE project. *Am J Public Health* 2010;100(1):108–114.

Simoni-Wastila L, Yang HK. Psychoactive drug abuse in older adults. *Am J Geriatr Pharmacother* 2006;4(4):380–394.

Zevin S, Benowitz NL. Drug interactions with tobacco smoking. An update. *Clin Pharmacokinet* 1999;36(6):425–438.

# CHAPTER 7

# Benzodiazepines and Other Sedative-Hypnotics in the Older Adult

*Arthur Robin Williams and Olivera J. Bogunovic*

## Introduction

Benzodiazepines are the most frequently prescribed class of psychotropic medications (Bisaga 2008). Importantly, prevalence of use increases linearly with age, with rates of use among females roughly twice that of males (Olfson 2015, Bogunovic 2004). Yet, until recently, there have been few studies investigating benzodiazepine-use disorders among older adults (Rosen, Engel et al. 2013).

Although benzodiazepines are the most widely used sedative-hypnotic medications due to their more favorable efficacy and safety profile, other agents will also be mentioned in this chapter. Sedative-hypnotics include benzodiazepines, barbiturates, and non-benzodiazepine hypnotics often referred to as "the Z-drugs" (Table 7.1). These medications share a sedative and often anxiolytic profile but differ in other properties such as their therapeutic index, pharmacokinetics, safety profile, and potential for misuse and dependence (Bisaga 2008). Compared to older sedative-hypnotics, the benzodiazepines are better tolerated, given lower rates of lethargy, confusion, and respiratory depression (than, for instance, barbiturates); however, there is growing concern about the long-term use of benzodiazepines, especially among older adults, concerning cognitive effects and fall risks (Madhusoodanan and Bogunovic 2004). The 2014 American Geriatrics Society's "Choosing Wisely" initiative (supported by the American Board of Internal Medicine Foundation) cautions against the use of any benzodiazepines or other sedative-hypnotics as initial treatments

*Table 7.1*  **Sedative-Hypnotic and Anxiolytic Medications, Clinically Equivalent Doses, and Pharmacokinetic Profiles**

| Compound (brand name) | Approximate equivalent oral dose (mg) | Onset speed of behavioral effect[a] | Duration of behavioral effect (hrs) | Elimination half-life[b] (hrs) [active metabolites] |
|---|---|---|---|---|
| *Benzodiazepines* | | | | |
| Alprazolam (Xanax) | 0.5 | Fast | 3–5 | 6–12 |
| Chlordiazepoxide[c] (Librium) | 25 | Intermediate | <??> | 7–13 [36–220] |
| Clonazepam (Klonopin) | 0.5 | Intermediate | 10–12 | 18–50 |
| Clorazepate[c] (Tranxene) | 15 | Intermediate | <??> | 2 [36–200] |
| Diazepam[c] (Valium) | 10 | Fast | 4–6 | 20–100 [36–200] |
| Estazolam (ProSom) | 2 | Slow | 6–8 | 10–24 |
| Flunitrazepam[c,d] (Rohypnol) | 1 | Fast | 6–8 | 18–26 [36–200] |
| Flurazepam[c] (Dalmane) | 20 | Fast | 7–10 | 50–100 [40–250] |
| Lorazepam (Ativan) | 1 | Fast | 4–6 | 10–20 |
| Midazolam (IV) (Versed) | 15 | Ultrafast | 0.5–1 | 2–4 |
| Oxazepam (Serax) | 20 | Slow | <??> | 4–15 |
| Prazepam[c,d] (Centrax) | 20 | <??> | <??> | [36–200] |
| Quazepam[c] (Doral) | 20 | Slow | 6 | 25–40 [40–100] |
| Temazepam (Restoril) | 20 | Intermediate | 5–6 | 8–22 |
| Triazolam (Halcion) | 0.5 | Fast | 0.5–1 | 1.5–5.5 |

*Non-benzodiazepine alpha-1 selective GABA_A agonists*

| | | | | |
|---|---|---|---|---|
| Eszopiclone (Lunesta) | 3 | Fast | <6 | 5–6 |
| Zaleplon (Sonata) | 20 | Fast | 0.5–4 | 1 |
| Zolpidem (Ambien) | 20 | Fast | 3–5 | 2 |
| *Barbiturates* | | | | |
| Pentobarbital (Nembutal) | 100 | Intermediate | 1–4 | 33 |
| Phenobarbital (Luminal) | 30 | Slow | 8–12 | 50–100 |
| Secobarbital (Seconal) | 100 | Fast | 1–4 | 30 |
| *Other* | | | | |
| Chloral hydrate (Somnote) | 500 | Intermediate | 4–8 | 0.5 [8–12] |
| Meprobamate (Miltown) | 800 | Intermediate | 4–6 | 10–11 |
| Carisoprodol (Soma) | 2,800 | Intermediate | 4–6 | 2.4 [10–11] |

*Note:* GABA = gamma-aminobutyric acid.

[a] Approximate onset of behavioral effect following oral administration: Fast (15–30 minutes), intermediate (30–60 minutes), and slow (60–120 minutes).

[b] Duration of clinical effects may not be directly related to the elimination half-life, due to rapid shifts in distribution out of the brain (e.g., diazepam has a long half-life but short clinical effect); clinical evaluation is better in determining frequency of dosing.

[c] Medications with metabolites that themselves are active benzodiazepines have half-lives that vary greatly among individuals and are usually greatly lengthened in the elderly.

[d] Medications not available on the U.S. market.

*Source:* Material adapted from Bisaga, A. (2008). Benzodiazepines and other sedatives. In M. Galanter and H. D. Kleber, Eds., *Textbook of Substance Abuse Treatment* (5th ed., 215–236). Washington, DC: American Psychiatric Publishing.

for agitation, insomnia, or delirium in older adults, yet their use remains wide-spread for these purposes (American Geriatric Society 2014).

Given the great variety of indications for sedative-hypnotics, including anxiety disorders, sleep disorders, seizure disorders, movement disorders, and muscle spasticity, the increasing prevalence of these disorders as patients age, and the fact that older adults are particularly prone to adverse reactions to sedative-hypnotics, concerns over responsible prescribing, screening for misuse, and the development of interventions to manage and treat sedative hypnotic-use disorders are gaining traction throughout the medical community. This chapter will summarize the evidence base for the responsible management of benzodiazepine use among older adults, while also emphasizing areas in most need of further study.

## Overview of Sedative-Hypnotics

Initially synthesized in 1832, chloral hydrate was the first medication considered a sedative-hypnotic. It is still used clinically today, but it has been associated with adverse gastrointestinal (GI) and behavioral effects, some associated with fatalities (Bisaga 2008). Bromide salts were introduced later in the 19th century. Initially used for treating epilepsy, they became better known for their sedative and anxiolytic effects; however, a narrow therapeutic index and problems with chronic use led to discontinuation of their use in the United States. Phenobarbital, the first barbiturate, was introduced in 1912 and continues to be widely used today (now mostly in the inpatient setting, for seizures, alcohol withdrawal, etc.). The abuse liability of barbiturates became well known by the mid–20th century as they produce an alcohol-like intoxication, including euphoria, leading researchers to look for safer alternatives.

Benzodiazepines were first discovered in the 1950s and became widely prescribed over the course of the 1960s. The first two benzodiazepines available on the market were chlordiazepoxide and diazepam in the early 1960s. In part due to a faster onset of action and positive subjective "drug-liking" effects, diazepam became the preferred drug among patients, therefore becoming the most prescribed medication in the United States. Growing concerns about the side-effect profile of longer-acting benzodiazepines due to the accumulation of both active drug and metabolites (i.e., diazepam is metabolized to nor-diazepam and to a lesser extent temazepam and oxazepam, all pharmacologically active) led to a change in prescribing practices, so that by the 1990s, alprazolam outpaced sales of diazepam (Bisaga 2008). As a result, concerns emerged that shorter-acting agents with a faster onset of action (alprazolam, lorazepam, triazolam) may be more likely to produce serious adverse effects such as amnesia, psychosis, and depression. (For a summary of pharmacokinetic profiles of sedative hypnotics, see Table 7.1.) Resultant efforts to reduce their use led to a steep reduction in the prescribing of triazolam in particular.

The discovery of the gamma-amino-butyric acid (GABA)-A receptor complex in the late 1970s led to the creation of non-benzodiazepine alpha-1 selective GABA-A agonists, including zolpidem, eszopiclone, and zaleplon (generally referred to as the "Z-drugs"). The GABA-A receptor complex is a ligand-gated ion channel activated by the neurotransmitter GABA, which acts as the primary inhibitory receptor in the central nervous system (CNS). Activation of the receptor leads to Cl- ion influx and hyperpolarization of the neuronal membrane, increasing the threshold required to produce an action potential. The GABA-A receptor has binding sites for GABA as well as benzodiazepines, barbiturates, neurosteroids, anesthetics, anticonvulsants, and ethanol (Mohler, Fritschy et al. 2002).

Almost two dozen receptor subtypes have been discovered, each with a different activity profile (affecting sedation, anxiolysis, learning, memory, anesthesia, and sensorimotor processing) based on subunit composition and distribution throughout the CNS. Each class of sedative-hypnotic binds to different subunit architecture, and in general, greater selectivity of a pharmacological agent active at the GABA receptor is associated with lower abuse liability (Bisaga 2008). For instance, zolpidem (as a representative Z-drug) preferentially binds to alpha-1 subunits of the GABA receptor affecting sedation and has fewer anxiolytic or muscle relaxant effects. Comparatively, benzodiazepines are less selective because they bind to any of the GABA receptor alpha units containing histidine, including alpha-1, alpha-2, alpha-3, and alpha-5.

Adverse effects of benzodiazepines stem from cognitive and psychomotor disruption and are typically dose-dependent. With escalating doses, the intoxidrome can encompass sleepiness, lethargy, weakness, dizziness, ataxia, confusion, disorientation, and anterograde amnesia (Bogunovic 2004, Bisaga 2008). Although tolerance to many of these effects develops with stable maintenance dosing, there is no comparable tolerance for memory impairment, which can persist for years following daily use (Lister 1985). Unlike the barbiturates, benzodiazepines used alone (even at high doses) typically do not lead to fatal respiratory depression unless combined with alcohol or other medications with synergistic effects such as opioids (Bisaga 2008). Given the risk of psychomotor side effects affecting balance and coordination, benzodiazepines may contribute to falls in the elderly, especially when given in combination with other medications (Leipzig, Cumming et al. 1999).

The abuse liability of sedative-hypnotics is thought to be less than that of other drugs of abuse or alcohol (Griffiths and Weerts 1997). In human laboratory studies examining the subjective effects of benzodiazepines, healthy persons (without symptoms of anxiety, for instance) often prefer placebo to active drug, given the latter's unpleasant effects such as sedation and amnesia (Dewit, H et al. 1989). However, well-controlled studies have shown that reinforcing effects emerge for all benzodiazepines and alpha-1 selective hypnotics when given at sufficiently high bio-equivalent doses (Rush et al. 1999). In particular, patients with a history of sedative or alcohol-use disorders are at greater risk for developing problematic patterns of use (Chutuape 1994). Greater risk of abuse is also conferred by intravenous administration and the use of benzodiazepines that have a faster onset of action (Griffiths et al. 1997). Barbiturates and meprobamate have an even greater risk of abuse or dependence; hence their relative lack of use in the outpatient setting today (Uhlenhuth et al. 1999).

## Sedative-Hypnotic Use Among Older Adults

Almost a third of all prescription drugs, many of them psychotropics, are prescribed for older adults (Bogunovic 2004). Since the 1980s, the benzodiazepine class has maintained a relatively constant share of all drug sales, with approximately 5–8% of all adults filling a benzodiazepine prescription in the past month (Woods and Winger 1995).

Studies of the prevalence of benzodiazepine use in the elderly are complicated by different data-collection methodologies and the type of population studied. Prevalence rates of benzodiazepine use differ, depending on the population studied and on the duration of use. A prototypical long-term user is an older widowed female with various health problems and psychiatric symptoms. Such patients generally use medical services frequently. The prevalence of benzodiazepine use in a community setting among the elderly varies between 10% and 41.6% (Llorente et al. 2003). In a cohort study of community-dwelling older adults in Quebec, the prevalence of continuous use was 19.8%, and of cumulative use, 1.9%. Rates of use are generally higher among patients who are homebound. However in the study of Morgan et al. (1988) the duration of use was 1–5 years in 13% of the sample, 5–10 years in 19%, and over 10 years in 25% of the sample.

Benzodiazepines are even more frequently prescribed for elderly patients who are institutionalized. Data from the United States National Nursing Home Survey indicated that, out of all psychotropic drug prescriptions for patients 65 years and older, 41% were antianxiety agents, mainly benzodiazepines. Since the introduction of the Omnibus Reconciliation Act of 1987 (OBRA 1987) in the United States, which deals with patient rights and quality of life in nursing homes, the pattern of benzodiazepine use has significantly changed, as more attention has been paid to assessing and managing the mental health needs of residents. A six-month study assessing psychotropic drug use found that the proportion of patients receiving benzodiazepines was 14.7% in Baltimore area nursing homes (data obtained from computerized monthly pharmacy reports) (Rovner et al. 199). Another study of psychotropic drugs in nursing homes showed that as many as 32% of prescriptions were anxiolytics (Holmquist et al. 2003).

Indications for the use of benzodiazepines are the same for the elderly and younger patients and include generalized anxiety disorder and other anxiety disorders, as well as adjustment disorder and insomnia. The prevalence of insomnia in the general population increases with age and ranges from 40–60%, making it an especially common indication for benzodiazepine use among older patients. Benzodiazepines improve sleep latency, reduce the number of awakenings, and increase total sleep time on a short-term basis. However, overall sleep quality often does not improve. Behavioral treatments have shown superior results, and there appears to be virtually no evidence to support chronic use of benzodiazepines for insomnia among older patients.

Benzodiazepines are typically prescribed as the first-line treatment for anxiety in the elderly. However, data suggest that serotonergic antidepressants are more appropriate than benzodiazepines, given the increased likelihood of adverse effects with benzodiazepine use in the elderly and the efficacy of serotonergic antidepressants for multiple types of anxiety as well as depression. Furthermore, depression often presents in the elderly with symptoms of anxiety rather than classic symptoms of depression.

Benzodiazepines have also been commonly used to treat behavioral disturbances associated with dementia. But the use of benzodiazepines for the treatment of these disorders is limited because of side effects such as disinhibition, gait disturbances, falls, and cognitive impairment.

Two decades ago, indications for benzodiazepine treatment were poorly documented in one-third of cases (Gold et al. 1995). Recent literature shows that benzodiazepines are now used more appropriately and that a multidisciplinary approach improves prescribing patterns (Tannenbaum et al. 2014).

## Differences Among Older Patients

With advancing age, the elderly are more sensitive to the potential side effects of benzodiazepines because of altered pharmacokinetics and pharmacodynamics (see Table 7.2). There are numerous studies indicating alterations in

*Table 7.2*  **Physiological and Pharmacokinetic Effects of Aging on Sedative-Hypnotics**

| *Physiological Changes* | *Pharmacokinetics* | *Clinical Implications* |
|---|---|---|
| • Increased total body fat<br>• Decreased lean body mass<br>• Decreased total body water<br>• Decreased GI motility<br>• Hypochlorhydria | Absorption:<br>• Unaffected for IV drugs<br>• Maximum plasma concentration may be lower, although time to maximum may be longer<br>Distribution:<br>• Reduced for water-soluble drugs and drugs bound to muscle<br>• Increased for lipid-soluble drugs | • May observe slight decrease in overall absorption (unlikely to be clinically significant)<br>• May require dose reduction of hydrophilic drugs<br>• May prolong elimination time of lipophilic drugs |
| • Decreased hepatic mass<br>• Decreased hepatic blood flow | Metabolism:<br>• Reduced first-pass metabolism<br>• Reduced Phase I metabolism | • Potential increase in bioavailability of drugs subject to extensive hepatic metabolism and increased drug exposure |
| • Decreased cardiac output<br>• Decreased blood flow kidneys and liver<br>• Decreased renal mass<br>• Decreased renal clearance | Elimination:<br>• Reduced renal elimination<br>• Increased elimination half-life | • Increased plasma concentration of drug (or metabolites)<br>• Increased duration of drug action |

the distribution and elimination of benzodiazepines in older age due to a multitude of mechanisms:

- Serum albumin levels may decrease by 15–20%, leading to an increase in pharmacologically active free-drug fraction and potentiation of the effects of benzodiazepines.
- Reduced hepatic blood flow can modify the plasma concentrations and increase peak concentrations.
- Particularly in older females, there is an increased volume of distribution, which is caused by increased proportion of total body fat to lean mass. As a

consequence, the peak plasma concentrations are lowered, and the plasma half-life is prolonged.

- Drug metabolism decreases with age and may be reduced by 30%. Benzodiazepines are metabolized in the liver by oxidation, nitro-reduction, and glucuronidation.
- Plasma clearance of benzodiazepines, which requires oxidative metabolism, is decreased in the elderly.
- Finally, older patients are more likely to be on multiple classes of medications (polypharmacy) and are subject to greater rates of drug–drug interactions.

Benzodiazepines may be divided into three different groups based on half-life: long, intermediate, and short-acting. Most of the long-acting benzodiazepines share a common intermediate metabolite that has an elimination life exceeding 60 hours or longer in the elderly. Benzodiazepines are primarily metabolized via the cytochrome P450 3A4 and 2c19 systems. A variety of drugs may increase the plasma levels and/or toxicity of oxidatively metabolized benzodiazepines. In summary, benzodiazepines with oxidative pathways and longer half-lives are more likely to accumulate, remain longer in the body, and cause prolonged sedation.

Furthermore, alterations in pharmacodynamics rather than pharmacokinetic changes in the elderly can be more important in explaining the altered response to benzodiazepines. Significant disturbances in daytime functionality often do not correlate with plasma concentrations of medications in older adults. Rather, the increased sensitivity of older people to benzodiazepines is probably due to age-related alterations in CNS receptors. Specifically, it is likely that benzodiazepine receptors in the brain become more sensitive, causing increased sedation.

Investigation of drug-related hospital admissions has shown that up to 10% of admissions may be directly or indirectly due to benzodiazepines. Adverse drug reactions may be experienced to a greater extent among benzodiazepine-dependent patients who use them over a prolonged period of time with greater amounts and escalating frequency of doses. The Boston Collaborative Drug Surveillance program reported an increase in incidence of adverse reactions in benzodiazepines with chronic use.

Intellectual and cognitive impairments have been associated with the use of benzodiazepines in the elderly. The findings of one longitudinal study indicate that long-term use of benzodiazepine is a risk factor for cognitive decline. Elderly patients with cognitive impairment often show improvement once the offending agent has been discontinued.

Additionally, the use of benzodiazepines in hospital settings has been associated with an increased risk of delirium. They can contribute to a higher risk of psychomotor impairment and diminished speed and accuracy of motor tasks. Several studies have shown that the use of benzodiazepines in the elderly increased the risk of hip fracture by at least 50%; this risk was secondary to the effects of benzodiazepines on cognition, gait, and balance (Madhusoodanan and Bogunovic 2004). Furthermore, exposure to long-half-life benzodiazepines in older drivers has been associated with a 30–50% increase in motor vehicle accidents (Neutel 1995).

Benzodiazepines at both high and low doses can produce discontinuation symptoms characterized by either rebound (symptom exacerbation) or withdrawal (similar to alcohol withdrawal, but it may be less predictable in older populations). Rebound symptoms include the intensified return of symptoms, most frequently insomnia. Symptoms of withdrawal in the elderly may differ from those seen in younger patients, requiring clinicians to be especially vigilant for subtle signs and to use a low threshold for escalating levels of care. In a prospective study of benzodiazepine use and withdrawal in elderly medical inpatients, confusion and disorientation with or without hallucinations were predominant symptoms of withdrawal after benzodiazepines had been abruptly discontinued (Foy et al. 1995).

## Sedative-Hypnotic Use Disorders in the Older Patient

An analysis from 2006 of the National Epidemiologic Survey on Alcohol and Related Conditions concluded that nonmedical use rates of sedatives or tranquilizers were 4.1% and 3.4%, respectively, among adults in the general population (Huang, Dawson et al. 2006). Pockets of high rates of misuse and dependence occur in select populations, often those with additional substance-use disorders. For instance, up to half of methadone maintenance patients are thought to misuse benzodiazepines (Iguchi, Handelsman et al. 1993; Gelkopf, et al. 1999). Similarly, National Epidemiologic Survey on Alcohol and Related Conditions (NESARC) data found that persons with alcohol-use disorders were roughly 14 times more likely to have sedative hypnotic-use disorders (Huang, Dawson et al. 2006). However, benzodiazepines are rarely a primary drug of choice among individuals seeking addiction treatment; under 1% of treatment admissions are thought to be for patients primarily abusing benzodiazepines (Bisaga 2008). This pattern holds true among older adults as well (Culberson and Ziska 2008).

Although benzodiazepine-use disorders typically occur among patients with other alcohol and substance-use disorders, the history or presence of a substance-use disorder is not an absolute contraindication to therapeutic benzodiazepine use (Posternak and Mueller 2001). At the same time, there is a growing literature investigating the "invisible epidemic" of prescription drug abuse among older adults (Kalapatapu and Sullivan 2010). Among older adults entering treatment who were tracked through the Treatment Episode Data System (TEDS) in 2007, there was a bimodal distribution of sedatives as drug of choice (a resurgence among those 65 and older), suggesting that, rather than aging out of abuse liability, older adults are likely to retain or increase in their propensity for developing benzodiazepine-use disorders with prolonged exposure (Fernandez and Cassagne-Pinel 2001, Bogunovic 2004). Data from a geriatric psychiatric outpatient clinic examined in the late 1990s found that 11.4% of patients had benzodiazepine dependence (Holroyd and Duryee 1997). Given that benzodiazepine-use disorders are often comorbid with other substance-use disorders and psychiatric conditions, they should be considered as clinical red flags that may suggest the presence of additional psychopathology (Bisaga 2008).

Older women in particular have been found to be at greater risk for prescription drug abuse (Kalapatapu and Sullivan 2010), which may reflect the lower rates of alcohol-use disorders among older women compared to older men, as well as what may be a bias among providers to overlook aberrant drug-taking behaviors of older women (Bogunovic 2004). Benzodiazepine-use disorders occur among patients who are typically twice as likely to be diagnosed with another mental illness as patients entering addiction treatment generally. Huang et al. (2006) found among NESARC data that individuals with nonmedical use of sedative hypnotics were more likely to have any additional mood, anxiety, or personality disorder (odds ration [ORs] = 3.7–6.6). The increased rates of anxiety and mood disorders among women may mediate their increased likelihood of developing benzodiazepine abuse or dependence as they age, especially when such disorders go untreated.

## Screening, Assessment, and Management of Sedative Hypnotic Use Disorders

The under-diagnosis of prescription drug-use disorders among older adults remains a systemic concern (Wetterling, Backhaus et al. 2002). The aforementioned difficulties and barriers to the timely diagnosis of sedative hypnotic-use disorders among older patients suggests that treatment is often withheld until they are further along in the disease course. For the same reasons older patients may elude traditional screening measures, they may require enhanced treatment modalities that can account for unique considerations in the treatment of older adults.

Currently, there is no gold standard for adapting substance-use disorder diagnostic criteria to older patients. Rather, efforts must be made to assess for dysfunction in domains of life relevant to the individual patient's context: for example, interference with social activities, instead of problems on the job. Conversely, older adults may be prone to physical side effects and medical problems complicated by prolonged exposure to benzodiazepines and related drug–drug interactions (e.g., falls), even in the absence of a primary substance-use disorder. However, in general, the DSM criteria for substance-use disorders are often less sensitive for an aging population.

Approaches to treating sedative hypnotic-use disorders in all adults are similar, irrespective of age. Most important are considerations of how to best individualize treatment that will tailor interventions specific to the patient and his or her circumstances.

Detoxification may be an area with the most notable differences for older patients. Generally, patients with more prolonged exposure to sedative hypnotics (i.e., years or decades of continuous use) are likely to have greater difficulty detoxing and ultimately ceasing use (Schorr and Robin 2014). Clinicians should therefore consider slower and longer tapers (over a span of several months or longer) to minimize rebound symptoms, withdrawal, and possible relapse. For patients who are being detoxed off benzodiazepines on an expedited time frame (such as days), care should be taken to choose benzodiazepines with shorter half-lives and no active metabolites such as lorazepam (Bisaga 2008). Ultimately, data are lacking, and more research will be needed to offer specific guidance on treatment interventions for clinicians working with older populations.

## Prevention and Education

The American Geriatrics Society's "Choosing Wisely" list cautions against the use of any benzodiazepines or other sedative-hypnotics as initial treatments for agitation, insomnia, or delirium in older adults (American Geriatric Society 2014). Yet benzodiazepines are the most frequently prescribed drugs in the elderly for insomnia and anxiety. They may be considered for short periods (2–4 weeks) for stressful emotional states (e.g., grief reactions) or for relief of severe and disabling anxiety. Other indications include time-limited or intermittent adjunctive treatment for psychotic disorders, alcohol withdrawal, movement disorders, and medical procedures. Benzodiazepines and Z-drugs should be prescribed in small doses and for short periods of time. There are other classes of medications that may be substituted for benzodiazepines (especially antidepressants), based on diagnosis. Shorter-acting benzodiazepines such as oxazepam and lorazepam are usually recommended because these medications don't accumulate in blood and are rapidly cleared. Additionally, whether for an indication of anxiety or insomnia, various behavioral, psychosocial, and psychotherapeutic interventions should be attempted when possible, to minimize exposure to unnecessary medication and polypharmacy in the older patient.

Benzodiazepine-use disorder us a serious problem in the elderly. Future research is needed to better understand the risk factors and potential markers for abuse. Clinicians should be aware of the risks associated with benzodiazepine-use disorders in this population in order to develop strategies for prevention, detection, and treatment.

# References

American Geriatrics Society. Ten things physicians and patients should question. 2014. At http://www.choosing wisely.org/doctor-patient-lists/american-geriatrics-society/. Accessed July 30, 2014.

Bisaga A. Benzodiazepines and other sedatives. In: Galanter M and Kleber HD, Eds., *Textbook of Substance Abuse Treatment*, 5th ed. Washington, DC: American Psychiatric Publishing; 2008:215–236.

Bogunovic OJ, Greenfield SF. Use of benzodiazepines among elderly patients. *Psychiatr Serv* 2004;55(3):233–235.

Chutuape MA, de Wit H. Relationship between subjective effects and drug preferences: Ethanol and diazepam. *Drug Alcohol Depend* 1994;34:243–251.

Culberson JW, Ziska M. Prescription drug misuse/abuse in the elderly. *Geriatrics* 2008;63(9): 22–31.

deWit H, Pierri J, Johansen CE. Reinforcing and subjective effects of diazepam in non-drug-abusing volunteers. *Pharmacol Biochem Behav* 1989;33(1):205–213.

Fernandez L, Cassagne-Pinel C. Benzodiazepines addiction and anxious and depressive symptoms in elderly persons. *Encephale—Revue de psychiatrie clinique biologique et therapeutique* 2001;27(5):459–474.

Foy A, O'Connell D, Henry DD, et al. Benzodiazepine use as a cause of cognitive impairment in elderly hospital patients. *J Gerontol* 1995;50:M99–M106.

Gelkopf M, et al. Characteristics of benzodiazepine abuse in methadone maintenance treatment patients: A 1-year prospective study in an Israeli clinic. *Drug Alcohol Depend* 1999;55(1–2):63–68.

Gold MS, Miller N, Stennie K, Populla-Vardi C. Epidemiology of benzodiazepine use and dependence. *Psychiatr Ann* 1995;25:146–148.

Griffiths RR, Weerts EM. Benzodiazepine self-administration in humans and laboratory animals—implications for problems of long-term use and abuse. *Psychopharmacology* 1997;134(1):1–37.

Holmquist IB, Svensson B, Hoglund P. Psychotropic drugs in nursing and old age homes: Relationships between needs of care and mental health status. *Eur J Clin Pharmacol* 2003;59:669–676.

Holroyd S, Duryee JJ. Substance use disorders in a geriatric psychiatry outpatient clinic: Prevalence and epidemiologic characteristics. *J Nerv Ment Dis* 1997;185(10): 627–632.

Huang B, Dawson DA, Stinson FS, et al. Prevalence, correlates, and comorbidity of non-medical prescription drug use and drug use disorders in the United States: Results of the National Epidemiologic Survey on Alcohol and Related Conditions. *J Clin Psychiatr* 2006;67(7):1062–1073.

Iguchi MY, Handelsman L, Bickel WK, Griffiths RR. Benzodiazepine and sedative use/abuse by methadone maintenance clients. *Drug Alcohol Depend* 1993;32(3):257–266.

Kalapatapu RK, Sullivan MA. Prescription use disorders in older adults. *Am J Addict* 2010;19(6):515–522.

Leipzig RM, Cumming RG, Tinetti ME. Drugs and falls in older people: A systematic review and meta-analysis: I. Psychotropic drugs. *J Am Geriatr Soc* 1999;47(1):30–39.

Lister RG. The amnesic action of benzodiazepines in man. *Neurosci Biobehav Rev* 1985;9(1):87–94.

Llorente MD, David D, Golden AG, et al. Defining patterns of benzodiazepine use in older adults. *J Geriatr Psychiatr Neurol* 2003;13:150–160.

Madhusoodanan S, Bogunovic OJ. Safety of benzodiazepines in the geriatric population. *Exp Opin Drug Saf* 2004;3(5):485–493. Review.

Mohler H, Fritschy JM, Rudolph U. A new benzodiazepine pharmacology. *J Pharmacol Exper Therapeut* 2002;300(1):2–8.

Morgan K, Dallosso H, Ebrahim S, et al. Prevalence, frequency, and duration of hypnotic drug use among the elderly living at home. *BMJ (Clin Res)* 1988;296:601–602.

Neutel CI. Risk of traffic accident injury after a prescription for a benzodiazepine. *Ann Epidemiol* 1995;5(13):239–244.

Olfson M, King M, Schoenbaum M. Benzodiazepine use in the United States. *JAMA Psychiatry* 2015;72(2):136–142.

Posternak MA, Mueller TI. Assessing the risks and benefits of benzodiazepines for anxiety disorders in patients with a history of substance abuse or dependence. *Am J Addict* 2001;10(1):48–68.

Rosen D, Engel RJ, Hunsaker AE, et al. Just say know: An examination of substance-use disorders among older adults in gerontological and substance abuse journals. *Soc Work Public Health* 2013;28(3–4):377–387.

Rovner BW, Edelman BA, Cox MP, Smuely Y. The impact of antipsychotic drug regulations on psychotropic prescribing practices in nursing homes. *Am J Psych* 1992;149(10):1390–1392.

Shorr RI, Robin DW. Rational use of benzodiazepines in the elderly. *Drugs Aging* 2014;4(1):9–20.

Tannenbaum C, Martin P, Tamblyn R, Benedetti A, Ahmed S. Reduction of inappropriate benzodiazepine prescriptions among older adults through direct patient education: The EMPOWER cluster randomized trial. *JAMA Intern Med.* 2014;174(6):890–898.

Wetterling T, Backhaus J, Junghanns K. Addiction in the elderly—an underestimated diagnosis in clinical practice? *Nervenarzt* 2002;73(9):861–866. German.

CHAPTER 8

# Assessment in the Older Patient

*Rahul Rao and Ilana Crome*

## Introduction

Assessment is the most fundamental component of clinical practice. A detailed assessment forms the basis for confidence in understanding a patient's condition. This, in turn, leads to a considered, analytical approach to the treatment options and management plans. During this process, there is the opportunity to ensure that the patient's engagement with care is sustained, and to be mindful of the patient's anxieties, ambivalence, and their attitudes in how they perceive their problem, its context, and the treatment. Assessment is continuous: there are likely to be inevitable and unpredictable changes in the patient's situation. Sometimes a repeat assessment may be brief; at other times it needs to be lengthy, and these decisions will be informed by experience and expertise. What follows is our suggestion for the building blocks for an overall protocol for an assessment that can be tailored to the individual's needs.

## Eliciting a Substance-Misuse History

Substance use often remains undetected in older people who are admitted to healthcare settings such as old age and addiction psychiatry, care of the elderly medicine, or primary care. However, in social care and the voluntary sector settings where professionals with senior roles within these organizations may have the remit and/or the experience in caring for older people with substance misuse, appropriate assessment procedures are required in social and welfare services. Even though this group may have multiple vulnerabilities, their substance problems are often missed.

Lack of identification of substance use occurs for many reasons, but if a detailed substance-use assessment is routinely undertaken, omission of much-needed clinical information is unlikely. Every single patient should be assessed for the nature and extent of their substance use. This is because substances may be directly or indirectly related to the physical and psychological problems with which the patient presents. A very frequent reason that substances are misused is for their psychoactive effect. Not only can assessment be conceptualized as the first part of the treatment journey, but it is also an ongoing process, which can sometimes be prolonged and should be recurrent so as to monitor and review changes and progress.

For the purposes of this chapter, the terms "drug" or "substance" refer to licit substances, tobacco and alcohol, illicit substances, central nervous system (CNS) depressants such as opiates, stimulants, lysergic acid diethylamide (LSD), khat, and magic mushrooms. "Drug" and "substance" will also be used in describing "street" use, use of prescription drugs (e.g., benzodiazepines) in a manner not indicated or intended by a medical practitioner, and similar use of over-the-counter preparations such as codeine-based products or drugs bought over the internet (Royal College of Psychiatrists 2011).

It can be very difficult to differentiate the effects of ageing from those of substance misuse. Healthcare professionals need to be proactive in drawing out the relevant features. The "Geriatric Giants," or five main areas that have a great impact on an older person's life are memory, instability, immobility, incontinence, and sensory impairment, all of which may be the result of, or lead to, substance use or a combination of both. Iatrogenesis (increased sensitivity of older people to drugs) is also a significant factor.

## THE INITIAL ASSESSMENT OF SUBSTANCE MISUSE IN OLDER PEOPLE

The suggested format below of an initial assessment draws on the Royal College of Psychiatrist Information Guide for Substance Misuse (Rao et al. 2015). This will include a comprehensive history, a physical and mental state examination, and biological tests.

### History
There are some general overarching assessment principles, which include the following:

- Adopting a non-judgemental and non-ageist approach, combined with a respect for dignity and individuality, is essential.
- Assess whether the patient is sufficiently fluent in the language in which the assessment is being conducted, and seek the support of an interpreter if necessary.
- Take into account the values and experiences of the patient.

- Adjust the tempo of the assessment according to the needs of the patient, taking into consideration factors such as seating position and comfort, sensory impairment, clouding of consciousness, level of comprehension, cognitive impairment, and privacy.
- Presentations can be atypical, and clues can be found in what is not mentioned but suspected in the way that they fit in with the rest of the clinical picture.
- Under-reporting may occur from denial, fear of stigma, lack of awareness, or memory impairment.
- Additional information from other sources is invaluable.
- Assessment will lead to a formulation and management plan that is weighted towards multiple comorbidity, functional abilities, the influence of loss events on mood state, cognitive state (including the influence of substances and physical disorders), and social support.
- Multiple assessments are often required to build up a clinical picture, including the need for vigilance around safeguarding the patient from the risks of abuse.

Thereafter a more systematic assessment is valuable:

- Age; sex; ethnicity; living arrangements; living environment (emphasizing the importance of home visits to gain a full clinical picture of disability and vulnerability)
- Presenting problem (may be masked and requires a flexible approach)
- Discuss substances separately (whether alcohol, nicotine, over the counter, prescribed, or illicit)
- Age at first use; weekend, weekly, and daily use
- Age of development of dependence syndrome
- Maximum use and when/for how long
- Pattern (quantity/frequency) over day/week
- Access to alcohol and other substances
- Drinking or drug-taking "environment" (e.g., home drinking, drinking partners, sharing medications)
- Route of use
- Cost/"funding"
- Abstinence/relapse and link to stability/life events
- Preferred substance(s)
- Treatment (dates, service, intervention, outcome)
- Past and family psychiatric history
- Occupational and psychosexual history
- Medical history (especially known complications from substance and effects on any existing age-related impairment; interactions with medications)

- History of sleep problems
- Forensic history (especially public order and acquisitive/theft offences)
- Risk of falls, social/cultural isolation, financial abuse
- Activities of daily living, statutory/voluntary/private care
- Level of nutrition: inability to prepare food or cook, dietary neglect, dental problems all affect daily intake
- Social support from informal caregivers and friends
- Social pressures—from debt, substance-using "carers," open drug dealing

### Collateral Information

Information from relatives, friends, and informal caregivers (taking account of information-sharing and confidentiality) can build up a picture of the person that can complement information from GP consultations and medication, hospital discharge summaries, home caregiver reports, day center reports, reports from housing officers/wardens of supported housing, criminal justice agencies, and results from previous investigations (including cognitive testing and neuroimaging).

### Assessment and Identification

Clinical staff should be able to detect the acute and chronic effects of substances, including intoxication, overdose, withdrawal, and dependence. Extra attention needs to be paid to physical disorders such as hypertension, diabetes mellitus, and disorders affecting mobility. Assessors should also vigilant over interactions with prescribed and over-the-counter medication. A protocol (Table 8.1) can support the practitioner in ensuring that major areas have been covered.

## Diagnosing Substance-Use Disorders

### CLASSIFICATION AND MAKING A DIAGNOSIS: CRITERIA FOR SUBSTANCE USE DISORDER (DSM-5) AND HARMFUL USE (ICD-10)

There are two systems used to make the diagnosis of Substance Use Disorder of Harmful and Dependent Substance Use (Table 8.2). These are:

1. DSM-5: *Diagnostic and Statistical Manual of Mental Disorders, 5th edition* (American Psychiatric Association 2013). In the DSM-5, "dependence" and "abuse" diagnoses are combined into "substance-use disorder," which has been expanded to include gambling disorder.
2. ICD-10: *International Classification of Diseases, 10th edition* (WHO 1992) is currently being revised for version 11. (World Health Organisation 1992)

*Table 8.1* **Protocol for Assessment of Substance Use and Misuse in Older People**

| Area of questioning | Questions to ask |
|---|---|
| Substance use<br><br>Ask the same questions for each substance in turn:<br>• Alcohol<br>• Amphetamines<br>• Benzodiazepines<br>• Cannabis<br>• Cocaine<br>• Ecstasy (XTC)<br>• Heroin and other opiates<br>• "Legal highs"<br>• Methadone<br>• Nicotine<br>• Over-the-counter medication<br>• Substances bought over the internet<br>• Prescribed medication<br>• Solvents/glue | • Age of initiation: first tried each substance<br>• Age of onset of weekend use<br>• Age of onset of weekly use<br>• Age of onset of daily use<br>• Pattern of use during each day, i.e., quantity/weight, frequency<br>• Route of use, e.g., oral, smoking, snorting, intramuscular, intravenous, subcutaneous ("skin popping")<br>• Age of onset of specific withdrawal symptoms and dependence syndrome features<br>• Current use over previous day, week, month<br>• Number of days of abstinence (reasons for this)<br>• Current cost of use<br>• Maximum use ever<br>• How substance use is funded<br>• Source of substances<br>• Periods of abstinence<br>• Triggers to relapse<br>• Preferred substance(s) and reasons<br>• If injecting, current injection sites, previous injection sites, any problems with these |
| Treatment episodes for substance misuse | • Dates, length of contact with service<br>• Type of services, and what was provided/types of interventions<br>• The outcome of each contact, what was achieved; did patient view it as successful or otherwise?<br>• Reason for discontinuing contact with the service<br>• Triggers to relapse, reasons for contact with the service again |

(*continued*)

*Table 8.1* **Continued**

| Area of questioning | Questions to ask |
| --- | --- |
| Family history | • Parents, siblings, grandparents, aunts, uncles, wife, husband, partner, children<br>• History of substance use within the family members mentioned and any related problems<br>• History of psychiatric problems, e.g., suicide, self-harm, depression, anxiety, psychotic illness, alcohol-related dementia |
| Personal history | • Educational attainment<br>• Separation, divorce, death<br>• Family relationships, conflict, support<br>• Occupational history<br>• Whether childhood was spent with biological parents or others |
| Social history | • Current living arrangements, e.g., home, hostel, care home; and with whom<br>• Cared for/caregiver<br>• Permanent, temporary<br>• Social network<br>• Future plans and current activities<br>• Housing support needs<br>• Benefits<br>• Any suggestions of vulnerability<br>• Typical day |
| Life style issues | • General physical state<br>• Sleep<br>• Diet<br>• Injecting practices, including risk to others<br>• Wound management<br>• Oral health<br>• Vaccination history<br>• History of breast, cervical cancer screening<br>• Sexual health issues |

*Table 8.1* **Continued**

| Area of questioning | Questions to ask |
|---|---|
| Medical history | • Past history—chronic conditions<br>• Current diagnosis, medications, treatment<br>• Episodes of acute or chronic illnesses: respiratory, infective, HIV, tuberculosis, cardiovascular, hepatitis, injury, accidents, surgery, overdose, disability—and whether any of these are related to substance use<br>• Any screening for blood-borne viruses (hepatitis B, C; HIV), dates and outcomes<br>• Falls, pain, constipation, sensory impairment<br>• Admission to hospital, dates, problems, treatment, length of admission, and outcome<br>• Current GP, care, condition/s, treatments |
| Psychiatric history | • Current signs and symptoms<br>• Current diagnosis, medication<br>• Assessment by GP for anxiety, depression<br>• Treatment by GP with psychoactive drugs<br>• Referral to specialist psychiatric services for assessment and treatment, dates, reasons, diagnosis, outcome (including inpatient admissions)<br>• Any Mental Health Act (UK) assessments |
| Criminal history | • Involvement in criminal activities, both related and not related to substance use<br>• Age at first contact with the criminal justice system, and reasons<br>• Cautions, charges, convictions<br>• Types of activity, shoplifting, theft, prostitution<br>• Imprisonment at any time<br>• Any current issues |
| Social background/Personality | • Ethnicity and cultural background<br>• Religious and spiritual beliefs<br>• Coping styles/resilience |

*(continued)*

*Table 8.1* **Continued**

| Area of questioning | Questions to ask |
|---|---|
| Financial status | • Mental Capacity over finances<br>• Debt<br>• Arrangements for budgeting and expenses |
| Biological measures | • Biochemistry: alcohol levels, drug screens, liver function tests<br>• Hematology<br>• Virology |
| Psychological measures | Brain MRI, liver ultrasound, endoscopy |
| Contact with other services (current and previous) | • Vulnerable adult<br>• Safeguarding risk to children (as grandparent) |
| Risk factors | • Social/cultural isolation<br>• Self neglect<br>• Recent losses<br>• Carer stress<br>• History of harm to self and others<br>• Elder abuse |
| Further information | • Carers, family, friends<br>• Other service providers |
| Perspective of patient | • Perception of problems<br>• Motivation for change—strengths, barriers, support |

*Source*: adapted from: Crome and Ghodse, 2007, and Society for Study of Addiction website, https://www.addiction-ssa.org 2015.

Coming to a diagnosis of mild, moderate, or severe substance-use disorder using DSM-5, or of harmful use or dependence using ICD-10, will crystallize the nature and severity of the substance problem and provide some indication of the relationship of the disorder to the mental and physical problems with which the patient presents. This is essential to determining the best treatment-management plan as well as aiding communication between professionals, family, and caregivers.

However, it is important to interpret the diagnostic criteria when applied to older people (Table 8.3), which highlights its limitations. These criteria were

*Table 8.2*  **Diagnostic Criteria for Substance-Use Disorder**

| DSM VI | CD 10 |
|---|---|
| The presence of at least 2 of these symptoms indicates Substance Use Disorder (SUD). The severity of the SUD is defined as | *Harmful use*: A pattern of psychoactive substance use that is causing damage to health; the damage may be to physical or mental health. |
| **Mild:** the presence of 2–3 symptoms<br>**Moderate:** the presence of 4–5 symptoms<br>**Severe:** the presence of 6 or more symptoms | *Dependence*: Diagnosis of a dependence should be made if three or more of the following have been experienced or exhibited at some time during the last year: |
| 1. The substance is often taken in larger amounts or over longer period than was intended | • A strong desire or sense of compulsion to take the substance |
| 2. There is a persistent desire or unsuccessful efforts to cut down or control substance use | • Difficulties in controlling substance-taking behavior in terms of its onset, termination, or levels of use |
| 3. A great deal of time is spent in activities necessary to obtain substances, use substances, or recover from their effects | • Physiological withdrawal state when substance use has ceased or been reduced, as evidenced by either of the following: the characteristic withdrawal syndrome for the substance of use of the same (or closely related) substance with the intention of relieving or avoiding withdrawal symptoms |
| 4. Craving, or a strong desire or urge to use a substance(s) [This is new to DSM-5] | • Evidence of tolerance, such that increased doses of the psychoactive substance are required in order to achieve effects originally produced by lower doses |
| 5. Recurrent substance use resulting in a failure to fulfil major role obligations at work, school or home | • Progressive neglect of alternative pleasures or interests because of psychoactive substance use and increased amount of time necessary to obtain or take the substance or to recover from its effects |

*(continued)*

*Table 8.2* **Continued**

| DSM VI | CD 10 |
|---|---|
| 6. Continued substance use despite having persistent, recurrent social or interpersonal problems caused or exacerbated by the effects of the substance | • Persisting with substance use despite clear evidence of overly harmful consequences (physical or mental) |
| 7. Important social, occupational, or recreational activities are given up or reduced because of substance use | |
| 8. Recurrent substance use in situations in which it is physically hazardous | |
| 9. Substance use is continued despite knowledge of having had a persistent or recurrent physical or psychological problem that is likely to have been caused or exacerbated by the substance | |
| 10. **Tolerance, as defined by either of the following:** <br> a) A need for markedly increased amount of substance to achieve intoxication or desired effect, or markedly diminished effect <br> b) A markedly diminished effect with continued use of the same amount of substance | |
| 11. **Withdrawal, as manifested by either of the following:** <br> a) The characteristic withdrawal syndrome for substance use <br> b) A substance is taken to relieve or avoid withdrawal symptoms | |

Table 8.3  **Diagnosing Substance Use Disorder in Older People**

| Criteria | | Special considerations for older adults |
|---|---|---|
| 1 | Substance taken in larger amounts or over a longer period that was intended | Cognitive impairment may interfere with self- monitoring |
| 2 | There is a persistent desire or unsuccessful efforts to cut down or control substance use | There may be reduced incentive to decrease harmful use, which includes fewer social pressures and also fewer personal and family pressures secondary to ageism |
| 3 | A great deal of time is spent in activities necessary to obtain substances, or recover from effects | Negative effects may occur at relatively low levels of use |
| 4 *New criterion:* | Craving or a strong desire or urge to use substances | Older people may not recognize the urges as cravings, or may attribute them to something else such as anxiety, depression, or boredom |
| 5 | Recurrent substance use resulting in failure to fulfil major role obligations of work, school, or home | The roles and expectations of older people and their families might have changed so that this is not acknowledged as a problem |
| 6 | Continued use despite having persistent or recurrent social or interpersonal problems caused or exacerbated by substance use | Older people deny or may not realize that the problems are associated with substance use |
| 7 | Important social occupational or recreational activities are given up or reduced due to substance use | Older people may have decreased activities due to physical and psychiatric comorbidities or 0 Social isolation and disabilities may detection more difficult |
| 8 | Recurrent use in situation in which it is physically hazardous | Older people may deny or not realize that a situation that was once safe has become physically hazardous |

*(continued)*

*Table 8.3* **Continued**

| Criteria | | Special considerations for older adults |
|---|---|---|
| 9 | Substance use is continued despite knowledge of having a persistent or recurrent physical or psychological problem that is likely to have been caused or exacerbated by substances | Older people may deny or not realize that these symptoms are substance-related Practitioners may not attribute some or all problems to substance abuse |
| 10 | Tolerance | Older people may not develop dependence |
| 11 | Withdrawal | Even low intake may cause problems |

*Source*: Adapted from Blow, 1998.

developed on an adult population so that, as Table 8.3 indicates, there may be reasons why older people may not fulfill the criteria as outlined in the classification systems. The criteria described remain pertinent, however, despite the changes in the DSM-5 classification. A low level of consumption may still have a damaging impact due to biological and functional changes; withdrawal symptoms may not be manifest as in younger people; older people may not be vigilant about the quantity of alcohol they are consuming and the effect; since there is a lesser expectation or need to fulfil obligations or roles at work or at home or in recreational activities, there is less motivation to reduce their consumption or less opportunity for the ill effects to be noticed. The threshold for a clinical decision in an older person may be different; i.e., the detrimental impact might be discerned even if the level of use is apparently low, when a decision about admission to a hospital is being made.

A thorough, systematic assessment is the lynchpin of a treatment management plan. A comprehensive history is fundamental, and it incorporates the physical, social, and psychological components of the patient's life so as to envision a care program that can be maximally beneficial. Further investigations may be futile if the possibility of substance use has been ignored and potential treatment for substance-related problems is not implemented.

DSM-5

The presence of at least two of these symptoms (Table 8.3) indicates a Substance Use Disorder (SUD). The severity of SUD is defined as *mild* (the presence of

2–3 symptoms); *moderate* (presence of 4–5 symptoms) or *severe* (the presence of 6 or more symptoms). However, this is based on a general adult population, rather than older adults. Special considerations for older adults are detailed in Table 8.3.

There are specific withdrawal symptoms that comprise a syndrome, and symptoms of intoxication for each substance. Knowledge about the different syndromes can often clarify the picture. For example, in ICD-10, the diagnosis of "F10.3 alcohol withdrawal" requires clear evidence of recent cessation/reduction in alcohol use and three or more of the following symptoms:

1. Tremor of tongue, eyelid, or outstretched hand
2. Sweating
3. Nausea, retching, vomiting
4. Tachycardia, hypertension
5. Psychomotor agitation
6. Headache
7. Insomnia
8. Malaise, weakness
9. Transient visual, tactile, or auditory hallucinations or illusions
10. Grand mal convulsions

## Clinical Assessment of Psychiatric and Physical Presentations

### MENTAL STATE EXAMINATION

Ideally, the Mental State Examination should be undertaken regularly as part of the assessment of substance consumption and when patients are abstinent, if feasible. It should also be noted that a low level of substance use may destabilize someone with a mental health problem. The basic elements of a mental state examination need to be undertaken: the patient's behavior and appearance, speech, mood, thoughts, perceptions, cognition, insight, and judgement. This is because the commonest presentations in the context of substance misuse in older people are delirium, mood disorders, cognitive impairment, and psychotic symptoms.

Delirium may be associated with intoxication or withdrawal states. Recognizing delirium tremens in acute hospital settings is especially important, as it has a high morbidity and mortality, and it is treatable. Those at risk before or in the earliest stages of withdrawal require appropriate detoxification plans and nutritional support.

Wernicke's encephalopathy may also present with, or be confused with, signs of delirium. Low mood and anxiety may accompany the misuse of a range of substances, particularly depressant drugs such as alcohol, sedatives, and hypnotics. It is not uncommon to find an atypical presentation of symptoms suggestive of a mood disorder. These include being "masked" by cognitive impairment or "somatized" by presenting as physical symptoms such as lack of energy.

The presence of multiple physical comorbidities may make the detection of depression and anxiety more difficult, particularly somatic symptoms of depression, which are also associated with many physical disorders such as rheumatological and neurological disease. Detecting mood disorders is determined by cognitive and behavioral symptoms such as poor concentration, pessimism, suicidal ideation, and irritability. The assessment of alcohol misuse is particularly important in older people who are at the highest risk of completed suicide, where alcohol misuse often accompanies the worsening of depressive symptoms and lowers impulse control, and is therefore likely to facilitate the suicidal act.

Cognitive impairment associated with alcohol misuse may present with alcohol-related brain injury in the form of amnestic disorders confined to memory impairment, or with alcohol-related dementia where there is a more global loss of cognitive function. In either case, screening cognitive functions using a tool covering a range of cognitive domains such as the Mini Mental State Examination (MMSE; Folstein et al. 1975) is required.

Psychotic symptoms can be associated with the acute effects of a variety of substances such as cannabinoids, stimulants, and hallucinogens; withdrawal states accompanying alcohol and/or sedatives and hypnotics are also commonly associated with transient psychotic symptoms. Chronic use of stimulant and depressant drugs can manifest as psychosis.

## PHYSICAL EXAMINATION

The following areas should be covered in a routine physical examination:

- Frailty (may not appear immediately obvious, especially when patients are fully clothed)
- Self-care and hygiene
- Gait and balance
- Use of walking aids
- Inspection of all the skin (including the genital areas) for any injury, pressure area breakdown, damage from incontinence, and ulceration

- Tar staining of the fingers and hair as evidence for tobacco use and nicotine addiction
- Stigmata of chronic liver disease, such as palmar erythema, spider nevi, and caput medusa or jaundice in alcohol misuse or exposure to hepatitis C virus from needle sharing. These stigmata may also be accompanied by a macronodular liver, liver tumor, or ascites.
- Psoriasis is associated with alcohol misuse, as is increased risk of skin carcinomata and porphyria cutanea tarda (also prevalent in hepatitis C).
- Injected drugs of abuse are associated with thrombosis of superficial and deep veins, ulceration, and sinus formation. In bacterial endocarditis, which can be as a result of injecting drugs, immune complex deposits can lead to nail-fold infarcts, splinter hemorrhages, and Osler's nodes in the pulps of the digits. Janeway lesions (tender nodules in the palms or soles) are due to septic emboli.
- HIV infection in older intravenous drug misusers is associated with cutaneous manifestations such as a macular rash in seroconversion; increased rates of bacterial, viral, and fungal infections; higher rates of skin cancers; higher rates of drug reactions, and specific reactions to anti-retroviral therapy. Psoriasis and seborrheic dermatitis are also seen.
- Poor nutrition in substance misuse may be evident from gum disease and dental caries, or the corkscrew-shaped body hair seen in scurvy (vitamin C deficiency). Methamphetamine use is particularly associated with dental problems.
- Respiratory complications from tobacco and cannabis often present as chronic obstructive pulmonary disease (COPD), with purse-lipped breathing, barrel-shaped chest, or pulmonary hypertension.
- Hypertension may coexist with smoking, as may alcohol, and both increase the likelihood of ischemic heart disease, vascular disease, heart failure, and stroke. Some stimulant drugs, particularly cocaine, can induce myocardial infarction and stroke.
- Rectal examination may reveal the pale stools of malabsorption associated with pancreatic insufficiency.
- Complications such as HIV and hepatitis C are also common and diverse.
- Neurological manifestations of alcohol and drugs are associated with traumatic intracerebral bleeding, sometimes without evidence of external injury.
- Pain is commonly associated with substance misuse. Substances can be used to manage the pain, and the effects of substances may produce pain from infection (e.g. cellulitis or septicemia) or injury.
- Alcohol may be associated with injuries in acute intoxication, as well with cerebellar syndrome and peripheral neuropathy, seen in harmful drinking and alcohol dependence.

Functional status is a necessary accompaniment to any comprehensive assessment of an older person, given the impact of ill health on both acute and chronic functional status. Such an assessment should cover both personal and instrumental (domestic) activities of daily living (ADLs); complemented by an account of a typical day.

## ASSESSMENT OF COMORBIDITY

The term *comorbidity* (or "dual diagnosis") is used to describe the co-occurrence of two or more disorders. It is important to understand the many mechanisms by which substance use can be associated with psychological and physical symptoms and syndromes, and to be able to differentiate between symptoms and disorders. It is also necessary to bear in mind that substance use is rarely limited to one substance, and that is can be problematic to reach a conclusion about which condition or conditions developed first. Social problems may also be part of the picture: older people are often very vulnerable, with histories of deprivation, poor educational attainment, and trauma experiences, which may even involve violence. For example, approximately 40% of people with psychosis misuse substances at some point in their lifetime. This is at least double the rate seen in the general population. Those with coexisting mental health and substance-misuse problems have a higher risk of relapse and hospitalization (National Institute of Clinical Excellence [NICE] 2011).

The interrelationship between comorbidity and substance use can be complex:

- Substance use (even one dose) may produce psychiatric or physical symptoms or disorders.
- Harmful use may produce psychological and physical symptoms or syndromes.
- Dependent use may produce psychological and physical symptoms or disorders.
- Intoxication from substances may produce psychological and physical symptoms.
- Withdrawal from substances may lead to psychological and physical symptoms, or psychiatric and physical diagnoses.
- Substance use may exacerbate a pre-existing psychiatric disorder.
- Psychological morbidity that does not amount to a disorder may precipitate substance-use disorder.
- Primary psychiatric or physical disorders may lead to substance-use disorders.

• Primary psychiatric or physical disorders may precipitate substance-use disorders, which may, in turn, lead to psychiatric syndromes.

## Comorbid Psychiatric Disorders

In older people with alcohol misuse, acute intoxication may be followed by or associated with acute withdrawal symptoms in the dependent patient and should be recognized early, so that these patients can be treated in an appropriate hospital setting. It may mask the development of the potentially life-threatening Wernicke's encephalopathy, which causes brain damage and is thought to be caused by a lack of the vitamin thiamine due to poor diet and/or absorption at a time of increased requirement for the vitamin. Untreated Wernicke's encephalopathy may lead to Korsakoff's psychosis, in which there is lasting damage to areas of the brain involved with memory (So et al. 2012). Although Wernicke's and Korsakoff's may appear to be two different disorders, they are generally considered to be different stages of the same disorder, which is called Wernicke-Korsakoff syndrome. Wernicke's encephalopathy represents the "acute" phase of the disorder, and Korsakoff's amnesic syndrome represents the "chronic" phase. The acute effects of a variety of substances such as cannabinoids, stimulants, and hallucinogens can include an acute psychosis, while the withdrawal states accompanying alcohol and/or sedatives/hypnotics are also commonly associated with transient psychotic symptoms. Other substances such as nicotine, opiates, stimulants, and cannabis also have distinct withdrawal symptoms (Crome et al. 2015).

Delirium tremens is a severe form of alcohol withdrawal that can manifest as a severe mental or nervous system disorder. It is a medical emergency. It is characterized by hallucinations, disorientation, tachycardia, hypertension, fever, agitation, convulsions, and diaphoresis (sweating) and typically sets in following acute reduction/cessation of alcohol. It typically begins 48–96 hours after the last drink, and in the absence of complications, it can last for up to seven days (Mayo Smith et al. 2004).

Delirium tremens is usually a clinical diagnosis. Acute alcohol withdrawal can be managed by fixed-dosing medication regimes or by giving an initial "loading" dose (front-loading) in conjunction with a symptom-triggered or "as required" regimen.

Comorbid psychiatric disorders in older people with substance misuse pose challenges in meeting the needs of both substance misuse and mental disorders. Comorbid mental disorders (termed "co-occurring disorders" or "dual diagnosis") in older people are any accompanying mental disorder, but most often depression and cognitive impairment; with the latter mostly referring to alcohol-related brain injury. Comorbid psychiatric disorders ranges from

21–66%, with higher rates seen across inpatient settings for those with more severe mental health problems (Bartels et al. 2006). Older adults with depression are three to four times more likely to have alcohol-related problems than those without (Devanand 2002), with higher risk of suicide and social and functional impairment (Davis et al. 2008).

The 80–84 age group have the highest suicide rate (Office of National Statistics 2014a). In the under-65 population, the "baby boomers," born between 1946 and 1964, have had higher suicide rates at any given age than earlier or later cohorts. The upper end of this cohort is already over 65, and there is expected to be a rapid growth in the over-65 population over the next few decades (Conwell et al. 2011). Risk factors for suicide cluster in risk profiles and include male gender, family history of psychiatric disorder, previous attempted suicide, more severe depression, hopelessness, as well as comorbid anxiety and alcohol misuse (Hawton et al. 2013).

In older people, low mood may be downplayed, misattributed to cognitive impairment by clinicians (so-called pseudodementia) and masked by either physical illness or alcohol intoxication. Older people are more likely to "somatize" their depression through complaints such as worsening pain or abdominal discomfort. Older people do not commonly present with the classic depressive symptoms seen in their younger counterparts, such as feeling low and being tearful. Rather, they present with feeling "down in the dumps," "fed up," or "lonely." Similarly, given the restricted lifestyle of some older people, it is difficult to gauge loss of interest.

Other symptoms such as loss of appetite and sleep disturbance may be shared with both physical health problems and alcohol misuse, as may loss of energy. However, the diagnosis is made clearer by the presence of pessimism, hopelessness, thoughts of life not being worth living, and suicidal ideation.

Once feelings of hopelessness have been established, it is essential to explore suicidal ideation, particularly the severity and frequency of suicidal thoughts; as well as factors driving this ideation and those holding the person back from attempting suicide. This is particularly important when assessing older people who have presented with an act of self-harm. In such cases, the presence of depression, with or without alcohol misuse, may (under certain circumstances, in the UK) require the use of legal detention under the Mental Health Act.

As mentioned previously, the MMSE is commonly used as a screen of general cognitive function. However, it should be borne in mind that this screening tool does not assess frontal lobe function, which is known to be more sensitive than other brain areas to the initial effects of alcohol toxicity (Zahr et al. 2011). If a more comprehensive assessment of cognitive function is required, the Addenbrookes Cognitive Examination offers such a screen (Mioshi et al. 2006).

*Comorbid Physical Disorders*

Acute hazards from intravenous injections are associated with damage to veins, infection, and overdose, with such damage representing the most common harm from misuse of cocaine. Bacterial endocarditis and hepatitis C can also arise as a result of injecting drugs.

Other systemic effects of substances include gastrointestinal disease (e.g., damage to the liver and pancreas from alcohol misuse); respiratory disorders (e.g., COPD and lung cancer from tobacco smoke, and chronic nasal inflammation from crack cocaine); low blood sugar (from misuse of cocaine and alcohol); and cardiac disease (from alcohol and cocaine misuse, as well as intravenous drug use)

The use of certain illegal or controlled substances has been shown to increase the risk of stroke, particularly hemorrhagic stroke, with a range of substance implicated. These include alcohol, cannabis, cocaine, amphetamines, phencyclidine (PCP or "angel dust"), and LSD.

Falls represent a particular risk in older people. Physiological changes associated with age, sensory deficits, postural imbalance, chronic health problems, substance misuse, and environmental hazards have all been identified as fall risk factors. Loss of balance, coordination, and judgement; risk-taking, autonomic neuropathy, peripheral neuropathy, cardiac disease, osteoporosis, and myopathy, may all conspire to make a fall more likely. There is increased prevalence of falls among elderly individuals with substance misuse, and this should always be considered in differential diagnosis.

# Limitations of Screening

Screening and assessment are separate processes, with the former carried out using a brief series of questions conducted on all new and ongoing patients at regular intervals. The goal of substance-abuse screening procedures is to document "use." In the assessment stage, the aim is to make a diagnosis of substance abuse or dependence and use relevant aspects of the history and examination to inform the treatment plan.

## ALCOHOL USE

Screening for alcohol-use disorders (AUDs) includes asking about the quantity and frequency of use, frequency of heavy drinking, symptoms of abuse or dependence, and indirect proxy questions (Berks and McCormick 2008). There is also an increasing number of biomarkers to detect recent or chronic use. Screening can also be accomplished by direct interview, pencil and paper, and electronic methods.

There are two primary alcohol-use questions. The first inquires about the frequency of use, and the second about quantity (Bradley et al. 1998; Bradley et al. 2007). The time frame is generally limited to the past year, and one "drink" is equivalent to 14 grams of pure alcohol (8 grams in the UK).

Using the US National Institute on Alcohol Abuse and Alcoholism (NIAAA) criteria, it is recommended that men and women 65 years or older not drink more than seven drinks a week and no more than one drink per day (NIAAA 2007). The NIAAA also suggests no alcohol use in older adults with certain comorbid disorders (e.g., hypertension, severe depression, diabetes, elevated lipids) or who are taking medication that interacts with alcohol (e.g., sedatives, regular doses of acetaminophen).

Proxy questions are included in the CAGE (acronym for Cut down, Annoyed by criticism, Guilty about drinking, Eye-opener drinks) questionnaire. A positive response to one or more questions suggests a lifetime history of an alcohol-use disorder, but it is primarily used a proxy measure for dependence.

Symptoms of abuse or dependence in older people are measured using two screening/assessment pencil-and-paper questionnaires. These include the Alcohol Use Disorders Identification Test (AUDIT) and the geriatric version of the Michigan Alcohol Screening Test (MAST-G). The AUDIT consists of three questions on alcohol use, three questions related to alcohol dependence, two questions on morbidity (injury and blackouts), and two further questions on family member concern. It has been validated in older populations (Roberts et al. 2005), with greatest sensitivity and specificity being shown with a cut-off point of 5 for older men and 3 for older women. Shorter versions of the AUDIT include the AUDIT-5 (5-item version) and the AUDIT-C (3-item version). A cut-off point of 4 has been suggested for both the AUDIT-5 (Philpot et al. 2003) and AUDIT-C (Aalto et al. 2011). However, these studies have not undergone extensive replication in older people. The Short Michigan Alcoholism Screening Test–Geriatric version [SMAST-G] (Blow et al. 1998) has shown the greatest validity and use in older populations.

## ALCOHOL BIOMARKERS

Although traditional liver-function tests such a gamma-glutamyl transferase (GGT) are neither sensitive nor specific, several new markers have been developed. Blood alcohol levels have limited value as a screening test as most people metabolize alcohol at the same rate, irrespective of blood alcohol level. Recently developed alcohol biomarkers include carbohydrate deficient transferase (CDT), ethyl glucuronide (ETG), ethyl sulfate (ETS), and phosphatidyl ethanol (PET) (Peterson 2005.)

## ILLICIT DRUG USE

An estimated 4.8 million adults aged 50 or older, or 5.2% of adults in that range, have used an illicit drug in the past year (Substance Abuse and Mental Health Services Administration 2011). Although the use of illicit drugs is a problem for individuals of all ages, it may be of particular concern for older adults, because they experience physiological, psychological, and social changes that place them at greater risk of harm from illicit drug use. However, there are no current screening tools for illicit drug use that have been validated in older people.

## PRESCRIPTION DRUG USE

A recent study conducted in a sample of 1,000 patients receiving opioids from a primary care physician found that a history of four or more aberrant behaviors was associated with prescription drug abuse (Fleming et al. 2007.). Aberrant behaviors most strongly associated with medication abuse include: requested early refills, felt intoxicated, increased dose on own, purposefully oversedated themselves. Other aberrant drug behaviors included seeking medication from more than one physician, hoarding medication, using an opioid for other reasons than prescribed, and losing medication or prescriptions.

For a comprehensive assessment, screening is only the initial component of a process that builds up a picture of how substance-misuse behavior interacts with other addictions and is influenced by personality, gender, culture, values, life experience, other substances and prescribed medications, mental health, physical health, social function (including vulnerability, activities of daily living, and social support), as well as current states of both mental and physical health.

Within the assessment process, there are certain areas that require a specific focus. These are coexisting mental and physical disorders, social functioning, and cognitive impairment.

# Distinctive Aspects of Assessment

In older people, there is comparatively less emphasis on forensic (legal) history (e.g., domestic violence, public order offences, offences against the person, and driving offences associated with substance use) and occupational history than in younger people. Instead, greater attention is paid to the aspects that are associated more specifically with the aging process and the risks associated with particular vulnerabilities.

## PRESENTATIONS OF SUBSTANCE MISUSE IN OLDER PEOPLE

All practitioners should be aware of the range of clinical presentations that may occur in older people with substance misuse. These include the following:

### Physical Presentations
- Seizures
- Malnutrition and muscle wasting
- Liver function abnormalities
- Chronic pain or other unexplained somatic symptoms
- Incontinence, urinary retention, difficulty urinating
- Poor hygiene and self-neglect
- Dry mouth or dehydration
- Unexplained nausea and vomiting
- Motor incoordination and shuffling gait
- Frequent falls and unexplained bruising and head injuries

### Psychiatric Presentations
- Sleep disturbances
- Cognitive impairment with memory problems
- Persistent irritability or anxiety
- Change in mood with depression
- Labile affect
- Unusual restlessness and agitation
- Unusual fatigue
- Daytime sedation
- Changes in eating habits
- Difficulty in concentration
- Difficulty in orientation

## MENTAL CAPACITY

Under the Mental Capacity Act (MCA) 2005 in the United Kingdom, a "lack of capacity" is defined in relation to a specific matter if a person is unable to make a decision for him/herself in relation to a matter because of an impairment of, or a disturbance in the functioning of, the mind or brain. Such incapacity may change over time.

The complex nature of problems associated with substance use in older people means that there are particular risks around mental capacity, especially when there is a conflict between capacity and the role of the practitioner in encouraging the older person to give up substance use (Hazelton et al. 2003).

This is especially relevant given that one of the core features of dependence syndromes is the persistence of substance misuse in spite of the user's being aware of the harm from the substance being taken. Using the core feature of harm awareness, an assessment of mental capacity in substance use can help distinguish an unwise decision from a lack of mental capacity on its own.

Under the MCA, a four-stage assessment of decision-making ability is required to prove that an individual is able to make a specific decision at that specific time:

- Possessing a general understanding of the decision and why they need to make it
- Possessing a general understanding of the likely consequences of making/ not making a decision
- Possessing an ability to understand, retain, use, and weigh up the information relevant to this decision
- Possessing an ability to communicate their decision

Capacity can vary over time and change for different decisions. For substance misusers, this becomes an even more crucial issue, as their states of incapacity may fluctuate according to their level of intoxication or delirium. Capacity should, therefore, be seen as decision-specific. If a person is deemed to be "lacking capacity," it means that they lack capacity to make a particular decision or take a particular action for themselves at the time the decision or action needs to be taken.

The MCA applies to anyone who has "an impairment of or disturbance in the functioning of the mind or brain," rather than to a particular mental disorder, which may not be appropriate to a person with substance-abuse problems.

Lack of capacity is distinct from making unwise decisions. The MCA acknowledges that individuals who have the capacity to make their own decisions may make what may be "unwise" decisions. In many cases, this applies to risk-taking, such as gambling, forming relationships, and choosing a certain type of lifestyle. In the case of substance misuse, individuals may choose to continue to use a substance in spite of being aware of its harmful effects.

If that individual is deemed as having the capacity to make a decision for themselves—i.e., if that individual is shown as being able to weigh up the consequences of their decision and still choosing to use a particular substance— the MCA safeguards that individual's decision-making capacity by suggesting that decisions otherwise deemed "unwise" are legally acceptable.

If capacity is an individual's ability to make decisions, "consent" can be seen as granting permission or agreeing to the decisions themselves. In relation to consent, the MCA covers the three areas: of substituted decision-making powers, best-interest principles and independent decision-makers.

Substituted decision-making is implemented through Advance Care Planning (ACP) in three forms:

1. Statements of wishes and preferences for future care that an individual would want; made *before they lost capacity*
2. Advance decisions to refuse certain treatment or intervention; made *before they lost capacity*
3. Granting a trusted friend or relative Lasting Power of Attorney (LPA) to cover health and welfare decisions; made *before they lost capacity*

Best-interest decision-making includes a checklist, which takes into account key indicators of an individual's well-being. In complex cases, such as working with older people with substance-misuse problems, assessing impaired capacity may not be straightforward, and there may be additional criteria to take into account. Hazelton et al. (2003) suggest delaying significant decisions for as long as possible, or at least until the acute effects have passed, as well as differentiating between alcohol-related cognitive deficits and addiction-related denial. Using the least restrictive option is also always recommended.

Independent decision-makers also have a role in decision-making. Family networks of older people with a history of substance misuse may be absent, chaotic, and challenging to engage. A relationship between the older person and their family relative may not be based on trust or prior knowledge of preferences of the individual. The MCA defines the role of an Independent Mental Capacity Advocate (IMCA), or someone who can step into the role of substitute decision-maker, to make major decisions regarding treatment or accommodation for a person with impaired capacity (UK Ministry of Justice 2007).

## ELDER ABUSE

There is no universally accepted definition of elder abuse, but the most common is "a single or repeated act or lack of appropriate action occurring within any relationship where there is an expectation of trust, which causes harm or distress to an older person or violates their human and civil rights" (World Health Organization [WHO] 2002). Elder abuse is generally categorized as physical, psychological (or emotional), financial, sexual, and neglectful. One or several of these abusive acts or omissions may be experienced in a person's own home, in community settings, or in settings such as long-term care facilities and hospitals.

In its more general sense, "elder abuse" refers to the ill-treatment of an older person by commission (abuse) or omission (neglect). Such abuse warrants further investigation. In England, the term *safeguarding* is used to describe multi-agency arrangements to prevent and respond to the abuse of "vulnerable" (generally meaning frail or disabled) adults. Use of this term marks a shift in emphasis from reaction and rescue to prevention and harm minimization, in the hope that outcomes for the older person might be better and of their own choosing (Manthorpe 2013). In other parts of the world, the terminology referring to the organization of professionals working to investigate and respond to elder abuse may include "adult protective services."

Up to 10% of older people experience some form of elder abuse, but only one in 25 of these is reported to social services (Dong 2012). Substance-misuse abuse is more likely to occur in the perpetrators of the abuse than in the person suffering abuse (Anetzberger 2005), and older women with neurological or mental disorders who misuse drugs or alcohol are at highest risk of experiencing elder abuse (Friedman 2011).

In the United States, substance dependence among perpetrators is a recognized risk factor (Anetzberger 2005). Risk of physical and verbal abuse appears to depend more on problematic characteristics associated with the perpetrator—particularly their physical and mental health (including dementia), but notably, in many studies, their consumption of and reliance on alcohol.

The World Health Organization (WHO 2005) review of elder abuse and alcohol outlined how the relationship between elder abuse of and harmful alcohol use in an older person may interact:

- Physical injury, financial problems, social withdrawal, malnourishment, and emotional and psychological problems, including depression and cognitive and memory impairments. As older people are often physically weaker, physical violence may result in greater injury or their convalescence may take longer.
- Since older people often have lower incomes and less opportunity to replace money, the economic consequences of financial abuse may be severe.
- Reduced life expectancy or depression may occur. In some cases harmful alcohol use becomes a coping strategy but leads to other life limiting health problems, such as cardiovascular diseases, cancers, and unintentional injuries. Wider impacts of alcohol use in older people are substantial, including self-neglect, suicidal ideation/behavior.

## PROVISION OF CULTURALLY APPROPRIATE SERVICES

Older people from black and minority ethnic (BME) backgrounds face major challenges in accessing substance-misuse services. These may include language barriers (Crome and Crome 2005). Individuals from some BME backgrounds have higher levels of alcohol misuse and resulting health problems than the general population, such as older Irish and South Asian (Sikh) male migrants to the United Kingdom (Rao 2006). Both alcohol misuse and ethnicity are bound to social disadvantage.

In the United Kingdom, the clustering of first-generation Irish people in areas of socioeconomic deprivation may explain, at least in part, their higher prevalence of alcohol use (Rao et al. 2008). Diversity also applies to older lesbian, gay, and bisexual alcohol misusers.

In the United States, cultural competence is equally important for African, Hispanic, and Asian Americans, as well as for other groups such as American Indians. Each racial/ethnic group is not homogenous, and may include many subcultures that may be influenced by cultural values such as traditional beliefs, family structure, lifestyle preferences, gender roles, degree of assimilation, and religious belief.

## Factors Influencing the Impact of Substance Use in Older People

The following factors influencing the impact of substance use in older people should be reflected in the assessment process.

### GENERATIONAL EFFECTS

The number of patients over the age of 50 expected to require treatment for substance misuse in the United States will increase from 1.4 million in 2000–2001 to 4.4 million in 2020 (Gfroerer et al. 2003; Colliver et al. 2006; Han et al. 2009). In Europe and the United Kingdom, it is estimated that the number of people over 65 with a substance use problem or needing treatment will more than double between 2001 and 2020 (European Monitoring Centre for Drugs and Drug Addiction 2008; National Health Service [NHS] Information Centre 2009a).

Alcohol is now by far the most commonly misused drug by people of all ages. In 2008, 21% of older men reported drinking more than 4 units of alcohol on at least one day a week, and 7% more than 8 units; 10% of older women said they drank more than 3 units of alcohol on at least one day in the week, and 2% of this age group drank at least 6 units (NHS Information Centre 2010).

In comparison, in 2001, 18% of older men said they drank more than 4 units of alcohol on at least one day a week, and 5% drank at least 8 units; 5% of older women reported drinking more than 3 units of alcohol on at least one day in the week, and 1% of this group drank at least 6 units (UK Office of National Statistics 2003).

Between 2005 and 2013, the percentage of men in the United Kingdom drinking 8 or more units of alcohol on any one day in past week reduced by only 5% in those aged 65 and over, compared with a reduction of 12% or more in all other age groups (Office of National Statistics 2014b). The highest mortality rate for alcohol related deaths was in men aged between 55 and 74 (Crome et al. 2011).

The number of older people between the ages of 60 and 74 admitted to hospitals in England with mental and behavioral disorders associated with alcohol use has risen by over 50% more than in the 15–59 age group over the past 10 years. People aged 75 and over with mental and behavioral disorders associated with alcohol experienced longer periods of hospitalization than their younger counterparts. In addition, the number of people aged 60 and over admitted to hospitals in England with alcohol-related amnestic syndrome has risen by over 140% over the past 10 years, compared with a rise of less than 10% in the 15–59 age group (Rao and Draper 2015).).

The number of deaths in the United Kingdom linked to alcohol more than doubled between 1992 and 2008, from 4,023 to 9,031, with the highest death rates found in men aged 55–74. Among women, those aged 55–74 had the highest alcohol-related death rates (UK Office for National Statistics 2009). These overall findings cannot be explained purely by rising numbers of older people in the general population, given that the population of people aged 65 and above in England and Wales increased by 11% between 2001 and 2011 (Office of National Statistics 2012).

The prevalence of illicit drug use is on the rise among people aged 50 years and over, and is projected to increase as baby boomers age. Fueling this increase is the large number of boomers and the popularity of substance use when they came of age. Past-year cannabis use among older adults aged more than 50 years in the general U.S. population increased from 0.7% in 1985 to 4.7% in 2007–2009. In the 2011 national survey in the United States, 7.9% of adults aged 50–54, 7.0% of adults aged 55–59, 4.4% of adults aged 60–64, and 1.0% of elders aged 65 years and above reported cannabis use in the past year (Chapman and Wu 2014). Data from the United Kingdom also suggested an increased prevalence of drug use. Cocaine, following marijuana, was the second-most-used drug by older adults.

However, substance-abuse-treatment admission data suggested a changing pattern of drug misuse, with decreased use of cocaine and increased use of marijuana and methamphetamine. Use patterns varied by age and gender, with females and older adults aged 65 and over more likely to use prescription-type drugs nonmedically than illicit drugs. Illicit drug use increased more among blacks than whites (Chapman and Wu 2014). Research is needed to better understand correlates of illicit drug use and predictors for developments of drug abuse and addiction among older adults.

Smoking tobacco is the largest cause of premature death in the United Kingdom, causing 106,000 deaths every year (Department of Health 2006). Although people over the age of 60 have the lowest prevalence of smoking, 14% of men and 12% of women in that age group smoke (Office of National Statistics 2013).

Older people receive the highest proportion of the prescription medication dispensed in the United Kingdom, often as multiple prescriptions, and there is a 10% chance that this is potentially inappropriate (McGrath et al. 2005). About a third of men and women over the age of 65 in private households take four or more prescribed medicines daily (Falaschetti et al. 2002).

The prevalence of psychotropic drug misuse is four times higher in older women than older men, and the risk of dependence is enhanced if the woman happens to be widowed, less educated, of lower income, in poor health, and/or with reduced social support (Simoni-Wastila and Yang 2006).

## PHYSIOLOGICAL CHANGES AND DRUG INTERACTIONS

Many age-related factors affect the way that drugs (including substances) interact with the body, either through the way the body affects drugs (pharmacokinetics) or the way in which drugs affect the body (pharmacodynamics). Both these processes may also affect the pharmacokinetics and pharmacodynamics of other drugs.

For example, older adults may have reduced and/or altered pharmacokinetics through kidney function (reduced renal blood flow and glomerular filtration rate), compromised liver function (reduced hepatic mass), as well as a decrease in total body water and reduced muscle mass (leading to a higher fat-to-water ratio) and a more permeable blood-brain barrier. In addition, age-related alterations in neurotransmitter function and receptor density can result in altered pharmacodynamics of substances on brain receptors (Jansen and Brouwers 2012).

### Alcohol

Older people are thought to be more sensitive to alcohol and show greater impairment than younger drinkers. However, it is unclear if these changes are due to pharmacokinetic or pharmacodynamic factors (Kalant 1998). Pharmacokinetic changes, including a decrease in volume of distribution, can result in increased alcohol levels, and therefore increased impairment, in older participants following standard doses of alcohol. Pharmacodynamic factors may include a decrease in sensitivity to the initial impairing effects or a decreased ability to develop tolerance to the effects of alcohol (Tupler et al. 1995).

## Opioids/Opiates

The primary route of elimination for opiates is via hepatic metabolism, with minor amounts excreted through urine or feces. Acute or chronic liver disease can therefore impair the metabolism of opiate drugs, with more pronounced side-effects, drowsiness, and depressed respiration.

## Benzodiazepines and Sedative-Hypnotics

Older individuals demonstrate an increased sensitivity to the effects of anxiolytics and hypnotics (Greenblatt et al. 1991). Decreased body water in older people can result in a prolonged duration of action for lipid-soluble medications like benzodiazepines. These drugs cause psychomotor and cognitive impairment (Buffett-Jerrott and Stewart 2002).

## Cocaine

Owing to cocaine's action on adrenergic and noradrenergic receptors, older people who use cocaine are at increased risk of serious adverse consequences, including cardiac arrhythmias, convulsions, and stroke.

## Cannabis

There remains a gap in our literature on the pharmacology of cannabis or its active compound (tetrahydrocannabinol [THC]) in older people. Given the increasing prevalence of cannabis use in this population, particularly as a result of increased prescription use of marijuana, there is a great need for improving knowledge in older populations.

## Alcohol–Drug Interactions

Alcohol interacts with numerous medications through pharmacokinetic and pharmacodynamic interactions. As alcohol is a central nervous system depressant, its sedative effect is enhanced by antidepressants, anxiolytics, anticonvulsants, opioid analgesics, and certain antihistamines, resulting in impaired balance, dizziness, and increased risk of injury. Risk of gastrointestinal bleeding increases with concomitant use of alcohol and non-steroidal anti-inflammatory drugs (NSAIDs). Alcohol affects the metabolism of various medications, mediated by the cytochrome P450 enzyme system, depending upon the type of drug and pattern of alcohol consumption.

Chronic heavy drinkers have been shown to have amplified CYP2E1 enzyme activity, which can enhance the metabolism of many drugs that are CYP2E1 substrates, including warfarin, phenytoin, propranolol, and isoniazid.

However, during acute heavy drinking, alcohol may compete with these drugs for liver enzymes, thereby decreasing the metabolism of the drugs. For example, acute alcohol consumption may increase anticoagulation by decreasing warfarin metabolism, whereas chronic alcohol intake decreases anticoagulation by increasing warfarin metabolism. Potentiation of blood-pressure-lowering effects may occur with anti-hypertensive drugs

Common interactions with alcohol in older people include arthritis and pain medications, H2-antagonists, antidepressants, and antihypertensive medications attributed to hazardous drinking. Pain medications are the most common medications used by at-risk drinkers (Moore et al. 2006).

Women are at particular risk of drug interactions with alcohol (Stockley's Drug Interactions 2012). Overall, women have a higher fat-to-water ratio than men. Women also let a higher amount of alcohol into their bloodstream after drinking a similar amount and concentration of alcohol when compared with men, so that a woman of the same weight as a man would end up with a 50% higher blood-alcohol level.

Commonly prescribed drugs that are known to interact with alcohol are listed next.

### Analgesics
Painkillers containing morphine and codeine-containing compounds can increase the effects of alcohol on attention and coordination, as well as on breathing, which has resulted in some fatalities, particularly with *dextropropoxyphene*. Alcohol has also been associated with the rapid release of morphine from extended-release preparations.

### Antibiotics
Alcohol can cause a small reduction in the absorption of *erythromycin*. "Disulfiram-like reactions" can occur in those who drink alcohol and take second-generation cephalosporins (*cefamandole, cefmenoxime, cefoperazone, cefotetan, latamoxef, sulfamethoxale/trimethoprim, metronidazole, isoniazid, and ketoconazole*).

*Disulfiram* (Antabuse) is sometimes used in the treatment of alcohol dependence (under specialist supervision), producing an unpleasant reaction after drinking small amount of alcohol. This includes flushing of the face, throbbing headache, palpitations, nausea, and vomiting. This reaction can last for several hours. Small amounts of alcohol such as those included in many oral medicines may be sufficient to precipitate a reaction—even toiletries and mouthwashes that contain alcohol should be avoided (British National Formulary 2014).

## Anti-allergic Drugs
Some drugs used to treat allergies can cause drowsiness, which can be increased by alcohol. These include *hydroxyzine, diphenhydramine,* and *promethazine.*

## Anticoagulants
Alcohol can affect the blood level of *warfarin* in two ways. Acute intake can increase blood levels of warfarin, and chronic drinking can reduce blood levels.

## Anti-emetics
*Metoclopramide* can increase the rate of alcohol absorption; thereby raising blood alcohol levels.

## Anti-epilepsy and Mood Stabilizing Drugs
Heavy drinking might increase the rate of which *carbamazepine* is cleared from the body, thereby lowering its level in the bloodstream. Acute intoxication from alcohol can be considerably increased by taking *meprobamate.*

## Anti-hypertensive Drugs
Drinking over recommended limits over a long period of time raises blood pressure and may reduce the effectiveness of drugs used to treat high blood pressure. Some people also experience low blood pressure, dizziness, and fainting shortly after having drunk alcohol. The risk of these interactions increases with age. Patients who take *glyceryl trinitrate* for angina pectoris while drinking alcohol may feel faint and dizzy.

## Food
Food and milk decrease the absorption of alcohol, and meals increase the metabolism of alcohol by the gut wall. The concentration and fizziness of alcoholic drinks can alter the rate of absorption of alcohol. Foods rich in serotonin (e.g., bananas) taken with alcohol might produce adverse effects such as diarrhea and headache.

## Nicotine
*Nicotine patches* may increase the effect of alcohol on heart rate and reduce the time taken to reach highest blood alcohol levels.

## Over-the-Counter Drugs
*Aspirin* can interact with alcohol to damage the stomach lining in people drinking over recommended limits over long periods of time, which may

lead to an increased likelihood of bleeding into the gut. This is also the case for other *non-steroidal anti-inflammatory drugs*. *Paracetamol* can interact with alcohol in people drinking over recommended limits over long periods of time and may lead to liver damage. *Panax ginseng* (*Asian ginseng*) increases the clearance of alcohol from the body and lowers blood alcohol levels.

## Psychotropic Drugs

All drugs that may cause drowsiness have the potential to enhance the effects of alcohol in this sensation; these include *amitriptyline, clozapine, mirtazapine, olanzapine, quetiapine, trazadone,* and *zuclopenthixol. Benzodiazepines* and related drugs for anxiety and sleep problems increase the effect of alcohol on attention and coordination. Alcohol may also increase the plasma levels of *diazepam.*

## Opiate–Drug Interactions

There has traditionally been a clear distinction between opiates and opioids. *Opiates* are naturally occurring and are derived from morphine and codeine; *opioids* are synthetic or semi-synthetic drugs based on opiate structure. Although the two have been used interchangeably, it is now more common to refer to both as *opiates*.

### BUPRENORPHINE, METHADONE, AND LOPERAMIDE

These three are inhibited by antibiotics (*ciprofloxacillin, clarithromycin, erythromycin, itraconazole, ketoconazole,* and *ritonavir*), the anti-hypertensive *diltiazem, grapefruit juice,* and the antidepressant *nefazodone.*

They are induced by drugs for epilepsy (*carbamazepine, phenytoin, phenobarbitone*), the antibiotic *rifampicin,* and the herbal drug *St John's wort.*

### OXYCODONE, CODEINE, DIHYDROCODEINE, AND TRAMADOL

These drugs are inhibited by the antidepressants *fluoxetine* and *paroxetine,* the anti-emetic *metoclopramide,* and the anti-arrhythmic drug *quinidine.*

### PENTAZOCINE

This is inhibited by the anti-arrhythmic drug *amiodarone;* the beta-blocker *propranolol;* antibiotics *ciprofloxacillin* and *rifampicin;* antidepressants *duloxetine* and *fluvoxamine,* as well as the antipsychotics *olanzapine, clozapine.* Its metabolism is also inhibited by caffeine.

Morphine, naloxone, and naltrexone are minimally affected by these pathways and therefore have clinically insignificant drug interactions with non-substances.

### Nicotine–Drug Interactions

Nicotine alone has few interactions with other drugs. Its metabolism is inhibited by *ketoconazole, isoniazid,* and grape juice. *Phenobarbitone* and *rifampicin* are associated with enzyme induction. However, the most common exposure to nicotine is through tobacco smoke. This smoke contains polycyclic aromatic hydrocarbons (PAH), chemicals that affect the same enzyme pathway affected by metabolism of the drug *pentazocine.* However, in this case, smoking is associated with enzyme induction or inhibition of the drugs affecting the metabolism of this opiate. The metabolism of the anti-epilepsy drug *carbamazepine* is induced by *chronic smoking.*

### Drug Interactions with Anxiolytics and Sedative-Hypnotics

The sedatives and anxiolytics *benzodiazepines* and *buspirone,* as well as the benzodiazepine antagonist *flumazenil,* are metabolized by the same pathway as *buprenorphine, methadone,* and *loperamide* and are therefore induced and inhibited by the same drugs as these opiates. The same is true of the hypnotic drug zopiclone.

The increased presence of substances in the body at higher concentration levels suggests that older adults may be significantly more susceptible to substance-abuse problems at low dosage levels. This also includes alcohol (Crome et al. 2011). The threshold between use and abuse for the average adult may be simply too high for the aging adult.

An emerging body of literature predicts a rise in the use of alcohol and psychotropic medications among older adults in the future. A study of the National Health Interview and Examination Survey found that the prevalence of combined use of alcohol and psychotropic medication was 7.6% (Du et al. 2008). Considering the vulnerability of this population, it is imperative to take into account the impact of concurrent use of alcohol and medication in older adults.

## The Effect of Mental Health Problems on Treatment

It is recognized that people with comorbidity are beset with numerous predicaments. The problems they are faced with may have a long or brief history. Mental health problems can be the main reason for substance use in the first instance, can result from substance use, and could be responsible for lack of response to treatment.

Mental health problems may interfere with patients' complying with the logistics of treatment, whether this means getting to appointments, adherence to medication, insight, and judgement. Other considerations include:

- History of abuse (compounded by socioeconomic deprivation)
- Early onset of substance use is more likely to lead to continuation across the life course and is related to the development of mental health problems
- The patient's awareness of the relationship between substance use and their mental health
- Polysubstance misuse may result in unpredictability as a result of combinations of licit and illicit substance use taken impulsively
- Initiation of substance use later in life may be associated with depression, anxiety, psychosis, and cognitive dysfunction
- Non-response to treatment may reflect cognitive impairment or a missed diagnosis of depression
- Use of over-the-counter and prescribed medications in a way that is not in accordance with medical instructions, particularly in patients with chronic physical disorders

Whether the substance use predates the mental health problem or not, it is vital to ensure that patients are offered the variety of treatment options available for all conditions in an integrated and coordinated package of care. It is also fundamental that patients be monitored with regularity to ensure that, if their condition or situation changes, appropriate steps can be taken.

## Conclusion

This chapter has outlined a systematic approach to the assessment of older people presenting with substance misuse in its different forms and offering a broader overview that includes challenges inherent in the presentation and detection of substance misuse problems in later life.

Commenting on the assessment and treatment of alcohol misuse after establishing the very first treatment centers for alcohol misuse in the United Kingdom, Edwards (1967) noted,

> It would be too optimistic to suppose that the relative under-representation of subjects in the older age groups among clients of information centres is just explained by older people having generally got the treatment they required or having reverted to normal drinking; it seems likely that this finding is in part a hint of the diminished life expectancy of the alcoholic.)

Almost 50 years later, improvements in healthcare and welfare in the United Kingdom have increased longevity. In addition, the progressive increase in substance use in the baby boomer generation of older people who began to cross the age of 65 in 2011 now means a heavier clinical burden for clinical services.

At present, substance misuse in older people is still largely confined to alcohol, sedatives, hypnotics, nicotine, and opiates. However, the clinical field of substance misuse is likely to change again in another 50 years, particularly with rises in lifetime illicit drug use by younger people.

# References

Aalto M, Alho H, Halme JT, Seppa K. The Alcohol Use Disorders Identification Test (AUDIT) and its derivatives in screening for heavy drinking among the elderly. *Int J Geriatr Psych* 2011;26(9):881–885.

American Psychiatric Association. *Diagnostic and Statistical Manual of Mental Disorders* (5th ed.). Washington, DC: American Psychiatric Association; 2013.

Anetzberger A. The reality of elder abuse. *Clin Gerontologist* 2005;28(1–2):1–25.

Bartels SJ, Blow FC, Van Citters AD, et al. Dual diagnosis among older adults: Co-occurring substance abuse and psychiatric illness. *J Dual Diagn* 2006;2(3):9–30.

Berks J, McCormick R. Screening for alcohol misuse in elderly primary care patients: A systematic literature review. *Int Psychogeriatr* 2008;20(6):1090–1103.

Blow FC, Gillespie BW, Barry KL, Mudd SA, Hill EM. Brief screening for alcohol problems in elderly populations using the Short Michigan Alcoholism Screening Test–Geriatric Version (SMAST-G). *Alcohol Clin Exper Res* 1998;22(Suppl):131A.

Bradley KA, DeBenedetti AF, Volk RJ, Williams EC, Frank D, Kivlahan DR. AUDIT-C as a brief screen for alcohol misuse in primary care. *Alcohol Clin Exper Res* 2007;31(7):1208–1217.

Bradley KA, McDonell MB, Bush K, Kivlahan DR, Diehr P, Finn SD. The AUDIT Alcohol Consumption Questions: Reliability, validity, and responsiveness to change in older male primary care patients. *Alcohol Clin Exper Res* 1998;22(8):1842–1849.

Amin S, Clarke SE, Halai M, Fowlie K, Villen BG, & McFarlane AMG. *British national formulary*. London: BMJ Group & Pharmaceutical Press; 2014.

Buffett-Jerrot SE, Stewart SH. Cognitive and sedative effects of benzodiazepine use. *Curr Pharmaceut Des* 2002;8(1):45–58.

Chapman SLC, Wu L-T. Epidemiology and demography of illicit drug use and drug use disorders among older adults aged 50 and older. In Crome I, Wu L-T, Rao TR, Crome P, Eds., *Substance use in older people*. London: Wiley-Blackwell; 2014:91–208.

Colliver JD, Compton WM, Gfroerer JC, Condon T. Projecting drug use among aging baby boomers in 2020. *Ann Epidemiol* 2006;16(4):257–265.

Conwell Y, Van Orden K, Caine ED. Suicide in older adults. *Psychiatr Clin N Am* 2011;34(2):451–468.

Crome IB, Ghodse A-H. Drug misuse in medical patients. In G Lloyd & E Guthrie, Eds., *Handbook of liaison psychiatry*. Cambridge, UK: Cambridge University Press; 2007:180–220.

Crome I, Crome P. "At your age, what does it matter?" Myths and realities about older people who use substances. *Drugs* 2005;12, 343–347.

Crome I, Crome P, Rao R. Addiction and ageing—Awareness, assessment and action. *Age Ageing* 2011a;40(6):657–658.

Crome I, Dar K, Janikiewicz S, et al. *Our Invisible Addicts (College Report CR165)*. London: Royal College of Psychiatrists; 2011b.

Davis L, Uezato A, Newell, Frazier E. Major depression and comorbid substance use disorders. *Curr Opin Psychiatry* 2008;21(1):14–18.

Devanand DP. Comorbid psychiatric disorders in late life depression. *Biol Psychiatry* 2002; 52(3):236–242.

Dong X. Advancing the field of elder abuse: Future directions and policy implications. *J Am Geriatr Soc* 2012;60(11):2151–2156.

Du Y, Scheidt-Nave C, Knopf H. Use of psychotropic drugs and alcohol among non-institutionalised elderly adults in Germany. *Pharmacopsychiatry* 2008;41(6):242–251.

Edwards G, Fisher MK, Hawker A, Hensman C. Clients of alcoholism information centres. *BMJ* 1967;4(5575):346–349.

Gossop M. Substance use among older adults: a neglected problem."*Drugs in focus"—Briefing of the European Monitoring Centre for Drugs and Drug Addiction* (18). 2008.

Falaschetti E, Malbut K, Primatesta P. *The general health of older people and their use of health services (health survey for England 2000)*. London: The Stationery Office; 2002.

Fleming MF, Balousek SL, Klessig CL, Mundt MP, Brown DT. Substance use disorders in a primary care sample receiving daily opioid therapy. *J Pain* 2007;8(7):573–582.

Folstein MF, Folstein SE, & McHugh PR. "Mini-mental state": a practical method for grading the cognitive state of patients for the clinician. *J Psychiatr Res* 1975;12(3):189–198.

Friedman LS, Avila S, Tanouye K, Joseph K. A case-control study of severe physical abuse of older adults. *J Am Geriatr Soc* 2011;59(3):417–422.

Gfroerer J, Penne M, Pemberton M, Folsom R. Substance abuse treatment need among older adults in 2020: The impact of the aging baby-boom cohort. *Drug Alcohol Depend* 2003;69(2):127–135.

Greenblatt DJ, Harmatz JS, Shader RI. Clinical pharmacokinetics of anxiolytics and hypnotics in the elderly. Therapeutic considerations (Part II). *Clin Pharmacokinet* 1991;21(4): 262–273.

Edwards G, Fisher MK, Hawker A, Hensman C. Clients of alcoholism information centres. *BMJ* 1967;4(5575):346-349.

Hawton K, Casañas I, Comabella C, Haw C, Saunders K. Risk factors for suicide in individuals with depression: A systematic review. *J Affect Disord* 2013;147(1–3):17–28.

Hazelton L, Sterns GL, Chisholm T. Decision-making capacity and alcohol abuse: Clinical and ethical considerations in personal care choices. *Gen Hosp Psychiatry* 2003;25(2):130–135.

Jansen PA, Brouwers JR. Clinical pharmacology in old persons. *Scientifica*, 2012.

Kalant H. Pharmacological interactions of aging and alcohol, in alcohol problems and aging. In: Gomberg HA, Zucker RA, Eds., *NIAAA research monograph no. 33*. Bethesda, MD: National Institute of Health; 1998:98–4163.

Manthorpe J. Elder abuse. In: Dening T, Thomas A, Eds., *The Oxford Textbook of Old Age Psychiatry* (pp. pp.779–783). Oxford, UK: Oxford University Press; 2013.

Mayo-Smith MF, Beecher LH, Fischer TL, et al. Management of alcohol withdrawal delirium: an evidence-based practice guideline. *Arch Intern Med* 2004;164(13):1405-1412.

McGrath A, Crome P, Crome IB. Substance misuse in the older population. *Postgrad Med J* 2005;81(954):228–231.

Ministry of Justice. *MCA code of practice*. London: Ministry of Justice; 2007.

Mioshi E, Dawson K, Mitchell J, et al. The Addenbrooke's Cognitive Examination Revised (ACE-R): A brief cognitive test battery for dementia screening. *Int J Geriatr Psych* 2006;21(11):1078–1085.

Moore AA, Giuli L, Gould R, et al. Alcohol use, comorbidity, and mortality. *J Am Geriatr Soc* 2006;54(5):757–762.

National Collaborating Centre for Mental Health. Psychosis with Coexisting Substance Misuse: The NICE Guideline on Assessment and Management in Adults and Young People (No. 120). Washington, DC: RCPsych Publications; 2011.

National Institute on Alcohol Abuse and Alcoholism. *Helping patients who drink too much: a clinician's guide*. Bethesda, MD: Department of Health and Human Services, National Institutes of Health, National Institute on Alcohol Abuse and Alcoholism; 2007.

NHS Information Centre. *Statistics on drug misuse: England, 2009.* London: Health and Social Care Information Centre; 2009a.

NHS Information Centre. *Statistics on alcohol: England, 2008.* London: Health and Social Care Information Centre; 2010.

Office of National Statistics. *Statistics on Alcohol: England, 2001.* London: Office of National Statistics; 2003.

Office of National Statistics. Alcohol deaths: UK rates increase in 2008. 2009. At http://www.statistics.gov.uk/cci/nugget.asp?id=1091 (accessed February 7, 2015).

Office of National Statistics. *2011 census, population and household estimates for the United Kingdom.* London: Office of National Statistics; 2012.

Office of National Statistics. *General lifestyle survey 2011.* London: Office of National Statistics; 2013.

Office of National Statistics. *Suicides in the United Kingdom, 2012 registrations.* London: Office of National Statistics; 2014a.

Office of National Statistics. *Statistics on alcohol.* London: Office of National Statistics; 2014b.

Peterson K. Biomarkers for alcohol use and abuse—a summary. *Alcohol Res Health* 2005;28(1):30–37.

Philpot M, Pearson N, Petratou V, et al. Screening for problem drinking in older people referred to a mental health service: A comparison of CAGE and AUDIT. *Aging Ment Health* 2003;7(3):171–175.

Rao R. Alcohol misuse and ethnicity: hidden populations need specific services—and more research. *BMJ* 2006;332(7543):682.

Rao R, Draper B. Alcohol-related brain damage in older people. *Lancet* 2016;2(8):674–675.

Rao R, Crome I, Crome P, et al. *Substance misuse in older people: an information guide.* London: Royal College of Psychiatrists; 2015.

Rao R, Wolff K, Marshall EJ. Alcohol use and misuse in older people: a local prevalence study comparing English and Irish inner-city residents living in the UK. *J Subst Use* 2008; 13(1):17–26.

Roberts AM, Marshall EJ, Macdonald AJD. Which screening test for alcohol consumption is best associated with "at risk" drinking in older primary care attenders? *Prim Care Ment Health* 2005;3:131–138.

Simoni-Wastila L, Yang HK. Psychoactive drug abuse in older adults. *Am J Geriatr Pharmacother* 2006;4(4):380–394.

Society for the Study of Addiction website. At www.addiction-ssa.org. (Last accessed February 2015.)

Baxter K. *Stockley's drug interactions.* London: Pharmaceutical Press; 2012.

Substance Abuse and Mental Health Services Administration. *The NSDUH report: illicit drug use among older adults.* Rockville, MD: SAMHSA; 2011.

Tupler LA, Hege S, Ellinwood EHJr. Alcohol pharmacodynamics in young-elderly adults contrasted with young and middle-aged subjects. *Psychopharmacol (Berl)*, 1995;118(4): 460–470.

World Health Organization. *ICD-10 Classifications of Mental and Behavioural Disorder: Clinical Descriptions and Diagnostic Guidelines.* Geneva: World Health Organization; 1992.

World Health Organization. *Missing voices: views of older persons on elder abuse.* Geneva: World Health Organization; 2002.

World Health Organization. *Elder abuse and alcohol.* Geneva: World Health Organization; 2005.

Zahr NM, Kaufman KL, Harper CG. Clinical and pathological features of alcohol-related brain damage. *Nat Rev Neurol* 2011;7(5):284–294.

# CHAPTER 9

# Sex Differences in Late-Life Substance-Use Disorders

*Elizabeth Evans and Maria A. Sullivan*

## Introduction

Sex differences in research were largely ignored until the 1970s. In part prompted by the women's rights movement, researchers and the federal government began to focus more attention on the need for, and importance of, research and treatment for women (Lex 1991, Zweben 2009, Brady and Randall 1999). In the 1980s, the U.S. Public Health Service created its Women's Task Force, with the purpose of correcting the "imbalance in knowledge" in substance-use research in women versus men (Ray and Braude 1986). In 1986, the National Institutes of Health (NIH) developed specific guidelines regarding the inclusion of women as subjects in clinical research (NIH 1986).

While there is now a growing understanding of the important biological and psychosocial differences between women and men, the literature on sex differences in late-life substance use remains relatively sparse (Hamilton and Grella 2009, Szwabo 1993). As the population ages, and particularly with the aging of the "baby boomers," clinicians will be seeing an increasing number of older adults of both genders with substance-use disorders. One recent study estimated that the number of adults aged 50 and older with substance-use problems will double, from 2.8 million (annual average) in 2002–2006 to 5.7 million in 2020 (Han et al. 2009). Understanding sex differences specific to older adults, therefore, is an area of increasing relevance for clinicians.

Older adults, and specifically older women, represent a particularly vulnerable group, with increased exposure to prescription drugs with abuse potential (Wu and Blazer 2011), a tendency to develop addiction more quickly than their male counterparts (National Center on Addiction and Substance Abuse Columbia 1998), and higher rates of mortality as a result of substance use (National Center on Addiction and Substance Abuse Columbia 1998). Yet addiction in women aged 50 and older is often underestimated (Koechl et al. 2012), undetected, and undertreated, with one study estimating that only 0.6% of older women who may benefit from treatment are actually receiving treatment (National Center on Addiction and Substance Abuse Columbia 1998).

This chapter will provide an overview of what is currently known about sex differences in late-life substance use, including the epidemiology of alcohol, prescription medications, illicit drugs, and nicotine. We will discuss risk factors, comorbidities, illness course, and treatment specific to this population. The aim is to help clinicians better identify substance use in this population, as well as to plan, tailor, and implement effective treatment interventions for older adults.

## Epidemiology

While prevalence rates of substance use in older adults are increasingly being reported (Blow and Barry 2009), data about gender differences in this population remain less evident, with many studies and surveys failing to look at rates in women versus men. Rates also vary widely across research studies, surveys, and reports, which may in part stem from varying definitions of "older adult," as well as varying definitions of "misuse" or "use disorder." Additionally, rates are typically derived using screening and assessment instruments developed for younger populations, and therefore may be underestimated. This issue may be particularly relevant for older women, as their symptom profiles may not be well addressed by the standard screening instruments (Blow 2000). For the purposes of this chapter, we will define "older adult" as 50 years old and above.

### ALCOHOL

As noted, varying definitions may have led to differing estimates of alcohol misuse in older adults. While the *Diagnostic and Statistical Manual of Mental Disorders* (DSM) offers criteria for alcohol abuse and dependence, and most recently with DSM-5, alcohol use disorder, many surveys utilize consumption-based measures (Sacco et al. 2009) to identify problem drinking. In 1995, the National Institute on Alcohol Abuse and Alcoholism (NIAAA) defined moderate drinking for persons aged 65 and older as no more than one drink a day (NIAAA 1995), with standards that may be stricter for older women; i.e., less than one drink per day and a maximum of four drinks per week (Sacco et al. 2009). However, more recent guidelines provided by the NIAAA are less strict and recommend that adults over age 65 who are healthy and do not take medications should not have more than three drinks a day or seven drinks a week (NIAAA 2015).

Older men report higher rates of alcohol use than older women. Data from the National Survey on Drug Use and Health (NSDUH) found that 66% of males and 55% of the females (at least 50 years old) reported alcohol use during the past year (Blazer and Wu 2009). In the 2001–2002 National Epidemiologic Survey on Alcohol and Related Conditions (NESARC), 37% of women and 55% of men aged 65 and older reported "current" alcohol use (defined as consuming at least 12 drinks in the past year) (Balsa et al. 2008). A multi-site primary care study of over 5,000 individuals aged 60 and older found that 15% of men and 12% of women regularly drank in excess of limits recommended by the National Institute of Alcohol Abuse and Alcoholism (defined at that time as more than seven drinks per week for women and more than 14 drinks per week for men) (Adams et al. 1996). In the same cohort, when using the CAGE questionnaire, the authors found that 3.1% of women screened positive within the past three months for "alcohol abuse" (defined as two or more affirmative answers); lowering the cut-off to one or more affirmative answers, 8.6% of women and 19.6% of men were CAGE-positive (Adams et al. 1996). A survey conducted by the National Center on Addiction and Substance Abuse (CASA), at Columbia University, found that primary care physicians estimated that 7% of their female patients over the age of 59 might have abused alcohol, although they did not query specifically if this was based on DSM-IV criteria for alcohol abuse (National Center on Addiction and Substance Abuse Columbia 1998). NESARC data from 2001–2002 looking at criteria met for DSM-IV diagnosis of abuse or dependence in older adults revealed smaller percentages, with 12-month prevalence rate for a DSM-IV diagnosis of alcohol abuse or dependence in men aged 65 and older of 2.75%, and for women aged 65 and older, 0.5% (Grant et al. 2004). When a broader definition of "older adults" (50 years or older) was used, a recent epidemiological study found that 5% of men and 1.4% of women had a past-year alcohol use disorder (Wu and Blazer 2014).

In most Western countries, alcohol consumption among women and older adults continues to increase. Geels et al. (2013) found that the previous gap between age of initiation of alcohol use, onset of regular drinking, and first alcohol intoxication has almost entirely closed. These findings highlight the importance of increased clinical focus on the issue of alcohol-use disorder in older women.

Results from a European household survey reveal that both male gender and higher socioeconomic status are independently associated with higher alcohol consumption (Nuevo et al. 2015). Similarly, an Australian study of adults aged 45 and over found that factors associated with alcohol use alone were age 45–64, male gender, higher socioeconomic status (SES), lower psychological distress, and no recent depression treatment (Bonevski et al. 2014). While fewer older women than men drink over the recommended limit, and women have lower rates of abuse and dependence, older women may be adversely impacted by smaller amounts of alcohol and therefore may not meet consumption-based cutoffs for at-risk drinking, but may still experience problems due to alcohol (Blow 2000, National Center on Addiction and Substance Abuse Columbia 1998). At all ages, women tend to experience the negative consequences of alcohol at lower levels of consumption and after much shorter periods of time, a concept known as *telescoping* (Zweben 2009). Older women may be particularly vulnerable and sensitive to the effects of alcohol, in part due to a decrease in total body mass relative to their male counterparts, and changes in metabolism that occur with age (Blow and Barry 2002). Finally, older women are more likely than men to develop alcohol problems for the first time later in life (Blow 2000, Gomberg 1995, National Center on Addiction and Substance Abuse Columbia 1998, Gomberg 1994); approximately half of all cases of alcoholism among older women begin after age 59, versus only a quarter among men (National Center on Addiction and Substance Abuse Columbia 1998).

## PRESCRIPTION DRUGS

Abuse of prescription medications is an escalating problem. The two classes of medications most subject to abuse in older adults, which we will focus on in this chapter, are the benzodiazepine sedative hypnotics and the opioid analgesics (Simoni-Wastila and Yang 2006). Stimulants and non-benzodiazepine sedative hypnotics are also medications with abuse potential; however, there are few data specific to older adults. Older adults are a particularly vulnerable population; about a quarter to a third of all prescribed medications, often including opioids and benzodiazepines, are prescribed to adults over the age of 65 (Gossop and Moos 2008, Culberson and Ziska 2008, Simoni-Wastila and Yang 2006). They are also subject to higher rates of polypharmacy and exposure to potentially inappropriate medications, compared to younger people. Moreover, older adults with opioid use disorders (OUD) are more likely to die from any cause than younger adults with OUD, and drug-related mortality rates to not decline with advancing age (Larney et al. 2015).

Women are prescribed psychoactive medications more than men. One study using data from the National Medical Expenditures Survey (NMES) found the rate of prescription drug use in women to be 70.9%, versus 52.5% in men, and that being female increased the odds of using any abusable prescription medication by 48% (Simoni-Wastila 2000). Data from the Addiction Severity Index–Multimedial Version Connect database found that women of all ages were more likely than men to report use of any prescription opioid (28% females vs. 21% males) and abuse of any prescription opioid (15.4% versus 11.1%) in the past month (Green et al. 2009). Older women are specifically more likely than men to be prescribed narcotics and benzodiazepines, and are more likely to be long-term users of these substances (Simoni-Wastila 2000, Simoni-Wastila and Yang 2006). CASA's physician survey found that 11%, or 2.8 million, women aged 60 and older may be abusing prescription medications (National Center on Addiction and Substance Abuse Columbia 1998).

## ILLICIT DRUGS

Clinicians will be confronted with increased rates of illicit drug use in older adults, not only because of the general increase in the population size due to the aging of the baby boomers, but also because of the cohort-specific effect that the baby boomers have much higher rates of illicit drug use (Johnson and Gerstein 1998, Han et al. 2009). Data from the 2011 National Survey on Drug Use and Health (NSDUH) revealed that, among adults aged 50–59, the rate of current (past-month) illicit drug use increased from 2.7–5.8% between 2002 and 2010. Among adults aged 50–54, the rate increased from 3.4% in 2002 to 7.2% in 2010, with rates in those aged 55–59 years old increasing from 1.9–4.1% during the same time period (Substance Abuse and Mental Health Services Administration 2012). Of note, the NSDUH definition of illicit drugs includes not only marijuana/hashish, cocaine/crack, heroin, hallucinogens, and inhalants, but also prescription psychotherapeutics used non-medically. While the numbers of women using illicit drugs may be expected to grow, as noted, the current data reveal that very few older women use illicit drugs. Data from CASA's analysis of the National Household Survey on Drug Abuse in 1995 reported only 3.8% of older women (versus 7.6% of older men) say they have ever tried illegal drugs (National Center on Addiction and Substance Abuse Columbia 1998). CASA's survey of physicians found that, on average, physicians reported only 2% of their older female patients had problems with illicit drug use (National Center on Addiction and Substance Abuse Columbia 1998). Among those women abusing illicit substances, data suggest that they may have higher rates of polysubstance use (Grella and Lovinger 2012, National Center on Addiction and Substance Abuse Columbia 1998).

Among older adults, substance use has increased and is associated with unprotected intercourse (Brennan-Ing et al. 2014). Aging HIV-positive populations have high rates of substance use than their non-infected peers. In a sample ($n = 239$) of HIV-positive bisexual and gay men aged 50 and older, bisexual men were more likely to report cigarette, cocaine, crack, and heroin use compared to gay men. However, bisexual men were less likely to use "club drugs" (e.g. ecstasy, ketamine, *gamma*-Hydroxybutyric acid [GHB]), crystal methamphetamine, or nitrate inhalers than gay men. In particular, a logistical regression analysis found that nitrate inhalers ("poppers") and erectile dysfunction (ED) medications, used at higher rates by gay men, were associated with an increased rate of unprotected intercourse in this population (Brennan-Ing et al. 2014).

## NICOTINE

In the United States, approximately 17% of older women are addicted to nicotine, compared to about 20% of older men (National Center on Addiction and Substance Abuse Columbia 1998). The rates are lower for older adults of both sexes than for their younger cohorts (NSDUH 2012, CASA 1998, Giovino et al. 1995). Across all ages, males have higher rates of use than females; however, the difference between the two sexes becomes less pronounced with age (NSDUH 2012). One out of nine older women and one out of six older men smokes at least a pack per day (National Center on Addiction and Substance Abuse Columbia 1998). Interestingly, while rates for both adult men and women have decreased from 1965 to the present, rates of women aged 65 and older have remained around 10–13% (National Center on Addiction and Substance Abuse Columbia 1998, Husten et al. 1996, King et al. 1990). Furthermore, there are some data suggesting that fewer older women quit smoking, with one study estimating 73.3% of older women who have ever smoked have quit, compared to 77.5% of such men (National Center on Addiction and Substance Abuse Columbia 1998, King et al. 1990).

## Risk Factors

Older women face a number of social, psychological, and medical problems that may specifically impact their risk of substance-use disorders. Women of all ages experience more stigma and societal disapproval for this activity than their male counterparts (Blume 1986, Beckman and Amaro 1986). Alcoholic women are more likely than alcoholic men to have a family history of alcoholism and to be married to an alcoholic spouse (Lex 1991, Brady and Randall 1999). Furthermore, one study by McKenna and Pickens found that female alcoholics are more than twice as likely as male alcoholics to have been raised by two alcoholic parents (McKenna and Pickens 1981). Wilsnack and colleagues found that women who reported being sexually abused in childhood were more likely than other women to have experienced alcohol-related problems and to have one or more symptoms of alcohol dependence (Wilsnack et al. 1997). Another study found that women in treatment for alcohol abuse were significantly more likely to report childhood sexual abuse and a history of physical violence compared with women in the general population (Miller et al. 1993).

Women have longer life expectancies than men, are more likely to live alone than men at an older age, are more likely to be widowed, and are more likely to suffer financial troubles, and therefore may be at a greater risk for substance-use disorders than older men (Blow and Barry 2002, National Center on Addiction and Substance Abuse Columbia 1998). Social isolation has also been identified as a risk factor for developing a substance-related disorder later in life (Koechl et al. 2012), and both social isolation and female sex have been found to be risk factors for prescription drug abuse in older adults (Wastila and Yang 2006). Women who have been widowed may increase their alcohol intake for at least the first year after the loss (Gomberg 1994), and among older women, psychoactive drug use is associated with recent divorce and widowhood (Simoni-Wastila and Yang 2006). In CASA's analysis of the National Household Survey on Drug Abuse, older women who were widowed were more likely to smoke cigarettes (21.2%) than were married women (13.9%), although the sample size was small, and this was not statistically significant (National Center on Addiction and Substance Abuse Columbia 1998). Despite this finding, there are some data that spouse-specific events may be more likely to influence older men's alcohol consumption than older women, which is consistent with a belief that the loss of wife for a male is more socially isolating than the loss of husband for an older female (Glass et al. 1995). Retirement has also been found to represent a risk factor for increased alcohol consumption in older men, whereas a similar association was not observed among women (Wang et al. 2014). And while stressful life events are associated with older men and women, an analysis of Wave 2 (2004–2005) NESARC data found that older men with alcohol use disorder (AUD) are at increased risk for crime victimization. In addition, perceived stress appears to have a dampening effect on alcohol use among older women and a positive association with AUD among older men (Sacco et al. 2014). In contrast, in a sample of late–middle-aged adults, residing in neighborhoods with more psychosocial hazards was more associated with binge drinking for females but not for males (Rudolph et al. 2013). These findings highlight gender-specific differences in alcohol consumption as a behavioral response to subjective stress and adverse environmental conditions in older adults.

Gender differences in coping with, and expressing, anxiety and distress may contribute to women's greater psychotropic use; there are some data that women in particular tend to rely on psychoactive drugs, or a combination of alcohol and psychoactive drugs, to cope with stress (Mellinger et al. 1978, Mellinger et al. 1984, Simoni-Wastila 2000, National Center on Addiction and Substance Abuse Columbia 1998). In younger women, low self-esteem in pre-teen and teenage girls has been identified as a risk factor for becoming a later problem drinker; this was not seen in their male counterparts (Blume 1986). (Psychiatric comorbidities will be discussed in depth in the next section of this chapter, "Comorbidity.")

Numerous studies have documented that women are more likely than men to be exposed to psychoactive prescription drugs with abuse potential (Simoni-Wastila et al. 2004). In a 2000 study, Simoni-Wastila found that women were 41% more likely to receive a narcotic analgesic (e.g., morphine, acetaminophen with codeine, propoxyphene), and that, controlling for other factors, being female rather than male increases the likelihood of anx-iolytic (e.g., diazepam, alprazolam, triazolam) use by 51% (Simoni-Wastila 2000). In particular, older women are more likely than older men to receive prescriptions for benzodiazepines (Blow and Barry 2002). Furthermore, the prescribing of potentially inappropriate medications, including but not limited to psychoactive drugs, contributes to adverse outcomes in the el-derly and may also contribute to abuse and addiction (Beers et al. 1991, The American Geriatrics Society 2012, Spore et al. 1997, National Center on Addiction and Substance Abuse Columbia 1998). In 1991, Beers et al., using expert-based consensus, published a comprehensive set of explicit criteria for inadequate prescribing, and focused on medications that pose potential risks outweighing potential benefits for people 65 and older (Beers et al. 1991). In 2012, an update of the Beers criteria was published in partner-ship with the American Geriatrics Society (American Geriatrics Society 2012). Potentially inappropriate medications, however, continue to be pre-scribed, despite poor outcomes. Estimates from studies in ambulatory and long-term care settings found that 27% of adverse drug events in a primary care setting, and 42% of adverse drug events in long-term care facilities, were preventable (American Geriatrics Society 2012, Gurwitz et al. 2005, Gurwitz et al. 2003). At least 20%, and in one study up to 40%, of nursing home residents receive an inappropriate prescription; in the United States, approximately 71% of all nursing home residents are women (Beers et al. 1992, Jones et al. 2009).

While exposure to drugs with abuse potential may be a contributing factor in abuse of and addiction to prescription medications, there is also evidence that pain, and under-management of pain, plays a role in opioid misuse (Cicero et al. 2012, National Center on Addiction and Substance

Abuse Columbia 1998). Pain is a common symptom for older adults (Sawyer et al. 2006), with estimates ranging from 45–85% of older adults reporting chronic pain in various settings (Gianni et al. 2009). There is evidence that physicians, perhaps in part due to fear of addiction or fear of adverse drug effects, fail to adequately control pain in chronic-pain geriatric patients (Culberson and Ziska 2008, Levi Minzi et al. 2013). One study with nursing home residents found that 49% had persistent pain, of whom 83% were female, and a quarter received no analgesics (Won et al. 2004). Furthermore, Cicero et al. used a large medical insurance claims database to identify groups based on opioid use and found that women were substantially over-represented in the chronic pain group and used a much greater share of all medical services than males, particularly as they aged (Cicero et al. 2009). Chronic pain has been found by some to be a factor associated with prescription drug misuse (Becker et al. 2009, Havens et al. 2008). There are also data that those most likely to progress from opioid misuse to abuse have significant levels of, often untreated, pain (Cicero et al. 2009, Cicero et al. 2012, Levi Minzi et al. 2013, Ziska 2008). Thus, pain syndromes, pain management, and the potential relationship to misuse and abuse of opioids may be particularly relevant risk factors for older women, and they highlight the particular importance when treating older women of suing careful prescribing practices to treat pain while also monitoring for misuse.

Finally, biological and physiological changes that occur with age, many of which are more prominent in older women than in older men, function as risk factors for intoxication and adverse effects (Blow and Barry 2002, Brady 1999). Women of all ages have lower total body water than men of comparable size, and total body water also decreases with age and will therefore result in higher blood alcohol concentrations than their male or younger counterparts (Blow and Barry 2002, Brady 1999). Changes in lean muscle mass that occur with age have an impact on the metabolism of alcohol; women have less lean muscle mass than men throughout adulthood (Blow and Barry 2002). Women of all ages may have lower concentrations of gastric alcohol dehydrogenase, the most prominent enzyme in alcohol metabolism (Frezza et al. 1990). There is evidence that women metabolize nicotine more slowly than their male counterparts do (Brady and Randall 1999). Aging also interferes with the development of tolerance (Blow 1998). Older adults may, therefore, exhibit certain effects of alcohol at lower doses than younger individuals whose tolerance increases with increased consumption, and as a result, elders may experience adverse consequences if there is no change in their drinking pattern (Blow and Barry 2002, Blow 1998).

## Comorbidity

There is evidence that substance-use disorders are highly likely to be co-morbid with psychiatric disorders in both men and women, and that the comorbidities may differ between the sexes across all ages (Goldstein et al. 2012, Kessler et al. 1997, Compton et al. 2000). Kessler et al. reported significantly larger odds ratios (ORs) among women of all ages in the National Comorbidity Study (NCS) for lifetime DSM-III alcohol abuse with lifetime mood, anxiety, and additional substance-use disorders (Kessler et al. 1997). Studies of comorbid psychiatric disorders in opioid and cocaine abusers have also found a higher percentage of affective and anxiety disorders in women compared to men (Brooner et al. 1997, Rounsaville et al. 1991). In a 1989 study of hospitalized cocaine users, women were more likely than men to have an Axis I DSM-III-R diagnosis comorbid with their substance use (Griffin et al. 1989). Depression was more frequently reported by these women, and the severity of their depression on admission, and one month after, was more severe than that of men (Griffin et al. 1989). Goldstein et al. looked at sex differences across all ages, among data obtained from Wave 2 of the National Epidemiologic Survey on Alcohol and Related Conditions (NESARC) (Goldstein et al. 2012). They found that, across the diagnoses of alcohol abuse and dependence, women had higher rates of mood and anxiety disorders, as well as paranoid, histrionic, borderline, and avoidant personality disorders (Goldstein et al. 2012). In addition, alcohol abuse was positively associated with major depressive disorder with a modestly larger odds ratio for women than for men (Goldstein et al. 2012). Men with alcohol abuse and dependence in the NESARC sample had higher rates of narcissistic and antisocial personality disorders (Goldstein et al. 2012). Among respondents with drug abuse or dependence, women had significantly higher rates of mood and anxiety disorders, while men had higher rates of alcohol dependence and narcissistic and antisocial personality disorders (Goldstein et al. 2012).

There are fewer data specific to older adults. However, Grella et al. concluded that among their sample ($n$ = 343) of older adults with heroin dependence, women had poorer mental health than men, based upon significantly higher scores on the Beck Depression Inventory (BDI), and the Symptom Checklist–56 (Grella and Lovinger 2012). Moreover, the women in this sample had significantly higher rates of lifetime suicidal ideation and suicide attempts, with about half of them reporting a history of suicidal ideation and one-third a history of suicide attempt (Grella and Lovinger 2012). In another study of active prescription opioid abusers across all ages, those aged 45 and older were significantly more likely to have a psychiatric disorder relative to younger individuals, and the odds of women's having a comorbid psychiatric disorder was significantly greater than for men (Cicero et al. 2012). Additionally, males and females older than 45 meeting DSM-IV criteria for (prescription) opioid abuse had greater odds of comorbid alcoholism, although there was no clear gender difference (Cicero et al. 2012). In this same study, Cicero et al. found that the older men and women who misused prescription opioids were more psychiatrically symptomatic than those who did not, and this was more pronounced in older women (Cicero et al. 2012). Finally, in a study of older adults (over the age of 50) enrolled in a methadone maintenance clinic, women were more likely to experience depression and anxiety disorders, with depression (44% vs. 27%) and agoraphobia (21% vs. 10%) approaching statistical significance ($p$ 0.06 and $p$ 0.07, respectively) (Rosen et al. 2008). Thus, across all ages and substances of abuse, there is some evidence that women are more likely to have comorbid anxiety or affective illness. Therefore, it is important for healthcare providers to be aware of the potential for comorbid affective illness when screening and treating older women with substance-use disorders.

Chronic medical illness is often comorbid with, and may predispose older adults to, substance-use disorders (Ross 2005, Blow and Barry 2002, Blow and Barry 2009). Older adults who develop late-onset problem drinking, or relapse after having early problem drinking, often do so to medicate uncomfortable physical states (Ross 2005). Insomnia and chronic pain are often linked to initiation and/or maintenance of alcohol-use disorders in older adults (Ross 2005). Cicero et al. found that in their sample of adults meeting criteria for prescription drug abuse or dependence, those aged 45 and older were twice as likely to report moderate to very severe, non-withdrawal pain as their younger counterparts were (Cicero et al. 2012). Chronic pain patients of all ages are several times more likely to have a diagnosis of an alcohol-related disorder than those not taking opioids or taking them for acute, short-term purposes (Cicero et al. 2009). In this same study, in which Cicero et al. divided individuals into three groups—non-opioid users, acute opioid users (one opioid prescription for fewer than 10 days of use) and chronic opioid users (180 days of use or more of a prescription opioid in one year)—they found that, as the intensity and persistence of reported pain increased, so did the percentage of females per group (Cicero et al. 2009). Furthermore, with increasing age, females became more prevalent, such that over 80% of the chronic pain sample were females aged 61 or older (Cicero et al. 2009). Thus, as previously noted in the "Risk Factors" section, pain conditions and pain management are particularly relevant to those providing treatment to older adults, especially older women, with substance-use disorders.

## Long-Term Consequences

Substance abusers have higher mortality rates than do age-matched non-abusers (Finney and Moos 1991, Moos et al. 1994). In a prospective follow-up study of alcoholic women, Smith et al. note that, while women in the general population have lower rates of death than men, alcoholism reduces this advantage, so that mortality is the same as or greater for women as for men (Smith et al. 1983). Furthermore, in their 11-year follow up study of 100 alcoholic women, Smith and colleagues found four times as many deaths in alcoholic women as expected in the general population; the lifespan of alcoholic women was shortened by over 15 years in their sample (Smith et al. 1983).

The misuse and abuse of substances is associated with medical consequences that may be more pronounced in older adults than in younger adults, and older women may be particularly vulnerable to some of these consequences. As described, women at all ages experience negative consequences of alcohol at lower levels of consumption and after shorter periods of time; this is known as "telescoping" (Zweben 2009). For example, women who drink alcohol are more likely to develop liver cirrhosis at lower levels of alcohol consumption than men (Deal and Gavaler 1994). Additional examples of adverse consequences of alcohol use that may develop more rapidly in women than men include malnutrition, anemia, and hypertension (Zweben 2009). In 2011, Chen et al. reported that even "moderate" alcohol consumption (3–6 drinks per day) was found to be an independent risk factor for developing breast cancer in older (over 40 years old) women (Chen et al. 2011).

Substance use may also indirectly result in negative medical consequences in older adults due to interactions with medications and reduced compliance with medication. One study looking at adherence to the National Cholesterol Educational Program by post-menopausal women found that failure to use lipid-lowering medications was associated with, among other factors, age, alcohol consumption, and current smoking (Schrott et al. 1997). In addition, alcohol and other substance use may degrade cognitive functioning, which may have consequences for older individuals' ability to care for their medical illness and may lead to unintentional medication errors in this highly vulnerable population (Trevisan 2008, Blow 2000). There are some data that cognition in women is affected negatively by alcohol after shorter and less severe drinking histories than in their male counterparts (Nixon 1994, Acker 1986).

Additional potential consequences in older adults abusing substances include accidents and injuries (Blow 2000). Increase in fall risk, and the resultant risk of injury, is a concern in elderly individuals, particularly among those who are abusing substances that may impair their balance and coordination. The number of hip fractures in women aged 65 and older attributable to heavy

(7 or more ounces per week) alcohol use may be large (Felson et al. 1988). In addition to the potential higher risk of accidents, older adults who are moderate and heavy alcohol drinkers are 16 times more likely to die by suicide (Grabbe et al. 1997, NIAAA 1998). Across all ages, 75–80% of deaths by suicide are in men, and the second highest suicide rate occurs in those aged 85 and older; alcohol and drug abuse is a key risk factor for suicide (American Foundation for Suicide Prevention). Thus, older males abusing substances may be at a significantly elevated risk of suicide.

## Screening and Detection

Substance use in the elderly can be difficult to assess, and it is often missed. In one study, of 400 primary care physicians presented with patient scenarios involving older women with symptoms indicating possible substance abuse problems, only 1% suggested substance use as a possible diagnosis. When the sex of the older adult was changed from female to male, 4% suggested substance use as a possible diagnosis, a difference that was not statistically significant (National Center on Addiction and Substance Abuse Columbia 1998). Many factors contribute to the under-detection, and ultimately under-treatment, of substance use in older adults. Older adults rarely self-refer for substance use. While 87% of elderly adults regularly see a physician, only a minority of older adults seek treatment specifically for problems related to alcohol use, providing a challenge to identification (Blow and Barry 2009, Ross 2005). Shame and guilt often contribute to the lack of self-referral (Blow and Barry 2002, Ross 2005), and this effect may be more prominent in older women, who are more likely to hide their drinking (Blow 2000). Older adults may also be more sensitive to the stigma of having a substance-use problem (Ross 2005). Asking screening questions in an empathetic, non-judgmental manner, avoiding potentially stigmatizing terminology such as "alcoholic," and asking substance-use questions in the context of other health variables (e.g., exercise, weight) are strategies to keep in mind when interviewing older adults, particularly women (Ross 2005, Blow and Barry 2012). Cognitive impairment may be an additional factor interfering with the older adult's ability to accurately self-report use; obtaining collateral information from family members, friends, and caregivers is, therefore, essential when screening older adults (Trevisan 2008, Ross 2005, Simoni-Wastila and Yang 2006).

Another potential barrier to screening and diagnosis of older adults is that current diagnostic criteria may be less appropriate or relevant to older adults, particularly those focusing on fulfillment of major role obligations and decreased social, occupational, or recreational activities as a result of substance use (Trevisan 2008, Wang 2013, Johnson 1989). Women drink less often in public places and are therefore less likely to drive while intoxicated, and "problem behaviors" may not be as readily notable (Blow 2000, Waller 1997). Additionally, older adults, and particularly older women, are more likely to experience problems with relatively small amounts of substances due to increased sensitivity, slower metabolism, and decreased volume of distribution (Trevisan 2008, Blow and Barry 2012, Simoni-Wastila 2004). Thus, screening questions relying solely upon quantity are not sufficient, particularly in older women. Furthermore, older women are more likely to use alcohol in combination with prescribed psychoactive drugs; thus, problems may be amplified or experienced at lower "doses" (Blow 2000). It is important to note psychoactive drug misuse and abuse by older adults is often unintentional, and that women may be at an elevated risk (Simoni-Wastila and Yang 2006, Blow and Barry 2012). The "brown bag approach"—asking a patient to bring in all of his/her medications—is one strategy to better assess prescription drug use in this population (Blow and Barry 2009), and it may be particularly effective in identifying patients who are unintentionally misusing medications.

The rise of prescription opioid misuse and abuse in older adults presents a new challenge in screening for substance use. Older adults abusing prescription opioids are more likely to obtain opioids from doctors (rather than a dealer or by theft) their younger counterparts are; women of all ages are less inclined to use a dealer, favoring medical channels (Cicero et al. 2012). The use of state database and prescription-monitoring programs, where available, provides an opportunity to determine potential drug misuse and may be a particularly relevant and useful tool in the evaluation of older women and men.

The Center for Substance Abuse Treatment (CSAT) recommends that everyone aged 60 and older be screened yearly for alcohol and prescription drug use and abuse as part of regular healthcare services, and rescreened if there are major life changes that could precipitate increased use and problems (e.g., retirement, death of a partner/spouse) (Blow 1998). The CAGE questionnaire (Mayfield et al. 1974) is a widely used alcohol screening test; however, it has not been well validated in women and older adults (Blow and Barry 2009). There are some validated screening instruments for use in older adults, including the Short Michigan Alcoholism Screening Test–Geriatric Version (SMAST-G) (Blow et al. 1992) and the Alcohol Use Disorders Identification Test (AUDIT) (Saunders et al. 1993), both of which are useful tools, although notably specific to alcohol, and therefore should be used in conjunction with questions about use of other substances, including prescription drugs. The SMAST-G includes questions that address risk factors that may be particularly relevant for older women; e.g., "Do you drink to relax or calm your nerves?" (Blow et al.1992). The Alcohol, Smoking and Substance Involvement Screening Test (ASSIST), modified for older adults to address psychoactive prescription use, is another screening tool for older adults (WHO Working Group 2002).

## Treatment

Relatively few older adults with substance-use disorders seek treatment specifically for substance abuse (Gossop and Moos 2008). Women at all ages are less likely to enter treatment over the course of a lifetime (Hamilton and Grella 2009), and younger women may be more likely to seek treatment in a non–substance-use treatment setting (Brady and Randall 1999). However, many older adults, both men and women, have regular contact with healthcare providers for other reasons. Older adults, and women in particular, may be particularly motivated to stop drinking because of health problems (Satre and Arean 2005). Thus, primary care and other healthcare providers are valuable resources for screening as well as potentially treating this population.

Older women may feel more shame and guilt about their substance use than men do (Blow 2000). Approaching older adults, particularly women, in an empathic, respectful, and straightforward manner, and avoiding pejorative terms, is imperative to the engagement process (Ross 2005). Working with older adults at a slower, age-appropriate pace, sensitive to potential slower cognitive processing times, is also necessary. Individualizing treatment plans with age-appropriate content is equally important. Older adults may also do better in age- and sex-segregated treatments (NIAAA 1998).

In treating older adults of both sexes, it is important to keep in mind the potential comorbidities, both medical and psychiatric, as well as recent stressors (e.g., loss, bereavement) and barriers to treatment (e.g., transportation); alcohol and substance-use problems tend not to occur in isolation in these groups. As discussed earlier in this chapter, women may be more susceptible to developing medical consequences from their substance use at lower doses and more quickly than men, and this must be taken into account when creating a treatment plan, including the setting of treatment as well as the choice of medication. In older adults, opioid and alcohol detoxification may need to be conducted in a medical setting and over a longer period of time, due to its potential for exacerbation of medical comorbidities. In addition, choice of pharmacotherapy may be different in older adults than in younger. For example, disulfiram (Antabuse) is not recommended in older adults because of the higher risk of adverse cardiovascular effects and hepatic toxicity (Ross 2005, Caputo et al. 2012). The long-acting injectable form of naltrexone (Vivitrol) may be a better choice in older adults with memory or cognitive impairment for whom taking a daily medication proves challenging (Johnson 2010). Thus, screening for medical comorbidities, including cognitive and physical, that may potentially interfere with treatment, and awareness that women may have more severe complications of their substance use at time of presentation, is essential in developing an appropriate plan.

Motivational brief interventions and brief therapies for substance use have been found effective in a variety of clinical settings, including primary care, mental health, and senior centers (Barry 1999). These interventions tend to include personalized feedback based on responses to screening questions, motivational interviewing, and goal setting (Blow and Barry 2012). While the majority of these studies have been done in younger adults, there are two studies that suggest that brief interventions with older adults are also effective, and perhaps particularly so with older women (Fleming et al. 1999, Blow and Barry 2000). Fleming et al. found that women were more likely than men to reduce their drinking and follow recommended guidelines, and in a study by Blow and Barry, women were more likely to change drinking patterns based upon screening questions, compared to men (Fleming et al. 1999, Blow and Barry 2000). The data therefore suggest that brief interventions, done in a variety of non–substance-abuse-treatment settings, can be quite effective in women. Blow and Barry, and Schonfeld et al., also found that cognitive behavioral approaches with a focus on teaching older adults skills necessary to re-build support networks and providing tools to overcome depression, grief, and loneliness were successful in reducing or stopping alcohol use (Blow and Barry 2000, Schonfeld et al. 2000). It is important to recognize that older adults do respond to treatment, and in fact, may be more likely to complete treatment than younger patients are (Schuckit 1977, Wiens et al. 1982–1983).

In summary, healthcare providers should discuss alcohol and drug use with older patients as part of routine care. Healthcare providers should be non-judgmental, avoiding pejorative terms, and counseling should include medical conditions common to older adults that could emerge from, or be worsened by, alcohol or other drug use. Treatment plans should be individualized, taking into account the likelihood of comorbidities, particularly in women. Interventions should be tailored to the level of risk, and providers should refer to specialized treatment when appropriate. It is important to keep in mind that treatment for alcohol and substance-use disorders is effective in this population and can be successful in a variety of settings (e.g., in primary care settings), and that older women may be particularly responsive to brief interventions.

## Conclusions

Sex differences in late-life substance-use disorders are particularly under-studied. Older women appear to be an especially vulnerable population, with unique risk factors and medical and psychiatric comorbidities. Older women are more likely than men to experience late-onset alcohol use disorder, and their patterns of alcohol consumption are often not well detected by standard screening instruments. Alcohol and substance use in older women is often undetected and untreated by clinicians. It is, therefore, important to screen older women regularly for alcohol and prescription drug use and abuse, to ask screening questions in a non-judgmental manner, to be sensitive to potential slower processing times, and to utilize collateral information from family/caregivers when possible. Motivational brief interventions and therapies can be quite effective in older women and should be utilized when risky use is identified. Finally, individualizing treatment plans with age-appropriate content is essential when treating older women with substance-use disorders.

# References

Acker C. Neuropsychological deficits in alcoholics: the relative contributions of gender and drinking history. *Br J Addict* 1986;81:395–403.

Adams WL, Barry KL, Fleming MF. Screening for problem drinking in older primary care patients. *JAMA* 1996;276(24):1964–1967.

American Foundation for Suicide Prevention. Facts and figures. N.d. Retrieved from http://www.afsp.org/understanding-suicide/facts-and-figures. Accessed on March 30, 2015.

American Foundation for Suicide Prevention. Suicide risk factors. N.d. Retrieved from http://www.afsp.org/understanding-suicide/suicide-risk-factors. Accessed on March 30, 2015.

American Geriatrics Society, 2012 Beers Criteria Update Expert Panel. American Geriatrics Society updated Beers criteria for potentially inappropriate medication use in older adults. *J Am Geriatr Soc* 2012;60:616–631.

Balsa AI, Homer JF, Fleming MF, French MT. Alcohol consumption and health among elders. *Gerontologist* 2008;48(5):622–636.

Barry KL. Brief interventions and brief therapies for substance abuse. Treatment Improvement Protocol (TIP) Series No. 34. Rockville, MD: U.S. Department of Health and Human Services, Public Health Service, Substance Abuse and Mental Health Services Administration, Center for Substance Abuse Treatment; 1999.

Becker WC, Fiellin DA, Gallagher RM, Barth KS, Ross JT, Oslin DW. The association between chronic pain and prescription drug abuse in veterans. *Pain Med* 2009;10(3):531–536.

Beckman LJ, Amaro H. Personal and societal difficulties faced by women and men entering alcoholism treatment. *J Stud Alcohol* 1986;47(2):135–145.

Beers MH, Ouslander JG, Fingold SF, et al. Inappropriate medication prescribing in skilled-nursing facilities. *Ann Intern Med* 1992;117(8):684–689.

Beers MH, Ouslander JG, Judge J, Reuben DB, Brooks J, Beck JC. Explicit criteria for determining inappropriate medication use in nursing home residents. *Arch Intern Med* 1991;151:1825–1832.

Blazer DG, Wu LT. The epidemiology of at-risk and binge drinking among middle-aged and elderly community adults: National Survey on Drug Use and Health. *Am J Psychiatry* 2009;166:1162–1169.

Blow FC. Substance abuse among older adults. Treatment Improvement Protocol (TIP) Series, #26. DHHS Publication No. (SMA) 98–3179. Rockville, MD: SAMHSA; 1998.

Blow FC. Treatment of older women with alcohol problems: meeting the challenge for a special population. *Alcohol Clin Exper Res* 2000;24(8):1257–1266.

Blow FC, Barry KL. Older patients with at-risk and problem drinking patterns: new developments in brief interventions. *J Geriatr Psych Neurol* 2000;13(3):115–123.

Blow FC, Barry KL. Use and misuse of alcohol among older women. *Alcohol Res Health* 2002;26:308–315.

Blow FC, Barry KL. Treatment of older adults. In: Ries RK et al., Eds., *Principles of Addiction Medicine* (4th ed.). Philadelphia, PA: Lippincott Williams & Wilkins; 2009:479–492.

Blow FC, Barry KL. Alcohol and substance misuse in older adults. *Curr Psychiatry Rep* 2012;14:310–319.

Blow FC, Brower KJ, Schulenberg JE, Demo-Dananberg LM, Young JP, Beresford TP. The Michigan Alcoholism Screening Test–Geriatric Version (MAST-G): a new elderly-specific screening instrument. *Alcohol Clin Exper Res* 1992;16:372.

Blume SB. Women and alcohol: a review. *JAMA* 1986;256:1467–1470.

Bonevski B, Rega, T, Paul C, Baker AL, Bisquera A. Associations between alcohol, smoking, socioeconomic status and comorbidities: evidence from the 45 and Up Study. *Drug Alcohol Rev* 2014;33(2):169–176.

Brady KT, Randall CL. Gender differences in substance use disorders. *Addict Disord* 1999;22(2):241–252.

Brennan-Ing M, Porter KE, Seidel L, Karpiak SE. Substance use and sexual risk differences among older bisexual and gay men with HIV. *Behav Med* 2014;40(3):108–115.

Brooner RK, King VL, Kidorf M, Schmidt CW, Bigelow GE. Psychiatric and substance use comorbidity among treatment-seeking opioid abusers. *Arch Gen Psychiatry* 1997;54(1):71–80.

Caputo F, Vignoli T, Leggio L, Addolorato G, Zoli G, Bernardi M. Alcohol use disorder in the elderly: a brief overview from epidemiology to treatment options. *Exper Gerontol* 2012;47:411–416.

Chen WY, Rosner B, Hankinson SE, Colditz G, Willet WC. Moderate alcohol consumption during adult life, drinking patterns and breast cancer risk. *JAMA* 2011;306(17):1884–1890.

Cicero TJ, Surratt HL, Kurtz S, Ellis MS, Inciardi JA. Patterns of prescription opioid abuse and comorbidity in and aging treatment population. *J Subst Abuse Treat* 2012;42:87–94.

Cicero TJ, Wong G, Tian Y, Lynskey M, Todorov A, Isenberg K. Co-morbidity and utilization of medical services by pain patients receiving opioid medications: data from an insurance claims database. *Pain* 2009;144:20–27.

Compton WM, Cottler LB, Ben Abdallah A, Phelps DL, Spitznagel EL, Horton JC. Substance dependence and other psychiatric disorders among drug dependent subjects: race and gender correlates. *Am J Addict* 2000;9(2):113–125.

Culberson JW, Ziska M. Prescription drug misuse/abuse in the elderly. *Geriatrics* 2008;63:22–31.

Deal SR, Gavaler JS. Are women more susceptible than men to alcohol-induced cirrhosis? *Alcohol Health Res World* 1994;18(3):189–191.

Felson DT, Kiel DP, Anderson JJ, Kannel WB. Alcohol consumption and hip fractures: the Framingham study. *Am J Epidemiol* 1988;128(5):1102–1110.

Finney JW, Moos RH. The long-term course of treated alcoholism: I. Mortality, relapse and remission rates and comparisons to community controls. *J Stud Alcohol* 1991;52:44–54.

Fleming MF, Manwell LB, Barry KL, Adams W, Stauffacher EA. Brief physician advice for alcohol problems in older adults: a randomized community-based trial. *J Fam Pract* 1999;48(5):378–384.

Frezza M, di Padova C, Pozzato G, Terpin M, Baraona E, Lieber CS. High blood alcohol levels in women. The role of decreased gastric alcohol dehydrogenase activity and first-pass metabolism. *N Engl J Med* 1990;322(2):95–99.

Geels LM, Vink JM, Van Beek JH, Bartels M, Willemsen G, Boomsma DI. Increases in alcohol consumption in women and elderly groups: evidence from an epidemiological study. *BMC Public Health* 2013;13:207.

Gianni W, Ceci M, Bustacchini S, et al. Opioids for the treatment of chronic non-cancer pain in older people. *Drugs Aging* 2009;26(Suppl 1), 63–73.

Giovino GA, Henningfield JE, Tomar SL, Escobedo LG, Slade J. Epidemiology of tobacco use and dependence. *Epidemiol Rev* 1995;17:48–65.

Glass TA, Prigerson H, Kasl SV, & Mendes de Leon CF. The effects of negative life events on alcohol consumption among older men and women. *J Gerontol B: Psychol Sci Soc Sci* 1995;50(4):S205–S216.

Goldstein RB, Dawson DA, Chou SP, Grant BF. Sex differences in prevalence and comorbidity of alcohol and drug use disorders: results from Wave 2 of the National Epidemiologic Survey on Alcohol and Related Conditions. *J Stud Alcohol Drugs* 2012;73(6):938–950.

Gomberg ES. Risk factors for drinking over a woman's life span. *Alcohol Health Res* 1994;18:220–227.

Gomberg ES. Older women and alcohol. Use and abuse. *Recent Dev Alcohol* 1995;12:61–79.

Gossop M, Moos R. Substance misuse among older adults: a neglected but treatable problem. *Addiction* 2008;103 347–348.

Grabbe L, Demi A, Camann MA. The health status of elderly persons in the last year of life: a comparison of deaths by suicide, injury, and natural causes. *Am J Public Health* 1997;87(3):434–437.

Grant BF, Dawson DA, Stinson FS, Chou SP, Dufour MC, Pickering RP. The 12-month prevalence and trends in DSM-IV alcohol abuse and dependence: United States, 1991–1992 and 2001–2002. *Drug Alcohol Depend* 2004;74(3):223–234.

Green TC, Grimes Serrano JM, Licari A, Budman SH, Butler SE. Women who abuse prescription opioids: findings from the Addiction Severity Index–Multimedia Version Connect Prescription Opioid Database. *Drug Alcohol Depend* 2009;103(1–2):65–73.

Grella CE, Lovinger K. Gender differences in physical and mental health outcomes among an aging cohort of individuals with a history of heroin dependence. *Addict Behav* 2012;37:306–312.

Griffin ML, Weiss RD, Mirin SM, Lange U. A comparison of male and female cocaine abusers. *Arch Gen Psychiatry* 1989;46:122–126.

Gurwitz JH, Field TS, Harrold LR, et al. Incidence and preventability of adverse drug events among older persons in the ambulatory setting. *JAMA* 2003;289:1107–1116.

Gurwitz JH, Field TS, Judge J, Rochon P, Harrold LR, Cadoret C, et al. The incidence of adverse drug events in two large academic long-term care facilities. *Am J Med* 2005;118:251–258.

Hamilton AB, Grella CE. Gender differences among older heroin users. *J Women Aging* 2009;21:111–124.

Han B, Gfroerer JC, Colliver JD, Penne MA. Substance use disorder among older adults in the United States in 2020. *Addiction* 2009;104:88–96.

Havens JR, Walker R, Leukefeld CG. Prescription opioid use in rural Appalachia: a community-based study. *J Opioid Manag* 2008;4(2):63–71.

Husten CG, Chrismon JH, Reddy MN. Trends and effects of cigarette smoking among girls and women in the United States, 1965–1993. *JAMWA* 1996;52:11–18.

Johnson BA. Medication treatment of different types of alcoholism. *Am J Psychiatry* 2010;167(6):630–639.

Johnson RA, Gerstein DR. Initiation of use of alcohol, cigarettes, marijuana, cocaine, and other substance in US birth cohorts since 1919. *Am J Public Health* 1998;88:27–33.

Jones AL, Dwyer LL, Bercovitz AR, Strahan GW. The National Nursing Home Survey: 2004 overview. National Center for Health Statistics. *Vital Health Stat* 2009;13(167).

Kessler RC, Crum RM, Warner LA, Nelson CB, Schulenberg J, Anthony JC. Lifetime co-occurrence of DSM-III-R alcohol abuse and dependence with other psychiatric disorders in the National Comorbidity Survey. *Arch Gen Psychiatry* 1997;54(4):313–321.

King AC, Taylor CB, Haskell WL. Smoking in older women: is being female a "risk factor" for continued cigarette use? *Arch Intern Med* 1990;150:1841–1846.

Koechl B, Unger A, Fischer G. Age-related aspects of addiction. *Gerontology* 2012;58(6):540–544.

Larney S, Bohnert AS, Ganoczy D, et al. Mortality among older adults with opioid use disorders in the Veteran's Health Administration, 2000–2011. *Drug Alcohol Depend* 2015;147:32–37.

Levi Minzi MA, Surratt HL, Kurtz SP, Buttram ME. Under treatment of pain: a prescription for opioid misuse among the elderly? *Pain Med* 2013;14:1719–1729.

Lex BW. Some gender differences in alcohol and polysubstance users. *Health Psychol* 1991;10:121–132.

Mayfield D, McLeod G, Hall P. The CAGE Questionnaire: validation of a new alcoholism screening instrument. *Am J Psychiatry*, 1974;131(10):1121–1123.

McKenna T, Pickens R. Alcoholic children of alcoholics. *J Stud Alcohol* 1981;42(11):1021–1029.

Mellinger GD, Balter MB, Uhlenhuth EH. Prevalence and correlates of the long-term regular use of anxiolytics. *JAMA* 1984;251:375.

Mellinger GD, Balter MB, Manheimer DI, Cisin IH, Parry HJ. Psychic distress, life crisis, and use of psychotherapeutics. *Arch Gen Psychiatry* 1978;35:1045–1052.

Miller BA, Downs WR, Testa M. Interrelationships between victimization experiences and women's alcohol use. *J Stud Alcohol Suppl* 1993;11:109–117.

Moos RH, Brennan PL, Mertens JR. Mortality rates and predictors of mortality among late middle-aged and older substance abuse patients. *Alcohol Clin Exper Res* 1994;18:187–195.

National Center on Addiction and Substance Abuse (CASA) Columbia. (1998, June). Under the rug: substance abuse and the mature woman. At http://www.casacolumbia.org/addiction-research/reports/under-the-rug-substance-abuse-mature-woman. Accessed January 16, 2016.

National Institute on Alcohol Abuse and Alcoholism. The Physicians' Guide to Helping Patients with Alcohol Problems. Bethesda, MD: U.S. Dept. of Health and Human Services, Public Health Service, National Institutes of Health, National Institute on Alcohol Abuse and Alcoholism; 1995.

National Institute on Alcohol Abuse and Alcoholism. Alcohol and aging. (1998). *Alcohol Alert*, 40, 1–3. At http://pubs.niaaa.nih.gov/publications/aa40.htm. Accessed on January 17, 2015.

National Institute on Alcohol Abuse and Alcoholism. Older adults. (2015). Retrieved from http://www.niaaa.nih.gov/alcohol-health/special-populations-co-occurring-disorders/older-adults. Accessed on March 30, 2015.

National Institutes of Health (NIH). Inclusion of women in study populations. *NIH Guide for Grants and Contracts*, 1986;15(22):1.

Nixon SJ. Cognitive deficits in alcoholic women. *Alcohol Health Res World* 1994;18(3):228–232.

Nuevo R, Chatterji S, Verdes E, Naidoo N, Ayuso-Mateos JL, Miret M. Prevalence of alcohol consumption and pattern of use among the elderly in the WHO European region. *Eur Addict Res* 2015;21(2):88–96.

Ray BA, Braude MC. Women in Drugs: A New Era for Research. National Institute on Drug Abuse (NIDA) Research Monograph Series 65. Rockville, MD: NIDA; 1986.

Rosen D, Smith ML, Reynolds CF. The prevalence of mental and physical health disorders among older methadone patients. *Am J Geriatr Psych* 2008;16(6):488–497.

Ross S. Alcohol use disorders in the elderly. *Primary Psychiatry* 2005;12(1):32–40.

Rounsaville BJ, Anton SF, Carroll K, Budde D, Prusoff BA, Gawin F. Psychiatric diagnoses of treatment-seeking cocaine abusers. *Arch Gen Psychiatry* 1991;48:43–51.

Rudolph KE, Glass TA, Crum RM, Schwartz BS. Neighborhood psychosocial hazards and binge drinking among late middle-aged adults. *J Urban Health* 2013;90(5):970–982.

Sacco P, Bucholz KK, Harrington D. Gender differences in stressful life events, social support, perceived stress, and alcohol use among older adults: results from a National Survey. *Subst Use Misuse* 2014;49(4):456–65.

Sacco P, Bucholz KK, Spitznagel EL. Alcohol use among older adults in the National Epidemiologic Survey on Alcohol and Related Conditions: a latent class analysis. *J Stud Alcohol Drugs* 2009;70:829–838.

Satre DD, Arean PA. Effects of gender, ethnicity, and medical illness on drinking cessation in older primary care patients. *J Aging Health* 2005;17:70–84.

Saunders JB, Aasland OG, Babor TF, de la Fuente JR, Grant M. Development of the Alcohol Use Disorders Identification Test (AUDIT): WHO Collaborative Project on Early Detection of Persons with Harmful Alcohol Consumption–II. *Addiction* 1993;88(6):791–804.

Sawyer P, Bodner EV, Ritchie CS, Allman RM. Pain and pain medication use in community-dwelling older adults. *Am J Geriatr Pharmacother* 2006;4:316–324.

Schonfeld L, Dupree LW, Dickson-Euhrmann E, et al. Cognitive-behavioral treatment of older veterans with substance abuse problems. *J Geriatr Psych Neurol* 2000;13:124–129.

Schuckit MA. Geriatric alcoholism and drug abuse. *Gerontologist* 1977;17(2):168–174.

Schrott HG, Bittner V, Vittinghoff E, Herrington DM, Hulley S. Adherence to National Cholesterol Education Program treatment goals in postmenopausal women with heart disease. The Heart and Estrogen/Progestin Replacement Study (HERS). The HERS Research Group. *JAMA* 1997;277(16):1281–1286.

Simoni-Wastila L. Gender and psychotropic drug use. *Med Care,* 1998;36(1):88–94.

Simoni-Wastila L. The use of abusable prescription drugs: the role of gender. *J Women Health Gender Based Med* 2000;9(3):289–297.

Simoni-Wastila L, Yang KL. Psychoactive drug abuse in older adults. *Am J Geriatr Pharmacother* 2006;4:380–394.

Simoni-Wastila L, Ritter G, Strickler G. Gender and other factors associated with the non-medical use of abusable prescription drugs. *Subst Use Misuse* 2004;39(1):1–23.

Smith EM, Cloninger CR, Bradford S. Predictors of mortality in alcoholic women: a prospective follow-up study. *Alcohol Clin Exper Res* 1983;7(2):237–243.

Spore DL, Mor V, Larrat P, Hawes C, Hiris J. Inappropriate drug prescriptions for elderly residents of board and care facilities. *Am J Public Health* 1997;87:404–409.

Substance Abuse and Mental Health Services Administration. Results from the 2011 National Survey on Drug Use and Health: Mental health findings, NSDUH Series H-45, HHS Publication No. (SMA) 12–4725. Rockville, MD: SAMHSA; 2012.

Szwabo PA. Substance abuse in older women. *Clin Geriatr Med* 1993;9:197–208.

Trevisan LA. Baby boomers and substance abuse. *Psychiatric Times.* (2008, July 1.) At http://www.psychiatrictimes.com/articles/baby-boomers-and-substance-abuse. Accessed January 16, 2016.

Wang X, Steier JB, Gallo WT. The effect of retirement on alcohol consumption: results from the US Health and Retirement Study. *Eur J Public Health* 2014;24(3):485–489.

Wang YP, Andrade LH. Epidemiology of alcohol and drug use in the elderly. *Curr Opin Psychiatry* 2013;26:343–348.

WHO Working Group. The Alcohol, Smoking and Substance Involvement Screening Test (ASSIST): DEVELOPMENT, reliability, and feasibility. *Addiction* 2002;97:1183–1194.

Wiens AN, Menustik CE, Miller SL, Schmitz RE. Medical-behavioral treatment of the older alcoholic patient. *Am J Drug Alcohol Abuse* 1982–1983;9(4):461–475.

Wilsnack SC, Vogeltanz ND, Kalssen AD, Harris TR. Childhood sexual abuse and women's substance abuse: national survey findings. *J Stud Alcohol* 1997;58(3):264–271.

Won AB, Lapane KL, Vallow S, Schein J, Morris JN, Lipsitz LA. Persistent nonmalignant pain and analgesic prescribing patterns in elderly nursing home residents. *J Am Geriatr Soc* 2004;52(6):867–874.

Wu LT, Blazer DG. Substance use disorders and psychiatric comorbidity in mid and later life: a review. *Int J Epidemiol* 2014;43(2):304–317.

Wu L, Blazer DG. Illicit and nonmedical drug use among older adults: a review. *J Aging Health* 2011;23(3):481–504.

Zweben JE. Special issues in treatment: Women. In Ries RK et al., Eds., *Principles of addiction medicine.* Philadelphia, PA: Lippincott Williams & Wilkins; 2009:465–477.

# CHAPTER 10

# Treatment Options for Older Adults with Substance-Use Disorders

*Stacy A. Cohen, Margaret M. Haglund, and Larissa J. Mooney*

## Introduction

This chapter reviews pharmacological and behavioral treatment options for substance use disorders (SUDs) in the "older adult" (here defined as age 60 and older). We first discuss the identification of SUDs among the elderly via screening, then describe available and recommended treatment settings for older adults with SUDs, from the lowest to the highest levels of care. Focusing on treatments for which an evidence base exists to support their utility in older patients, we discuss available behavioral and pharmacological interventions for SUDs. Given the relative scarcity of evidence-based treatments specific to older patients, we include common treatments applied in the general population, with special consideration given to how these might be modified to suit older individuals. Topics include alcohol use disorder, sedative/hypnotic use disorder, opioid use disorder, tobacco use disorder, and stimulant use disorder.

## Treatment Settings and Level of Care for Older Adults with Substance-Use Disorders

### SCREENING FOR SUDS IN THE OLDER POPULATION

Identifying those who need treatment for SUDs can be especially complicated in the elderly. Certain signs or symptoms that may be part of normal aging or other conditions commonly associated with older age may confuse the picture and prevent clinicians from recognizing addiction. For instance, symptoms of dementia and depression in the elderly, as well as increasing frailty and falls, are often attributed to normal age-related changes but may in fact be related to active substance use. Behavioral changes such as social isolation, irrational fears or delusions, and neglect of personal hygiene, which often accompany illnesses like dementia, can also be signs of ongoing addictive disorders.

In general, older individuals tend to visit their primary care physicians more regularly than younger adults do (Moy et al. 2011). Paradoxically, older adults with SUDs, in particular those with harmful drinking patterns, appear to be less likely to seek medical attention (Merrick et al. 2008). Older adults are also less likely than younger adults to report alcohol and drug use as problematic (Nemes et al. 2004). Additionally, whereas work-related problems are a primary impetus for middle-aged adults to seek treatment, retired individuals who are not impacted on that dimension are likely to be less motivated to present to seek help.

Non-traditional medical venues such as pharmacies and senior centers, which are likely to capture a wide swath of the elderly demographic, may be of utility in identifying older individuals with SUD in need of treatment. Pharmacies can prove particularly useful in identifying older individuals at risk of SUDs, given that older adults tend to be prescribed multiple medications, frequently from different doctors, and also often combine these medications with over-the-counter medications and dietary supplements (National Institute on Drug Abuse [NIDA] 2014). Homebound elderly individuals are also at risk of SUDs (Bersci et al. 1993) and have limited access to healthcare; it is therefore crucial to educate home health aides, visiting nurses, social workers, and assisted living personnel about the recognition of signs of SUDs and first steps in obtaining treatment.

The Consensus Panel of the Treatment Improvement Protocol (TIP) #26 recommends screening for alcohol and prescription drug abuse in adults over the age of 60 as a part of regular physical examinations [Center for Substance Abuse Treatment (CSAT) 1998]. Traditional screening instruments such as the CAGE questionnaire (which asks about efforts to Cut down, being Annoyed by criticism, feeling Guilty about drinking, and needing an Eye opener), and the Michigan Alcohol Screening Test (MAST) identify members of the general adult population with current or lifetime alcohol-use disorders. The modified CAGE questionnaire (which includes screening for other substances in addition to alcohol) has been shown to have high sensitivity but low specificity in older adults (Hinkle et al. 2001). The MAST-G is a modified version of the MAST developed specifically for the elderly (Menninger 2002). The Alcohol Use Disorders Identification Test (AUDIT) detects a broader spectrum of hazardous and harmful drinking by assessing the quantity of alcohol intake.

The age-related decrease in total body water and increase in body fat affect older adults' ability to absorb and metabolize alcohol, resulting in higher blood alcohol concentrations per amount of alcohol consumed (Adams & Cox 1995, Meier & Seitz 2008); additionally, as noted, elderly individuals are more likely to be on multiple medications and supplements, which can also impair alcohol metabolism. Thus, the AUDIT may underestimate alcohol-use disorder (AUD) severity in the older population by using the number of drinks per day as a criterion for alcohol-related problems. Furthermore, in older persons, alcohol-related safety hazards and health risks may be increased due to medical comorbidities and age-related cognitive and functional decline. Therefore, broadly used screening tools for the general population may be limited by their inability to address alcohol-associated risks unique to older people (Fink et al. 2002).

More recently developed screening tools such as the Alcohol-Related Problems Survey (ARPS) and the Short ARPS were created specifically for screening older adults, and have been found to be more sensitive than the AUDIT and the MAST-G in identifying at-risk older individuals (Moore 2002). The ARPS aims, not only to detect AUDs, but to identify problematic and at-risk drinking that is exacerbated by comorbidities, medications, and functional status (Fink et al. 2002). A screening and brief intervention project for older adults (The Florida Brief Intervention and Treatment for Elders [BRITE] project) has been found to increase the number of older adults accurately screened, identified, and treated for SUDs (Schonfeld et al. 2010). The DAPA-PC (the Drug and Alcohol Problem Assessment for Primary Care) is a computerized screening system for quickly identifying and addressing substance use issues in primary care settings (Nemes et al. 2004). While there is support for its use in patients over 55 years old, its utility may be limited in older adults who lack familiarity with computers (Nemes et al. 2004).

In summary, there is no single tool widely agreed upon to detect SUDs in the older adult; however, this is an area of active research, with increasing numbers of assessments being developed and validated. Achieving consensus on a small number of well-validated and easy-to-use tools will be an important step in improving screening for SUDs in older patients.

## TREATMENT SETTINGS: SELECTION AND OUTCOMES

The American Society of Addiction Medicine (ASAM) Patient Placement Criteria (ASAM PPC-2R, revised 2013) is the most widely used and comprehensive set of national guidelines for placement, continued stay, and discharge of patients with SUDs. This set of criteria has been designed and modified to meet a growing need for a variety of services to treat the range of severity of substance use and behavioral disorders, rather than using a "one size fits all" approach. The guidelines aim to help patients obtain access to quality treatment while conserving healthcare resources, as well as to assist clinicians in matching patients to appropriate treatment settings. While there are two major sets of guidelines for patient placement (one for adults and one for adolescents), there are no current guidelines specifically tailored to the older adult. Thus, the following section outlines general treatment-setting guidelines for the adult population, with considerations specific to older adults.

There are three levels of medical-based care for adults seeking SUD treatment. In increasing order of intensiveness, these include individual outpatient office-based treatment, intensive outpatient/partial hospitalization programs, and medically monitored and/or medically managed inpatient treatments. As outlined by the ASAM criteria, several factors influence selection of appropriate level of care, including whether acute intoxication or potential for withdrawal is present, presence of medical or psychiatric comorbidities, the patient's state of readiness to change, availability of a support network, and their living environment. In the older individual, medical comorbidities and their ability to care for activities of daily living are almost always a consideration, and these can have a major impact on selection of treatment level. Financial circumstances can also pose a particular challenge in older patients and can constrain the selection of treatment setting.

### Acute Treatment Settings for Intoxication and Withdrawal

Once an at-risk patient is identified, and prior to treatment referral, assessing for acute intoxication and for withdrawal potential is important in order to determine whether detoxification services are required. In the general population, detoxification can be conducted in a variety of settings, ranging from ambulatory detoxification with or without extended on-site monitoring, to clinically managed residential detoxification, and medically monitored or managed inpatient detoxification. In the elderly, given that intoxication and withdrawal generally pose graver medical risks, special attention should be paid to substance-specific intoxication and withdrawal complications, and, in general, more intensive monitoring is recommended. Acutely intoxicated older adults should be referred to medically monitored or medically managed treatment settings for safety. Benzodiazepine, alcohol, opioid, and stimulant intoxication can all be life-threatening, particularly in this population, and benzodiazepine, alcohol, and opioid withdrawal in particular necessitate careful detoxification due to their associated clinical risks. Older individuals are more likely to obtain benzodiazepines and opioids through doctors' prescriptions (Sproule et al. 2009) and to be using multiple substances, increasing risks associated with intoxication and withdrawal.

For alcohol detoxification, most sources recommend inpatient detoxification for older patients, given their increased sensitivity to detoxification symptoms, the potential adverse effects of medications, and varying pharma-cokinetics due to aging and comorbidity (O'Connell 2003); overall, severity and duration of alcohol withdrawal are greater in elderly patients (Brower et al. 1994). Due to physiological differences in the elderly, relatively lower daily intake of alcohol may be followed by more severe withdrawal symptoms than would be expected in younger adults (Benshoff & Harrawood 2003). Additionally alcohol consumption is associated with greater risk for injury in aging individuals, again leading to the recommendation to err on the side of cau-tion with inpatient monitoring (Resnick & Junlapeeya 2004). The American Medical Association's guidelines recommend inpatient treatment with close supervision and medication monitoring for older adults who are dependent on alcohol and at risk for withdrawal. Outpatient monitoring may be appro-priate for selected patients if symptoms are mild, if medical and SUD history is well known and does not include worrisome withdrawal symptoms, and if close daily monitoring is accessible (Kraemer et al. 1999). Inpatient treatment for detoxification from benzodiazepines is also generally recommended, given similar risks of seizures as with alcohol; there is also specific evidence suggest-ing that inpatient benzodiazepine detoxification in older adults reduces subse-quent medical and mental health services (Burke et al. 1995).

For detoxification from opioids, as with alcohol and benzodiazepines, more intensive detoxification treatment settings are generally recommended in the older population. Older individuals tend to be more likely to comply with and complete inpatient detoxification programs (Backmund et al. 2001) which puts them at an advantage for achieving abstinence (Digiusto et al. 2005). As with other substances, more intensive settings are generally recommended due to increased medical comorbidities and frailty in older individuals; spe-cific to opioid-use disorder, older patients tend to have more pain complaints, and thus are likely to have more difficulty tapering down on opioid-containing substances (Barry et al. 2013).

Once the patient is stabilized via treatment for intoxication and/or with-drawal, the process of transitioning to SUD treatment programs can begin. Those not requiring acute detoxification or hospitalization for intoxication can be referred directly to treatment programs.

## SUD Treatment Programs

Various organizations, including the Substance Abuse and Mental Health Services Administration (SAMHSA), the National Registry of Evidence-Based Programs and Practice (NREPP), the National Institute on Drug Abuse (NIDA), and various state agencies have delineated sets of criteria by which to gauge the quality of evidence for SUD programs, but there is no clear consensus on how to define "good evidence" for SUD treatment effectiveness (Glasner-Edwards & Rawson 2010). There is some evidence that older adults stay in treatment longer than younger adults (Weiss & Petry 2011); given that treatment retention is a primary predictor of treatment success, this is a factor that plays in favor of the older age group. However, a number of other factors (i.e., cognitive impairment, difficulty with mobility, comorbid medical conditions) can negatively affect treatment's effectiveness in the elderly adult and can confound the ability to create generalized treatment recommendations for this population based on limited studies. Furthermore, the demographics of older adults with SUDs is changing; increasing numbers of older adults are seeking treatment for combined alcohol and drug use or for drug use alone (Wu et al. 2011). Thus, limitations continue to arise regarding the application of recommendations to an ever-changing, complex population.

Studies regarding treatment outcomes in older adults focus primarily on alcohol-use problems. Those comparing treatment outcomes (i.e., post-discharge abstinence rates and quality-of-life improvements) in patients with AUD demonstrate that results are similar to those of middle-aged adults (Oslin et al. 2005). Older adults may improve with treatment substantially better than their younger adult counterparts (Blow et al. 2000, Lemke and Moos 2003). Specific variables such as gender and length of treatment may be associated with better outcomes. For instance, older women and patients with longer length of stay tended to have better outcomes (Satre et al. 2004, Oslin et al. 2005). These results may be limited due to small sample sizes of older participants in these studies (Blow et al. 2000).

SAMHSA and the Center for Substance Abuse Treatment (CSAT) have developed Treatment Improvement Protocols (TIPs), which outline the best-practice guidelines for the treatment of SUDs. TIPs #26 and #39 recommend that less intensive options for older substance abusers be explored first (CSAT 1998, 2004). Interventions that are integrated into primary care for the elderly have been shown to be more effective than intensive treatment programs (Bartels et al. 2004, Fink et al. 2005). Prior to any intervention, the clinician can assess readiness for change. The "stages of change" model proposed by Prochaska and DiClemente (1986) can help guide clinicians in addressing resistant or ambivalent patients.

There is evidence that, as is the case with other specialized groups, elderly adults may respond more favorably to brief interventions (Culberson 2006). "Brief interventions" are counseling tools that focus on changing behavior and the assessment of readiness to change, and are patient-focused. They can be conducted in ambulatory settings and include from one to five meetings lasting ten to thirty minutes, and offered at weekly or biweekly intervals. A workbook helps the provider, together with the patient, work through the various stages of change (Blow & Barry 2000). Elderly "late-onset" drinkers may fare particularly well with this minimally invasive intervention.

In cases where brief intervention is not sufficient, other tools are available. Levels of care vary from outpatient individual or group treatment (which can occur at a variety of intervals), to Intensive Outpatient Program/Partial Hospitalization Programs (IOP/PHP), to inpatient residential treatment. Regardless of the setting, TIPs specifically recommend the following approaches to treating elderly patients: cognitive-behavioral approaches, group-based approaches, individual counseling, medical/psychiatric approaches, marital and family involvement/family therapy, and case-management/community-linked services and outreach (CSAT 2005). Elderly-specific biological, psychological, and social considerations must be addressed when one is designing a treatment program. For instance, counselors should be trained and motivated to work with older adults. Some self-help, mixed-age groups, which are often incorporated into treatment, may be less appropriate for some older adults. Others may allow older individuals to use their life experiences to help others, thus increasing their sense of purpose and social interaction (Culberson 2006). Outpatient treatment settings may allow patients to seek treatment for SUDs while maintaining a certain quality of life outside of treatment. For instance, elderly patients in group homes or assisted living can retain their necessary accommodations at home and go to programs during the day, rather than finding inpatient programs with specific accommodations for functional limitations. Some older adult–specialty centers are starting to offer prescription drug addiction treatment to address the growing population in need (Rothrauff et al. 2011). However, when a residential level of care is deemed necessary, physicians should seek medically managed facilities that are equipped to deal with a variety of medical conditions and can address the needs of the elderly (Wu et al. 2011).

Promising outcomes have been achieved using elder-specific, inpatient residential rehabilitation programs. Results from one study found that older adults responded positively to inpatient alcoholism treatment tailored for older adults. The treatment program was established in response to clinical observations of older adults' dropping out of treatment and was designed to accommodate a variety of needs, including detoxification and medical treatment for comorbidities. Age-related issues such as loss, isolation, serious physical health problems, and other aging-related experiences were emphasized. Confrontational approaches were limited, cognitive-behavioral approaches employed, and positive therapeutic alliances with treatment staff were strongly emphasized. Over half the sample (55.9%) reported abstinence during a six-month follow-up period, while the rates of abstinence in younger persons are typically 25% after inpatient treatment (Blow et al. 2000).

Few inpatient treatment facilities are designed with older adults in mind (Schultz et al. 2003). They may not meet the specific needs of the elderly, such as the ability to address the limited mobility and lack of access to transportation. A nationally representative sample of private treatment centers in the 2006–2007 National Treatment Center Study indicated that only 18% provided special services for older adults (Rothrauff et al. 2011). Regardless, older adults may still benefit from age-integrated treatment. A study conducted within the Department of Veterans Affairs comparing older men who entered mixed-aged treatment programs with their younger and middle-aged counterparts found that older patients being treated for AUD have relatively good prognoses, receive comparable treatment, and responded similarly to their younger counterparts. Initial functioning upon entering the program was the strongest predictor of good discharge functioning and was more relevant than age regarding treatment outcome (Lemke & Moos 2002).

## Behavioral Treatments for SUDs in Older Adults: Cognitive Behavioral Therapy, Motivational Enhancement Therapy (MET), Family and Community-Based Treatment

Behavioral therapy techniques are generally a major component of SUD treatment. Despite growing evidence, there currently remains a scarcity of high-quality evidence available about the effectiveness of behavioral treatments for SUD in the general adult population (Klimas et al. 2014), let alone evidence tailored to older adults. There is evidence suggesting that behavioral treatment programs adapted and tailored for older adult populations may improve engagement and retention outcomes, compared to mixed-age behavioral programs (Kofoed et al. 1987). Behavioral programs have been designed for older adults and have been compared to treatment-as-usual. For instance, the Older Alcoholic Rehabilitation Program demonstrated improved abstinence at 6 and 12 months when compared to a standard, more confrontational mixed-age program (Kashner et al. 1992). SAMHSA has published a group therapy manual for older adults that incorporates relapse-prevention skills and self-management techniques entitled "Substance Abuse Relapse Prevention for Older Adults: A Group Treatment Approach" (CSAT 2005). Principles that may be preferable when tailoring treatment for older adults include use of supportive rather than confrontational approaches, enhancement of social support, and incorporating age-appropriate pace and content that reflects common medical comorbidities, social issues, and psychological problems in this population (CSAT 1998). Keeping in mind the lack of consensus and small evidence base overall, we will delineate the behavioral treatments currently thought to be most effective in treating SUDs among older adults.

## COGNITIVE BEHAVIORAL THERAPY

Cognitive behavioral therapy (CBT) employs behavioral counseling in individual and group settings and has been demonstrated to be effective in the treatment of SUD. CBT for SUD focuses to a large degree on relapse-prevention skills, including identification of relapse triggers, strategies to diminish cravings, and engagement in alternative non-drug activities (Vocci & Montoya 2009). There is some evidence that CBT's effectiveness in treating SUDs may operate via its enhancement of coping skills (Kiluk et al. 2010); specifically, the identification and employment of adaptive behaviors in the face of triggers to relapse. Of particular relevance in the older adult, cognitive impairment negatively affects the ability to acquire positive coping skills (Kiluk et al. 2011); the presence of specific cognitive impairments in attention, verbal learning, executive function, impulsivity, and decision-making both predisposes individuals to SUDs and reduces their ability to effectively learn CBT skills (Kalapatapu et al. 2013). Despite the higher likelihood of cognitive impairment in the older adult, however, there is some evidence to suggest that CBT can be of particular utility in older adults, at least with respect to alcohol use (Rice et al. 1993).

## CONTINGENCY MANAGEMENT

Contingency management (CM) has been shown to be effective in treating SUDs in the adult population (Vocci & Montoya 2009, Rawson et al. 2006, Roll, et al. 2006), especially when combined with other behavioral interventions such as CBT (Petitjean et al. 2014). CM is designed to shift decision-making incentives in substance users by monetarily rewarding desired behaviors (i.e., reductions in drug use, attendance at appointments). CM interventions appear to primarily impact treatment retention and to thereby improve outcomes. As noted, older individuals appear to stay in treatment for longer periods than their younger counterparts, which should be expected to predict better response to contingency management. Additionally, older individuals who often have financial constraints may be more responsive to financial rewards. However, there is no clear evidence to date as to whether older individuals derive greater or lesser benefit from contingency management treatment than younger individuals. Of note, a confounding element in interpreting such studies has been the use of a variety of age thresholds for categorization of older cohorts, with some researchers using age as low as 40 as the threshold for inclusion in the "older" category.

## MOTIVATIONAL INTERVIEWING OR MOTIVATIONAL ENHANCEMENT THERAPY

Motivational interviewing (MI), or motivational enhancement therapy, takes an approach designed to assist individuals in addressing any underlying ambivalence toward change and gaining their commitment to making and maintaining healthy changes (Miller 1996). In MI, the clinician takes an empathic and supportive stance yet challenges the patient through targeted questioning to recognize underlying conflicts, resistance and ambivalence toward change of problematic behaviors. The clinician also helps the patient find the inner desire and strength to make and maintain positive changes. Recovery from SUDs requires an individual's motivation to change as a key element, and MI has a relatively large evidence base in the treatment of SUD, in particular with respect to AUDs, especially when combined with other treatments such as CBT or CM techniques (Glasner-Edwards 2011). There is a small body of literature to support the use of MI in the older population with addiction (Chang et al. 2014), and further studies incorporating motivational interviewing sessions are underway (Coulton et al. 2008). A potential challenge when using motivational interviewing techniques in older adults is presented by one of the key elements of motivational interviewing, which calls on an individual's desire for future goals (i.e., family, career, homes, travel) in fostering motivation for change. Aging adults whose health is failing and who may have lost their spouses and friends may have difficulty envisioning attainable goals for the future that could motivate them to change current behaviors.

## FAMILY THERAPY

When providing treatment to older adults, at least some degree of participation by family members is common. Family therapy may be used to facilitate changes in interactions and relationships between family members and to optimize their support and involvement during SUD treatment. Family therapy has a long history in mental health treatment and focuses on assessment and intervention at the level of the entire family. Though the use of family therapy in the treatment of older adults with SUDs has not been extensively studied, family therapy may be useful to enhance support and outcomes in older adults and reduce feelings of isolation during the treatment process (CSAT 2004). Integrated models of family therapy include solution-focused therapy

(Berg & Reuss 1997), network therapy (Galanter 1993), and multi-systemic therapy (Cunningham & Henggeler 1999). When working with older adults, the family unit may consist of adult children, spouses, and/or siblings as the focus of therapy. Family members may learn skills to help facilitate abstinence, set goals, problem solve, and optimize support while maintaining appropriate boundaries. Issues relevant to working with older adult populations may include addressing specific treatment barriers (e.g., medical comorbidity, ageism, transportation issues) and integrating other relevant therapeutic issues such as grief, loss, or concerns about health or dying (CSAT 2004).

## MUTUAL SUPPORT, 12-STEP THERAPIES

Mutual support and self-help approaches such as "12 Step" programs (i.e., Alcoholics Anonymous [AA]) have been extensively studied, including their use in the elderly (e.g., Satre et al. 2004), comparing outcomes against those in younger individuals. While older adults may benefit from AA like younger adults, studies suggest they may be more reluctant to join AA and may require more support in facilitating entry into 12 Step therapies. Furthermore, practical barriers such as lack of transportation and physical disabilities, reluctance to go out in the evening, or greater dependence on spouses may limit this population further. In the Satre et al. (2004) study, older patients were less likely to report ever having attended AA when interviewed at intake to SUD treatment. At a five-year follow-up, participation in AA was similar in younger and older adult populations; however, older adults were less likely than middle-aged adults to consider themselves members of 12 Step groups or to call a member of a 12 Step group for help. In another study, by Lemke and Moos (2003), overall participation in 12 Step groups was similar for younger and older patients, and those who participated more in years 1 and 2 had improved drinking outcomes at five-year follow-up. Greater efforts during treatment to help older adults identify groups they are comfortable with and that are practical for them to attend may help enhance their attendance and participation in AA, thus improving drinking-related outcomes.

## THE MATRIX MODEL

The Matrix Model, originally developed with funding from NIDA and SAMHSA/CSAT for development and evaluation, respectively, is a hybrid behavioral treatment approach that incorporates principles of CBT and motivational interviewing in individual and group settings, family education, and encouragement of 12-Step meeting participation (Rawson et al. 2004). This model, organized into a set of manuals and published by SAMHSA, provides the structure and content for a multi-element, three-visit-per-week, 16-week outpatient treatment experience, followed by a weekly social support group for one year. In addition to CBT materials delivered primarily in group sessions, the Matrix Model emphasizes that clinicians should employ principles of motivational interviewing in their sessions with patients. Family members are involved in structured psychoeducation sessions as well as in joint sessions with the patient. The Matrix Model has been demonstrated to be more effective than "treatment as usual" in the treatment of methamphetamine addiction (Rawson et al. 2004) and other SUDs.

Although behavioral treatments have demonstrated efficacy in treating SUD in the adult population, and with some limited evidence in older adult populations, rates of relapse and dropout are high. Combining behavioral treatments with available pharmacotherapies will be discussed here; encouraging inpatient rehabilitation stays, for example, can help restrict access to alcohol and other drugs and to drug-using partners and environmental cues, maximizing effectiveness of behavioral treatments.

## Pharmacotherapies for Substance Use Disorders in Older Adults

Medication-assisted treatment (MAT) is the use of pharmacotherapy in combination with other treatment modalities, such as those described, in order to achieve better outcomes in the treatment of SUD. MAT helps integrate and individualize care by tailoring the medications to the treatment setting and the clinical considerations of a particular patient. Currently, the U.S. Food and Drug Administration (FDA) has approved pharmacotherapies for the treatment of alcohol, opioid, and nicotine use disorders. Medications for other SUDs, such as cannabis and stimulants, are still under investigation. In older adults, age-related factors such as comorbidities, changes in organ functioning, and medication interactions require specific considerations for appropriate prescribing of pharmacotherapy.

In general, there are two broad treatment categories for which pharmacotherapies are used to treat SUDS: (1) In the initial phase of treatment, medications may be used to treat acute withdrawal and to help attain initial abstinence during detoxification; (2) in ongoing treatment, MAT is used for relapse prevention and to help maintain abstinence. Maintenance therapies, in general, work either by blocking the effects of substances or by substituting a safer agent in lieu of the substance of abuse. With blocking agents (i.e., receptor antagonists), the reinforcing properties of illicit drugs are mitigated by competitive blockage. Therefore, both subjective and physiological effects of the substance are prevented, and use behaviors are no longer reinforced. Alternatively, replacement therapy (i.e., receptor agonists or partial agonists) employs cross-tolerance to a particular drug class by substituting a drug of abuse with a similar agent with less abusive properties. Still other medications target the complex pathways involved in motivation, reward, and learning (i.e., behavior) to alleviate the compulsion and craving common to addiction. All approaches aim to reduce cravings, use, and/or relapse by targeting both behavioral and physiological pathways of addiction.

Special considerations must be taken when prescribing to older adults, due to physiological and psychological differences. The changes in organ systems such as the kidneys and liver may require dose adjustments. Variables such as decreased blood flow to the gastrointestinal (GI) system, slower nephritic function, and age-related or disease-related changes in liver function can increase and prolong effects of drugs. These, plus other changes, such as a decrease in body mass and an increase in body fat, lead to increased concentrations of drugs in the body. Thus, typical adult dosages of many medications are too high for older individuals. In addition, older adults are more likely to experience cognitive impairments such as dementia. Mind-altering medications may worsen these conditions. Furthermore, cognitive impairment may lead to poorer medication compliance, which can be particularly worrisome when controlled substances are prescribed (Benshoff & Harrawood 2003).

The following sections review treatments for the most commonly abused substances, focusing mostly on evidence-based pharmacological treatments and special considerations for older adults.

## PHARMACOTHERAPIES FOR ALCOHOL USE DISORDER

Pharmacological treatment of AUDs includes both treatments for medical (i.e., physical) symptoms in the early phases like anxiety and tremors, and MAT for managing chronic (i.e., psychological or behavioral) symptoms such as craving and relapse. Alcohol withdrawal—the result of initial cessation of alcohol once physiological dependence has occurred—includes significant symptoms and risks when untreated. Dependence is classified by both tolerance to alcohol (greater amounts of alcohol are required to achieve the same effects) and withdrawal symptoms (physiological changes occurring in the absence of alcohol). Long-term alcohol use leads to compensatory changes in the brain's gamma-aminobutyric acid (GABA) and glutamate neurotransmitters and related receptors. These changes are disrupted abruptly as a result of sudden discontinuation of alcohol use. Medications diminish the discomfort and risks and of alcohol withdrawal symptoms, which arise as a result of hyperactivity of the autonomic nervous system. Autonomic hyperactivity includes symptoms such as anxiety, insomnia, tachycardia, and diaphoresis. More serious complications such as seizures or delirium tremens can occur when withdrawal is left untreated, with reported mortality rates of up to 8% (Goodson et al. 2014).

Alcohol withdrawal treatment settings are chosen and pharmacotherapy is administered based on prediction and measurement of withdrawal severity. The Clinical Institute Withdrawal Assessment of Alcohol Scale, revised (CIWA-Ar) is the most reliable and valid scale designed to objectively measure severity (Sullivan et al. 1989). The scale includes a measure of 10 symptoms associated with withdrawal and can be administered at standard intervals. Patients with CIWA scores greater than 15 are at increased risk for severe withdrawal symptoms. While these scales have successfully helped guide treatment in adults, their applicability to the elderly is still relatively unknown.

Risk factors such as comorbidities (i.e., infections, autonomic neuropathy), history of delirium and seizures may increase the risk of severe symptoms such as seizures, delirium, or hallucinations. For instance, one study of 539 withdrawal episodes noted that 55 patients over age 70 were at an increased risk for complications compared to those 70 and under (Foy et al. 1997). Commonly used medications such as beta-blockers may alter typical signs and symptoms of withdrawal, as well. Some studies suggest that older adults may have significantly more withdrawal symptoms and for a longer time. In one study, older adults had 6.8 vs. 5.6 symptoms, and their withdrawal symptoms lasted 9.0 vs. 6.5 days. The older group was also more likely to experience cognitive impairment, weakness, and high blood pressure (Brower et al. 1994). Although there is limited evidence regarding the differences of alcohol withdrawal in the elderly versus general adult populations, several observational studies suggest that there are more complications in older patients. A standardized supportive, non-pharmacological approach optimizing factors such as environment, nutrition, and elimination techniques was found to be supportive in certain patients, and can help mitigate risk factors related to pharmacotherapy in patients with mild to moderate withdrawal (Kraemer et al. 1999).

*Medications for Acute Alcohol Withdrawal*
While many medications have been described for alcohol withdrawal treatment, few have been specifically studied in the elderly. Universally, initial treatment includes fluid and electrolyte correction and thiamine administration to prevent Wernicke's and Korsakoff's syndromes. Older adults are more prone to hypomagnesaemia and are at greater risk for cardiac arrhythmias. Thus, magnesium replacement is recommended (2–4 mEq/kg intravenously on day 1, then 0.5–1 mEq/kg orally or intravenously on days 2–4). Thiamine is usually supplemented as 100 mg intravenously or orally on day 1, and

50–100 mg/day orally subsequently (Saitz & O'Malley 1997). The medications used to address withdrawal specifically are summarized here.

### Sedative Hypnotics

Sedative-hypnotic agents that are cross-tolerant with alcohol reduce the risk of delirium and mortality in alcohol withdrawal. Benzodiazepines, which act on the GABA-A receptors, are the most studied and most effective medications for preventing delirium and seizures (Mayo-Smith 1997). However, patients over 65 have been excluded from most studies of benzodiazepines, which pose significant risks in the elderly. Variables affecting pharmacokinetics and pharmacodynamics of benzodiazepines in the elderly require consideration when choosing both drugs and administration schedules to prevent complications like falls, sedation, or delirium.

Benzodiazepines are metabolized by the liver, then excreted in the urine. The liver metabolizes long-acting benzodiazepines by phase I oxidation followed by phase II glucuronidation. Desmethyldiazepam is the major phase I metabolite of these agents. Phase I oxidation is generally slower in the elderly, and the half-life of desmethyldiazepam is typically over 100 hours. Short-acting agents such as lorazepam, oxazepam, and alprazolam do not undergo phase I oxidation and are therefore more favorable. In contrast, long-acting benzodiazepines may be favored in younger patients to help promote self-tapering and to prevent seizures that may be associated with shorter-acting agents (Allen et al. 1980).

Pharmacodynamic effects account for greater sedation from all benzodiazepines in the elderly population at similar plasma levels. Tolerance may alter these changes. While shorter-acting agents are generally preferred, they paradoxically can create greater seizure risk during discontinuation and may also cause greater memory and cognitive impairments than longer-acting agents (Kraemer et al. 1999).

Benzodiazepine treatment regimens include fixed-schedule, front-loading, and symptom-triggered administration. Again, there are no studies comparing or assessing these regimens in the elderly. Each has advantages and disadvantages and should be tailored to the individual (Kraemer et al. 1999). Medications may be administered in standing regimens, defined by fixed dosages of benzodiazepines, tapering over 3–5 days. Front-loading and symptom-triggered schedules administer medications as needed based on symptoms checked every 1–2 hours. The difference between front-loading and symptom-triggered regimens is that symptom-triggered regimens have a threshold that must be met prior to medications' being administered. Using the CIWA-Ar scale, patients only receive medication if a certain score is met. Regardless of the dosing schedule, patients should be frequently reevaluated to tailor dosages to individual clinical pictures, and under-medicating and over-medicating should be avoided. Elderly patients should be monitored one hour after each dose is given, and for 24 hours after the last dose is given (Kraemer et al. 1999).

Barbiturates have also been used to control signs and symptoms of alcohol withdrawal. However, barbiturates carry risks such as higher abuse potential, increased risk for respiratory depression, and more drug–drug interactions than benzodiazepines. Furthermore, there are no short-acting barbiturates, which limits their use. Thus, barbiturates are not recommended for alcohol withdrawal in older adults (Bernus et al. 1997).

*Anticonvulsants*

Anticonvulsants have also been studied in the treatment of alcohol withdrawal (Malcolm et al. 2001, Eyer et al. 2011). Due to their limited sedating and cognitive effects, as well as low abuse potential, they may be considered safe alternatives to benzodiazepines in mild to moderate withdrawal (Ait-Doud et al. 2006), although they have not been studied in the elderly specifically. Carbamazepine has demonstrated superiority to placebo in rapid relief of symptoms such as tremor, sweating, palpitations, sleep disturbances, depression, anxiety, and anorexia (Stuppaeck et al. 1992). A major roadblock to their use as single agents is a recent meta-analysis with insufficient evidence that anticonvulsant monotherapy reduces seizures or delirium in alcohol withdrawal (Amato et al. 2011). Other limitations to anticonvulsant use include side effects (i.e., dizziness, nausea, vomiting), drug interactions (due to induction of the metabolism of hepatic cytochrome P450-3A4 substrates), and contraindications in those with severe hepatic and/or hematological disease.

Combining anticonvulsants with moderate doses of benzodiazepines can be effective for detoxification in patients with a history of alcohol withdrawal seizures or head trauma (Kasser et al. 1997). In these cases, the anticonvulsant should be administered at dosages that provide therapeutic blood levels and should be used in conjunction with benzodiazepines. The anticonvulsant is tapered within a week of completion of the benzodiazepine-assisted detoxification, assuming there is no prior seizure disorder requiring anticonvulsant medication. This approach may help limit benzodiazepine use in the elderly, if there are no contraindications to anticonvulsants. However, more evidence is needed in older adults to evaluate the safety and efficacy of this approach.

Other anticonvulsants, including vigabatrin and gabapentin, have been examined as adjunctive therapies for alcohol withdrawal (Myrick et al. 2009, 1998), but further studies are needed. Open-label studies have provided preliminary support for the use of levetiracetam in relieving symptoms of alcohol withdrawal (Müller et al. 2010). Gabapentin may alleviate withdrawal symptoms but may not be indicated for severe withdrawal (Bonnet et al.

2010). A 2009 study compared high-dose gabapentin to lorazepam for alcohol withdrawal symptoms. While symptoms were reduced in all three groups, they were most effectively treated with 1200 mg of gabapentin. Furthermore, those who received gabapentin were less likely to drink alcohol in the week following treatment than those who received lorazepam (Myrick et al. 2009). Finally, recent evidence supports the use of gabapentin in combination with naltrexone, an opioid antagonist, to ameliorate symptoms of early abstinence and improve drinking outcomes in alcohol-dependent individuals (Anton et al. 2011).

## Other Agents

Miscellaneous agents such as sympatholytic and antipsychotic pharmacotherapy have been used to reduce alcohol withdrawal symptoms. Sympatholytics such as beta-blockers (i.e., atenolol and propranolol) and alpha-2 agonists (clonidine) can be effective in adjunctive treatment when benzodiazepines alone are insufficient to reduce autonomic symptoms; however, they do not reduce the incidence of seizures and delirium (Baumgartner & Rowen 1987). The elderly can be particularly sensitive to side effects of these medications, such as delirium, hypotension, and postural changes, which limits their use in this population. On the contrary, many older adults with coronary artery disease already take these medications regularly. In these cases, they should be continued in order to prevent myocardial ischemia secondary to autonomic hyperactivity during withdrawal.

Antipsychotics such as haloperidol are often administered to agitated patients in hospital settings, and these can be effective in sleep cycle disturbances and for behavioral issues. While they may reduce some withdrawal symptoms, they have not been shown, however, to be effective in decreasing delirium and seizures. In fact, haloperidol lowers the seizure threshold and therefore should only be used at low dosages (0.25–1 mg) and as an adjuvant to benzodiazepines (Blum et al. 1976). Side effects such as orthostatic hypotension, tachycardia, delirium, and extrapyramidal adverse effects can complicate the clinical picture. Furthermore, antipsychotics have been shown to increase morbidity and mortality risks in the elderly (Barak et al. 2007). Thus, unless more is revealed in future studies to mitigate their apparent risks, their use is limited.

## Medications for Treatment and Management of Alcohol Use Disorder

Once the early phases of AUD have passed, maintenance treatment for AUD is addressed pharmacologically via complex pathways related to learning (behavioral) and reward systems. Recent developments in the general understanding of the neurobiological basis of addiction related to motivation and choice create a common thread that ties together otherwise distinct pharmacological treatment modalities. Research spearheaded by Nora Volkow involving imaging studies of those with SUDs has transformed the understanding of pathological brain changes that make it particularly difficult for those with SUDs to give up their addictions. Basic principles of these complex findings help explain how several agents with different mechanisms may all promote maintenance of AUD treatment. Increases in dopamine (DA) in the limbic system, including the nucleus accumbens (NAc), are related to the prediction of reward and salience (which refers to arousing stimuli and/or environmental changes that promote attentional-behavioral switching). Salience applies to both rewarding and aversive stimuli that affect motivation to seek anticipated rewards, thus facilitating conditioned learning even while the actual drug reward undergoes tolerance (Heilig et al. 2010). While some drugs (i.e., stimulants) increase dopamine directly, alcohol use indirectly increases dopamine by stimulating GABA receptors to modulate dopamine cell firing (Volkow and Li 2004).

While the neurobiology of classical reward systems has revolutionized our understanding of both natural and drug rewards, pharmacological treatments are still limited in number and efficacy. Current understanding of the role of the classical rewards pathway is perhaps least clear in alcohol addiction. Pharmacogenetic differences arise that create multiple distinct drinking patterns among those with AUDs and account for variability in alcohol effects and metabolism. For instance, brain stress and fear systems are pathologically activated in the later stages of alcoholism. Overall, alcohol modulates a wider range of neurotransmitter systems than do other addictive drugs. Therefore, pharmacological treatment of AUD is complex. Targets of MAT vary widely and may be most effective when personalized to unique factors, including genetics and history (Heilig et al. 2010).

Four FDA-approved medications for AUD (oral naltrexone, extended-release intramuscular naltrexone, acamprosate, and disulfiram) address three unique pathways influential in the neurobiological cascade of addictive behavior. Other agents such as topiramate, ondansetron, quetiapine, and gabapentin have some positive results, and still others are under investigation. Selective serotonin reuptake inhibitors (SSRIs) have also been studied, with mixed outcomes.

Naltrexone, a mu opioid receptor antagonist, is approved for the treatment of AUD. It is available in daily oral or monthly extended-release injectable formulations. Naltrexone blocks opioid receptors in the ventral tegmental area (VTA), which leads to downregulation of dopamine transmission. As a result, reward and salience related to alcohol use are decreased. Naltrexone has been shown to reduce alcohol consumption, craving, and relapse to heavy drinking (Bouza et al. 2004, Srisurapanont and Jarusuraisin 2005). Side effects include nausea, headache, vomiting, dizziness, and fatigue, and are usually mild (Srisurapanont and Jarusuraisin 2005). Naltrexone has been associated with dose-related hepatotoxicity in animal studies, but is not typically seen at recommended doses. As a precaution, naltrexone should be avoided in individuals with severe liver disease (Williams 2005). Naltrexone can precipitate opioid withdrawal in individuals taking opioid pain medications.

Naltrexone studies are limited in older adults. However, in the general population, naltrexone use appears to have a modest effect on short-term drinking outcomes, when used in combination with psychosocial support (e.g., Anton et al. 1999, 2006, Volpicelli et al. 1997, O'Malley et al. 1992). Longer-term studies have mixed findings (Krystal et al. 2001, West et al. 1999). A meta-analysis concluded that relapse risk was 28% in those taking naltrexone versus 43% in those taking placebo over the course of 12 weeks; however, 36% discontinued treatment prior to completing the study (Srisuraponont and Jarusuraisin 2005). One of the few studies focusing on older adults compared naltrexone to placebo in veterans over 50 years old. Naltrexone was well tolerated, and relapse to heavy drinking was significantly less frequent in the active treatment group than in the placebo group (Oslin et al. 1997).

One of the likely explanations for mixed outcomes with naltrexone use is genetic variability among those with AUD. Findings from several studies support differential treatment outcomes related to genetic polymorphisms, which are likely to be related to genetic factors that create variability in the response of the endogenous opioid system to alcohol (O'Brien 2005). Individuals with a family history of AUD or with an earlier onset of alcohol use have demonstrated improved outcomes with naltrexone, and various genetic polymorphisms have been identified that are associated with variable responses (Monterosso et al. 2001, Rubio et al. 2005, Oslin et al. 2003).

Monthly extended-release injectable naltrexone (XR-NTX) was approved for the treatment of alcohol dependence by the FDA in 2006 in order to address compliance issues with oral medications. Potential side effects are similar to those of oral naltrexone but also include injection-site reactions, which may involve pain, erythema, bruising, induration, or (rarely) tissue necrosis requiring surgical intervention. Older adults with slow wound healing may be more susceptible to these side effects. Site reactions are more likely when XR-NTX is inadvertently injected subcutaneously or into fatty tissue (CSAT 2009). In 2013, the black box warning regarding the impact of injectable naltrexone on the liver was lifted, as injectable naltrexone bypasses the liver due to lack of oral administration and GI absorption.

Alcohol's ability to acutely reduce tension (i.e., anxiolytic effects) via stimulatory inhibition on GABA transmission and inhibitory effects on the glutamate system probably contributes to the acute negative reinforcing effects of alcohol. Acamprosate is a synthetic analogue of homocysteic acid with a chemical structure similar to GABA, and has been reported to stimulate inhibitory GABA transmission and inhibit glutamate neurotransmitter systems (Williams 2005). As a result, acamprosate may act by reducing features of protracted abstinence such as restlessness, anxiety, and insomnia, symptoms that may predispose alcoholics to relapse (Littleton 1995). Acamprosate is given in 666 mg three times a day. It carries no abuse potential and is excreted unchanged by the kidneys, which may make it preferable to naltrexone in those with hepatic impairment. Side effects include gastrointestinal symptoms, especially diarrhea (Wilde & Wagstaff 1997). Multiple clinical trials in Europe have demonstrated the efficacy of acamprosate in reducing relapses and prolonging abstinence; however, two larger studies in the United States failed to demonstrate its benefits (Mann et al. 2004, Anton et al. 2006, Mason et al. 2006). The discrepancy may be due to variabilities in studies such as longer lead-in abstinence and greater severity of alcohol dependence in the European subjects (National Institute of Alcohol Abuse and Alcoholism [NIAAA] 2008). Though acamprosate has not been specifically studied in older adults, it may be particularly suitable for use in this population due to its relatively benign side-effect profile (Barrick & Connors 2002).

In a study comparing naltrexone, acamprosate, the combination of naltrexone and acamprosate, and placebo, both active drugs and the combination were associated with significantly longer time to first drink and relapse to alcohol use, relative to placebo. Additionally, there was a trend for more positive outcomes in the naltrexone-treated group relative to the acamprosate-treated group. The combination was more effective than placebo or acamprosate, but not better than naltrexone (Kiefer et al. 2003). The COMBINE study examined naltrexone and acamprosate alone and in combinations with cognitive behavioral treatment in alcoholics recently abstinent from alcohol and found that acamprosate was not effective alone or in combination with naltrexone; naltrexone, while effective at early stages of follow-up, did not work better when combined with acamprosate (Anton et al. 2006).

Disulfiram (Antabuse), a medication that inhibits aldehyde dehydrogenase, works by aversive conditioning. Aversive conditioning, a type of behavioral learning, involves pairing a noxious stimulus (e.g., physical sickness) with an unwanted behavior (drinking). Alcohol consumption in the presence of disulfiram causes an accumulation of acetaldehyde, which leads to flushing, nausea, vomiting, palpitations, and sweating (Wright & Moore 1990). More severe reactions include respiratory depression, hypotension, and cardiovascular collapse. In the general population, disulfiram can be helpful in motivated patients with monitoring of ingestion, or on an as-needed basis in situations that are more likely to trigger relapse (Garbutt et al. 1999, Allen and Litten 1992). Disulfram has limited use in the elderly, due to several contraindications.

Disulfiram is not recommended in those with severe cardiovascular disease, pulmonary disease, renal disease, diabetes, or psychosis. It also has several medication interactions such as warfarin, phenytoin, isoniazid, some benzodiazepines, and tricyclic antidepressants. Treatment of the disulfiram reaction includes hydration and oxygen (Elenbaas 1977).

Other medications, although not FDA-approved for AUD, may be effective. Topiramate is an antiepileptic medication that is believed to reduce alcohol's reinforcing effects by lowering glutamatergic activity and increasing GABA function, leading to inhibition of dopamine release (Johnson et al. 2003). While not studied specifically in older adults with AUD, topiramate has been studied in the elderly when used for seizures. Topiramate is shown to have a marked effect on cognition, including deficits in working memory and verbal fluency. Given the susceptibility of older adults to cognitive impairment and risk of falling, topiramate is rarely a first-line agent in epilepsy, and is probably not a strong candidate for AUD in this population (Sommer and Fenn 2010). Other agents such as SSRIs and second-generation antipsychotics (specifically quetiapine) have been studied, with varying results (Kranzler et al. 1995). Differential responses may be due to variations in efficacy in different alcoholic subtypes (Pettinati et al. 2000, Kampman et al. 2007).

Overall, while studies are limited in the elderly, some medications may be efficacious for AUD, as long as contraindications, side effects, and interactions are considered carefully. More data are needed to inform specific recommendations appropriate to the elder population with AUD. Because of the efficacy of non-pharmacological interventions in this population, medications that carry risks should be limited, especially when medications only appear to create modest improvements. Furthermore, in cases where MAT is utilized, it should remain part of an integrative plan with psychosocial support and other behavioral interventions.

## PHARMACOTHERAPIES FOR SEDATIVE, HYPNOTIC, ANXIOLYTIC USE DISORDERS

Long-term use of benzodiazepines and benzodiazepine receptor agonists (BzRAs) is particularly high in the elderly, specifically when used to treat insomnia. Although they are some of the most frequently prescribed medications in the United States for the treatment of anxiety and insomnia, few data establish their efficacy and safety in long-term use (Ancoli-Israel et al. 2005). While small improvements in sleep may occur, long-term use in the elderly is associated with increased risk of falls and cognitive impairment (Glass et al. 2005, Curran et al. 2003). Tolerance and physiological dependence may occur after long-term use (about 30 days), leading to increased dosages. Although no

FDA-approved pharmacological treatments are available for use disorders involving these drugs, sedatives and hypnotics affect \GABA receptors, similar to the action of alcohol, and carry similar withdrawal risks. They bind to a subunit of the GABA-A receptor and, like alcohol, enhance the effects of GABA. Thus, pharmacological treatment for disorders related to these medications in the elderly will be discussed briefly.

## Medications for Overdose

Although benzodiazepines and BzRAs carry a relatively low risk of toxicity compared to other sedative medications (i.e., barbiturates), there is still a risk of overdose leading to respiratory depression and coma. This risk can be elevated in the elderly due to decreased medication metabolism. Flumazenil is a competitive antagonist at the benzodiazepine receptor and causes reversal of benzodiazepine effects. It may be administered in 0.1–0.3 mg boluses as an antidote to benzodiazepine overdose. Precipitation of benzodiazepine withdrawal symptoms, including seizures, and re-sedation may occur after flumazenil administration (Weinbroum et al. 1997). Therefore, slow titration is recommended.

## Medications for Acute Withdrawal

Symptoms of benzodiazepine withdrawal are traditionally similar to those of alcohol. Interestingly, in some studies of long-term benzodiazepine us in the elderly, supervised withdrawal of these medications has led to an apparent reversal of impairments which proved to be drug-induced rather than solely age-related impairment (i.e., improved psychomotor and cognitive functioning). Withdrawal symptoms such as sleep disturbances and anxiety were lower in the elderly than some studies hypothesized, probably secondary to the altered metabolism of benzodiazepines in older adults (Curran et al. 2003). Patients even commented on their perceived alertness soon after withdrawing from benzodiazepines.

Benzodiazepine discontinuation may have significant benefits in this population, but the process can still be challenging, particularly in those who are taking high doses. Complications may occur that can be life-threatening, such as seizures, should tapering occur too rapidly. Therefore, benzodiazepines are tapered to avoid withdrawal-associated complications. Reports of tapering using both long-acting (e.g., diazepam) and various short-acting benzodiazepines (e.g., lorazepam) showed no superiority of one medication over another in the general adult population (Denis et al. 2006). Tapers of 20–50% every 1–2 weeks over durations of 4–12 weeks were reported. As with alcohol withdrawal, altered metabolism should be considered when tapering benzodiazepines.

When tapering low therapeutic doses of benzodiazepines in an outpatient setting, the taper may be conducted slowly to minimize withdrawal symptoms. Tapers are generally completed within 4–12 weeks and typically should not last more than 6 months. Other medications may be considered for benzodiazepine withdrawal. Adjuvant medications that have demonstrated benefit in improving taper outcomes after long-term benzodiazepine therapy in outpatient settings, but not in diminishing withdrawal severity, include trazodone, valproic acid, and carbamazepine (Rickels et al. 1999, Schweizer et al. 1991). Evidence is also emerging in support of newer anticonvulsants, such as pregabalin (Rubio et al. 2011), gabapentin (Himmerich et al. 2007), and oxcarbazapine (Croissant et al. 2008) in the treatment of benzodiazepine withdrawal.

## PHARMACOTHERAPIES FOR OPIOID USE DISORDER

### Treatment of Opioid Overdose

Opioid overdose is often a life-threatening medical emergency, and it is particularly dangerous in older adults. Elderly individuals tend to have reduced hepatic and renal function, increasing the peak concentration and duration of effect of opioids and their metabolites, and they are more likely to have underlying pulmonary disorders increasing the likelihood of life-threatening respiratory suppression (Pergolizzi et al. 2008; Pergolizzi et al. 2012). Thus, opioid overdose is a higher risk for older opioid-using individuals, and clinicians should be on high alert for the possibility of life-threatening overdose. As in the general adult population, naloxone is an effective medication for acute reversal of opioid overdose in the elderly. Naloxone works by displacing opioid agonists from mu receptors; it can be administered intravenously, intramuscularly, subcutaneously, and intranasally. It appears to be as safe and effective in the older population as it is in younger adults, following the general rule of thumb of using caution and administering lower doses in the elderly, out of concern for decreased clearance rates and the likelihood of drug–drug interactions.

### Treatment of Acute Opioid Withdrawal

Opioid withdrawal, while not usually life-threatening, causes significant discomfort and increased risk of relapse; in the elderly, opioid withdrawal symptoms are generally more severe. Additionally, older opioid-dependent individuals are more likely to have comorbid pain conditions (Barry et al. 2013), further exacerbating symptoms of opioid withdrawal. As with younger adults, the treatment of acute opioid withdrawal may involve non-opioid medications such as clonidine, gabapentin, and non-medications for sleep. In cases of severe withdrawal, atypical antipsychotics such as quetiapine may be used on a short-term basis. In general, the use of benzodiazepines should be avoided in the older population during opioid detoxification because of cognitive and sedating side effects, as well as increased risk of overdose mortality when combined with opioids. Detoxification from opioids can also effectively be accomplished using long-acting opioids (methadone or buprenorphine); however, lower initial doses and more careful monitoring should be initiated because of the generally increased risk of sedation and other side effects in older individuals (Chau et al. 2008). Buprenorphine appears to be well tolerated at low doses in older adults, with initial nausea and constipation appearing to be transient side effects, and buprenorphine may additionally have some anti-depressant effects (Karp et al. 2014). Buprenorphine may be a safer choice in the elderly, given lower rates of respiratory depression and sedation with opioid toxicity, as well as a shorter half-life than methadone (Lee et al. 2013); additionally, detoxification using buprenorphine tends to be associated with the highest rates of patient follow-up in post-detoxification maintenance treatment, thus increasing the appeal of using this medication (Digiusto et al. 2005).

"Ultra-rapid" detoxification, using heavy sedation or general anesthesia to achieve taper off opioids, is sometimes used in the general adult population to achieve abstinence within a matter of hours or days. However, it is not recommended for use in the geriatric population, given the increased risk of anesthesia-related complications in this population—which are significant even in younger adults (Rabinowitz et al. 2002).

Success rates for detoxification treatments have generally assessed only short-term outcomes, either becoming opioid-free or becoming opioid-free with concomitant naltrexone treatment, the latter which has not been widely adopted. Ling and colleagues (2009) showed low rates of opioid abstinence following completion of either a 7-day or a 28-day buprenorphine/naloxone taper in opioid-dependent individuals. Such results are common with other methods of opioid withdrawal as well, when ongoing pharmacotherapy is not utilized. Consideration should be given to maintaining recently detoxified patients on an opioid antagonist medication such as naltrexone because relapse rates to illicit opioid use following medical withdrawal are very high (over 90%) over a 6- to 12-month period without sustained outpatient treatment (Kleber 1981, Kosten and Kleber 1984). Methods for transferring those who are medically withdrawn from opioids using buprenorphine to naltrexone have been reviewed (Sigmon et al. 2012). In a study of methadone maintenance versus a 180-day methadone detoxification program with enhanced psychosocial treatment services, methadone maintenance therapy resulted in greater treatment retention and lower heroin use than did the enhanced detoxification treatment (Sees et al. 2000). Similarly, Kakko (2003) compared buprenorphine maintenance to medically supervised buprenorphine withdrawal, with both groups having access to enhanced psychosocial services. The entire sample of those randomized to buprenorphine withdrawal had dropped out of the study by 60 days, and four people in that sample died, although the causes of death were not described. These observations underscore the difficulty of successfully undertaking ópiate detoxification in opioid-addicted patients. Moreover, such observations speak to the need to increase the availability of opiate therapy programs that can provide long-term agonist or antagonist pharmacotherapy to this population.

*Maintenance Medications for Opioid Use Disorder in the Older Population*
In the general adult population, relapse rates to opioid abuse are high (greater than 70% within the first month) following opioid detoxification without continuation on medication maintenance therapy (Northrup et al. 2015). As mentioned previously in this chapter, older adults are consistently found to be significantly more likely to attend follow-up treatment, and in this regard they are particularly good candidates for opioid maintenance therapy. Additionally, untreated opioid use disorders in older adults are associated with significantly greater all-cause mortality than in younger adults with active opioid use disorders (Larney et al. 2015). Three medications are currently approved for use in the United States as maintenance pharmacotherapies, all of which can be used in older adults: naltrexone, buprenorphine, and methadone.

Naltrexone has a body of evidence for use in the treatment of older patients with alcohol dependence, and it has been found to be safe and well tolerated in the older adult (Oslin et al. 1997). While there is not a specific body of literature pertaining to the use of naltrexone for the treatment of older opioid-dependent adults, since the medication is well tolerated in older individuals with alcohol dependence, it can presumably be safely used in older opioid-dependent individuals as well.

Naltrexone is administered either orally or via long-acting depot by intramuscular injection, which has a duration of effect of approximately 30 days; both formulations are FDA-approved for the treatment of alcohol and opioid dependence. Given that it antagonizes the mu-opioid receptor, naltrexone is ideal in patients who want to achieve total abstinence from opioids. It is less useful in patients with comorbid chronic pain (more common in the older population), who may need some level of opioid pharmacotherapy over the long term (though, it should be noted, novel research is showing efficacy of low-dose naltrexone in some chronic pain conditions; see Younger et al. 2014). A risk in starting naltrexone therapy is causing precipitated opioid withdrawal; given that symptoms of opioid withdrawal tend to be significantly more severe in the older patient, particular caution should be used when starting naltrexone in this population. In general, one should wait 7–10 days from last use of short-acting opioids, and at least 10 days after last use of a long-acting agent such as methadone; in the older individual it is recommended to wait even longer, given reduced clearance of these drugs. An intramuscular "naloxone challenge" to detect presence of opioid can be a useful tool when there is doubt as to whether an individual is fully opioid-free.

The standard dosing of oral naltrexone is 50 mg daily, although this medication can also be administered less frequently at larger doses (100 mg every two days, or 150 mg every third day); doses of 100 mg have been studied in older individuals and have been well tolerated (Oslin et al. 1997), and there does not appear to be reason to decrease oral naltrexone dosing in the older patient. XR-NTX is available as "Vivitrol" in the United States, with a dose of 380 mg via monthly intramuscular injection. As with short-acting naltrexone, XR-NTX tolerability does not appear to differ in the older population; however, this has not yet been adequately studied. With both short-acting and long-acting naltrexone, there is a very small risk of hepatic toxicity, and liver enzymes should be monitored prior to and during treatment. Recent research suggests that XR-NTX can be safely started shortly after buprenorphine-assisted detoxification without precipitating withdrawal (Mannelli et al. 2014); these results are promising, given that buprenorphine detoxification and long-acting naltrexone maintenance therapies are among the most effective pharmacotherapies for opioid dependence. In a large multicenter trial, significantly greater opioid abstinence rates were achieved in participants treated with long-acting naltrexone (51%) than placebo (31%), and the medication was well tolerated (Krupitsky et al. 2011). This tolerability and effectiveness was observed across a wide range of demographic and severity characteristics (Nunes et al. 2015), and continued treatment proved to be effective for at least one year after initial study conclusion (Krupitsky et al. 2013).

For many patients, chronically recurring opioid relapses and/or a comorbid pain condition make opioid agonist maintenance treatment the best choice. Elderly patients may have decreased renal and hepatic function, leading to prolonged half-lives and elevated peak plasma concentrations of opioid medications relative to younger individuals; buprenorphine appears to be an exception to this rule (Pergolizzi et al. 2008). Methadone, however, carries increased risks in the older individual, including drug–drug interactions, potential for QTc prolongation, and overdose risk.

Therefore, given that the efficacies of buprenorphine and methadone appear largely equivalent as opioid-agonist-maintenance therapies, we suggest that the older patient in need of maintenance treatment should be considered for buprenorphine maintenance therapy. An additional benefit of buprenorphine over methadone in the elderly population is that buprenorphine can be prescribed in the clinician's office; older individuals with decreased mobility are likely to find it particularly challenging to manage the daily clinic attendance required with methadone maintenance programs. Buprenorphine inductions appear well tolerated in outpatients regardless of whether the opioid of abuse is short- or long-acting, and buprenorphine maintenance is also associated with pain relief, both important considerations in the elderly (Nielen et al. 2014, Rouxet al. 2013). Furthermore, recent analyses suggest that buprenorphine is currently more cost-effective than other maintenance treatments, including long-acting naltrexone, and that buprenorphine may be associated with better bone health and fewer fractures compared to other ongoing opioid use in the elderly (Jackson et al. 2015, Hirst et al. 2015).

## PHARMACOTHERAPIES FOR TOBACCO USE DISORDER (NICOTINE DEPENDENCE)

A variety of pharmacotherapies are FDA-approved for the treatment of nicotine dependence, including nicotine replacement therapy (NRT), the antidepressant bupropion, and varenicline, a nicotine receptor partial agonist. Second-line agents include clonidine and nortriptyline. These medications have repeatedly been shown to be effective in the general population for smoking cessation (Eisenberg 2008). Overall, 6- and 12-month quit rates observed in clinical trials remain low, with less than 25% abstinence observed in individuals receiving approved pharmacotherapies and 10% for placebo (McNeil et al. 2010). A recent review by Cawkwell and colleagues examined studies of pharmacological smoking-cessation therapies in adults over 60 years old. After exclusion criteria, only 12 studies were included in the review (Cawkwell et al. 2015). NRT has been the central pharmacological treatment studied in older people for smoking cessation. Data suggests that older adults who attempt to quit are more likely to be successful than their younger counterparts (Burns 2000). Among other benefits, men over 65 who quit smoking have been shown to live 1.4–2 years longer than those who continue, while women have been shown to live 2.7–3.7 years longer (Taylor et al. 2002). Thus, smoking cessation should be encouraged as soon as possible (Thomas 2013).

### Nicotine Replacement Therapy
Five NRT products have been approved by the FDA for smoking cessation treatment: transdermal patches, gums, lozenges, nasal sprays, and vapor inhalers. NRT, which replaces the nicotine from tobacco and in turn mitigates cravings and withdrawal symptoms, has been shown in clinical trials to improve quit rates relative to placebo (17% vs. 10%, respectively) (Stead et al. 2008) and to increase the odds of quitting smoking by 1.77 in the general population (Silagy et al. 2004). The largest study in elders, which occurred in

South Korea, showed a 57% quit rate among men over the age of 60, the largest quit rate of any age group, when they were given NRT plus behavioral counseling. In a large U.S. study designed specifically for those over 65, quit rates were closer to 10–20% (Joyce et al. 2008).

In one study, elderly patients with high-grade dependence had better results with NRT inhalers, while those with low-grade dependence had higher abstinence rates with the NRT patch (Elhassan et al. 2007). Guidelines recommend starting NRT on the target quit date (Raupach and van Schayck 2011) and limiting use to 12 weeks or fewer (Fiore et al. 2008), though initiating NRT earlier than the quit date may be associated with improved abstinence rates (Rose et al. 2009). Side effects common to all NRT formulations include nausea, dizziness, and headache. More specifically, the gum can cause mouth or dental irritation, the patch can cause skin irritation, and the spray can cause nasal irritation. In the elderly, practical limitations due to increased aspiration risks (i.e., patients who are recumbent or dysphagic) and dentures should also be considered when choosing the gum or lozenges.

Older adults have demonstrated significantly slower nicotine clearance than younger adults (Molander et al. 2001). However, this has not yet been shown empirically to affect the effectiveness of NRT (Kleykamp et al. 2011). Several transdermal formulations that deliver nicotine through the skin at a relatively stable rate are available (Henningfield et al. 2005). The recommended duration of patch use is generally ten weeks, beginning with six weeks at the highest dose, followed by two weeks each at the lower doses prior to discontinuation. Nicotine polacrilex (nicotine gum) is available over the counter in two doses: 2 mg or 4 mg. Recommended dosing is one piece every 1–2 hours for the first six weeks, followed by a reduction in dosing frequency every three weeks thereafter. The nicotine lozenge is also available without a prescription in 2-mg and 4-mg doses. The nasal spray permits more rapid delivery of nicotine than other NRTs, and the inhaler delivers nicotine via a mouthpiece and plastic cartridge, which releases a vapor in the mouth when "puffed." Use of the inhaler mimics the familiar hand-to-mouth ritual of smoking cigarettes that some users miss when they quit (Henningfield et al. 2005).

*Bupropion*
Sustained-release (SR) bupropion, an antidepressant with dopaminergic and noradrenergic properties, has demonstrated anti-smoking properties in multiple randomized clinical trials (RCTs) (Hurt et al. 1997, Hughes et al. 2007). The mechanism of action of bupropion in smoking cessation is not fully understood, but may be related to amelioration of nicotine withdrawal symptoms like dysphoria (Henningfield et al. 2005) and a reduction in reinforcing effects due to antagonistic effects at nicotinic receptors (Slemmer et al. 2000).

Bupropion has been used extensively as an antidepressant in the older population and is generally well tolerated (DasGupta 1998). In the general population, the effectiveness of bupropion treatment is at least equivalent to NRT's, with an approximate doubling of quit rates relative to placebo (Hughes et al. 2007). Although studies examining bupropion for smoking cessation in the elderly are limited, in one study investigating predictive factors for successful cessation with bupropion, advanced age (over 50) was a positive predictive variable (Dale et al. 2001).

The dose of bupropion SR used for smoking cessation is the same as that for depression (150 mg twice daily [BID]) in the general population, and it is recommended to begin medication 7–14 days prior to the target quit date. The half-life of bupropion may be prolonged in the elderly. Thus, toxic effects such as seizures and psychosis may occur from the accumulation of metabolites. Lower doses (such as 75–225 mg/day total) should be considered in those with renal or liver impairment or those with increased seizure risk (Howard and Warnock 2012). The duration of treatment is typically up to 12 weeks, but it may be extended. The most common side effects of bupropion include headache, insomnia, and dry mouth. In the study noted, older adults had greater efficacy with a 150-mg daily dose than the 300-mg total daily dose, despite a greater response in younger patients at the higher daily dose (Dale et al. 2001).

## Varenicline

Varenicline is a partial agonist at the α4β2 nicotinic acetylcholine receptor that alleviates nicotine craving and withdrawal symptoms while simultaneously inhibiting nicotine binding and diminishing the rewarding effects of smoking (McNeil et al. 2010). In prior clinical trials, varenicline has demonstrated greater efficacy in reducing cigarette smoking than both bupropion and NRT. A recent meta-analysis reported a 2.3 times greater likelihood of abstinence from smoking at six months or longer with varenicline than placebo and a 1.5 times greater likelihood of quitting at one year with varenicline compared to bupropion. Varenicline has not been studied specifically in the elderly for smoking cessation; however, safety and tolerability have been tested in this population. Varenicline is metabolized minimally by the liver and excreted primarily unchanged via the kidneys. When compared to younger smokers, older smokers (with normal renal function for age) experienced similar pharmacokinetic parameters. Thus, dose adjustment based on age alone is not necessary (Burnstein et al. 2006).

The standard duration of varenicline therapy is 12 weeks. Recommended dosing of varenicline is 0.5 mg daily, titrated gradually to 1 mg twice a day over eight days, starting seven days prior to the target quit date. The most common side effects include nausea, dizziness, and headache, which may be minimized by gradually titrating the dose (McNeil et al. 2010). Serious adverse reactions, including cardiovascular events and neuropsychiatric symptoms, have been reported to the FDA, prompting a safety warning issued in 2008 targeting serious behavioral symptoms, including suicidality. Subsequent research examining the causality of varenicline with serious cardiovascular events and neuropsychiatric symptoms has been inconclusive (Hays et al. 2012).

### Second-Line Agents

Other agents may be used off-label for smoking cessation. Clonidine, an α-2 noradrenergic receptor agonist, has demonstrated efficacy in the general population, but there is a lack of studies regarding its safety and efficacy in the elderly. Due to side effects such as hypotension and rebound hypertension, as well as dry mouth, dizziness constipation, and agitation, it remains a second-line agent. Nortriptyline, a tricyclic antidepressant, was found to reduce withdrawal symptoms compared with placebo in patients averaging 47 years of age (+/–14 years) (Prochazka et al. 1998). Neither clonidine nor nortriptyline is FDA-approved for smoking cessation.

### Combination Therapy

Multiple forms of pharmacotherapy may be combined in order to enhance smoking cessation rates. Literature supports the use of bupropion with NRT to improve smoking cessation outcomes (Jorenby et al. 1999, Shah et al. 2003). Nortriptyline has been shown to enhance cessation rates of NRT when used in combination with NRT in a study with participants of the average age of 41 years (+/–11 years) (Prochazka et al. 2004). The combination of varenicline with bupropion has been studied, indicating some potential efficacy (Ebbert et al. 2009); however, combining NRT with varenicline is not currently recommended and may increase the risk of side effects (McNeil et al. 2010). Combinations of the nicotine patch with other forms of NRT have also been shown more effective than either alone (Fagerstrom et al. 1993, Kornitzer et al. 1995, Piper et al. 2009).

## PHARMACOTHERAPIES FOR STIMULANT USE DISORDER

Stimulant drugs, including cocaine and amphetamines, act by increasing catecholamine levels in the brain, including dopamine and norepinephrine. Acute stimulant intoxication may be marked by autonomic hyperactivity (i.e., tachycardia, hypertension) and psychiatric symptoms such as anxiety, insomnia, agitation, or psychosis. Benzodiazepines and/or neuroleptics may be prescribed to treat agitation or psychosis, and sleep medications may be used to address insomnia (e.g., Shoptaw et al. 2009, Leelahanaj et al. 2005).

Withdrawal from stimulants may cause anxiety, depression, irritability, and hypersomnia, but the majority of symptoms typically resolve within several days (Newton et al. 2004). In cases of protracted depression or anxiety symptoms, antidepressants or other anxiolytics may be prescribed, in addition to sleep medications as indicated.

The majority of individuals seeking treatment for stimulant use disorder are younger and middle aged adults. Treatment studies have not been designed to address the specific needs of older stimulant users. To date, there are no FDA-approved medications for the treatment of stimulant use disorder. As such, evidence-based behavioral therapies such as cognitive behavioral therapy remain the gold standard for addressing ongoing cravings and reducing relapse risk. Multiple dopaminergic agents, antidepressants, and anticonvulsants have been studied as treatment agents for cocaine and methamphetamine addiction, but no medication has demonstrated conclusive evidence of efficacy.

Among cocaine users, topiramate has demonstrated preliminary efficacy in reducing relapse relative to placebo (Kampman et al. 2004, Johnson et al. 2013). Disulfiram, a medication approved for the treatment of alcohol dependence, has also been associated with reduced cocaine use in cocaine-dependent individuals in some studies (e.g., Carroll et al. 2000, Petrakis et al. 2000, Pani et al. 2010); effects on cocaine appear to be independent of those on alcohol use (Carroll et al. 2004). As a dopamine beta hydroxylase inhibitor, disulfiram raises dopamine levels and may increase the aversive effects of cocaine (Dackis 2004). Modafinil, a wakefulness-promoting agent approved to treat fatigue associated with certain sleep disorders, has reduced cocaine use in some studies (Dackis et al. 2005), but not all (Dackis et al. 2012, Anderson et al. 2009).

Bupropion, an antidepressant and smoking cessation agent with dopaminergic and noradrenergic properties, has been associated with reductions in relapse in methamphetamine-dependent adults (Elkashef et al. 2008). Though findings from prior studies have been mixed (Anderson et al. 2015), bupropion may act to reduce dysphoria commonly associated with methamphetamine use and early abstinence. Naltrexone, a mu opioid receptor antagonist, has demonstrated preliminary efficacy in reducing methamphetamine use and in minimizing subjective effects of methamphetamine (Jayaram-Lindstrom et al. 2008); this medication may minimize cravings and drug rewarding effects via its effects on the opioid reward system. The antidepressant mirtazapine has also demonstrated efficacy in reducing methamphetamine use relative to placebo in a select population of men who have sex with men (Colfax et al. 2011). A treatment approach under investigation is the use of stimulants as "replacement" therapy for stimulant use disorder; though findings have been mixed, preliminary support for the use of prescription stimulants to treat

methamphetamine or cocaine addiction has been evidenced in some studies (e.g., Grabowski et al. 2004, Tiihonen 2007, Galloway et al. 2011, Levin
et al. 2015).

## MONITORING AND SUPPORT DURING TREATMENT

Although there are challenges in the treatment of older adults with SUDs,
it appears that among those who are successfully treated, relapse rates may
be substantially lower than in younger adults (Barrick and Connors 2002).
Regardless, due to the tremendously negative consequences of SUDs and their
chronic nature, relapse prevention remains a high priority. Relapse prevention
involves identifying high-risk situations that might be followed by a return to
drug or alcohol use, employing strategies that have promoted abstinence in the
past, and engaging in various treatment techniques to mitigate relapse risk. In
the older adult, factors like anxiety, interpersonal conflict, loneliness, depression, and social isolation can be particularly risky triggers for relapse.

Relapse-prevention techniques are as effective in older adults as they are
in the general population (Barrick and Connors 2002). Treatments like cognitive behavioral therapy, self-help groups, and group counseling and family
therapy can be utilized, with particularly strong benefits derived from the
modalities that offer social support. Medicinal adjuncts, especially with medications having negligible adverse effects (i.e., naltrexone and acamprosate),
may be used for relapse prevention, provided solid compliance and monitoring are in place. Mindfulness-Based Relapse Prevention (MBRP), a specific
CBT focused on responses to high-risk situations coupled with skills training
and cognitive interventions, shows particular promise for maintaining abstinence (Bowen, et al. 2009). However, it has yet to be examined specifically in
the elderly. Aftercare programs, which may include monitoring (i.e., random
urine drug screens), group therapy, or 12-Step groups are offered following
intensive SUD treatment programs. Limitations like transportation should
be considered in the elderly. Finally, support groups for family members affected by those with SUDs, such as Al-Anon or other family support therapies,
may be useful to improve psychosocial support. Overall, combining treatment
strategies and individualizing techniques to patients' needs and preferences
are likely to show the greatest promise for reducing substance use and main-
taining/improving psychosocial functioning (Irvin et al. 1999).

## Conclusion

Substance use disorders are a growing problem in the elderly. Due to the co-
occurrence of multiple chronic medical issues, consequences of these disorders

can be particularly devastating. The treatment of older adults with SUDs is met with unique challenges, from screening and identification, to placement, to aftercare. Few guidelines exist to help providers, families, and patients outline appropriate treatment strategies. Programs and resources with special services for the elderly are limited. Thus, most treatment strategies involve identifying individual needs and limitations and utilizing resources that have proved effective in the general adult population. Certain programs and treatment strategies must be tailored to the older adult (i.e., creating behavioral programs with an older adult focus or adjusting medication dosages due to metabolic differences or drug interactions). Greater education and awareness are needed to help promote development of age-appropriate treatment options that will address unique challenges in this growing population.

# References

Adams WL, Cox NS. Epidemiology of problem drinking among elderly people. *Int J Addict* 1995;30:1693–1716.

Ait-Doud N, Malcolm RJ, Johnson BA. An overview of medications for the treatment of alcohol withdrawal and alcohol dependence with an emphasis on the use of older and newer anticonvulsants. *Addict Behav* 2006;31(9):1628–1649.

Allen JP, Litten RZ. Techniques to enhance compliance with disulfiram. *Alcohol Clin Exper Res* 1992;16(6):1035–1041.

Allen MD, Greenblatt DJ, Harmatz JS, et al. Desmethyldiazepam kinetics in the elderly after prazepam. *Clin Pharmacol Ther* 1980;28:196–202.

Amato L. Minozzi S, Davoli M. Efficacy and safety of pharmacological interventions for the treatment of alcohol withdrawal syndrome. *Cochrane Database Syst Rev* 2011;15(6), CD008537.

Ancoli-Israel S, Richardson GS, Mangano RM, Jenkins L, Hall P, Jones WS. Long-term use of sedative hypnotics in older patients with insomnia. *Sleep Med Rev* 2005;6:107–113.

Anderson AL, Li SH, Markova D, et al. Bupropion for the treatment of methamphetamine dependence in non-daily users: A randomized, double-blind, placebo-controlled trial. *Drug Alcohol Depend* 2015;150:170–174. doi:10.1016/j.drugalcdep.2015.01.036. [Epub Feb. 7, 2015.]

Anderson AL, Reid MS, Li SH, et al. Modafinil for the treatment of cocaine dependence. *Drug Alcohol Depend* 2009;104(1–2):133–139.

Anton RF, Moak DH, Waid LR, Latham PK, Malcolm RJ, Dias JK. Naltrexone and cognitive behavioral therapy for the treatment of outpatient alcoholics: Results of a placebo-controlled trial. *Am J Psychiatry* 1999;156(11):1758–1764.

Anton RF, Myrick H, Wright TM, et al. Gabapentin combined with naltrexone for the treatment of alcohol dependence. *Am J Psychiatry* 2011;168(7):709–717.

Anton RF, O'Malley SS, Ciraulo DA, et al., COMBINE Study Research Group. Combined pharmacotherapies and behavioral interventions for alcohol dependence: The COMBINE study: A randomized controlled trial. *JAMA* 2006;295(17):2003–2017.

Backmund M, Meryer K, Eichenlaub D, Schutz CG. Predictors for completing an inpatient detoxification program among intravenous heroin users, methadone substituted and codeine-substituted patients. *Drug Alcohol Depend* 2001;64:173–180.

Barak Y, Baruch Y, Mazeh D, Paleacu D, Aizenberg D. Cardiac and cerebrovascular morbidity and mortality associated with antipsychotic medications in elderly psychiatric inpatients. *Am J Geriatr Psych* 2007;15(4):354–356.

Barrick C, Connors GJ. Relapse prevention and maintaining abstinence in older adults with alcohol-use disorders. *Drugs Aging* 2002;19(8):583–594.

Barry DT, Savant JD, Beitel M, et al. Pain and associated substance use among opioid dependent individuals seeking office-based treatment with buprenorphine-naloxone: A needs assessment study. *Am J Addict* 2013;22(3):212–217.

Bartels SJ, Coakley EH, Zubritsky C, et al., PRISM-E Investigators. Improving access to geriatric mental health services: a randomized trial comparing treatment engagement with integrated versus enhanced referral care for depression, anxiety, and at-risk alcohol use. *Am J Psychiatry* 2004;161(8): 1455-62.

Baumgartner GR, Rowen RC. Clonidine vs chlordiazepoxide in the management of acute alcohol withdrawal syndrome. *Arch Intern Med* 1987;147(7):1223–1226.

Benshoff JJ, Harrawood LK. Substance abuse and the elderly: Unique issues and concerns. *J Rehabil* 2003;69(2):43–48.

Berg IK, Reuss N. *Solutions step-by-step: a substance abuse treatment manual.* New York: W.W. Norton; 1997.

Bernus I, Dickinson RG, Hooper WD, et al. Anticonvulsant therapy in aged patients: Clinical pharmacokinetic considerations. *Drugs Aging* 1997;10:278–289.

Blow FC, Walton MA, Chermack ST, Mudd SA, Brower KJ. Older adult treatment outcome following elder-specific inpatient alcoholism treatment. *J Subst Abuse Treat* 2000;19(1):67–75.

Blow FC, Barry KL. Older patients with at-risk and problem drinking patterns: New developments in brief interventions. *J Geriatr Psych Neurol* 2000;13(3):115–123.

Blum K, Eubanks JD, Wallace JE, et al. Enhancement of alcohol withdrawal convulsions in mice by haloperidol. *Clin Toxicol,* 1976;9, 427–434.

Bonnet U, Hamzavi-Abedi R, Specka M, Wiltfang J, Lieb B, Scherbaum N. An open trial of gabapentin in acute alcohol withdrawal using an oral loading protocol. *Alcohol Alcoholism* 2010;45(2):143–145.

Bouza C, Angeles M, Munoz A, Amate JM. Efficacy and safety of naltrexone and acamprosate in the treatment of alcohol dependence: A systematic review. *Addiction* 2004;99(7):811–828.

Bowen S, Chawla N, Collins SE, et al. Mindfulness-based relapse prevention for substance use disorders: A pilot efficacy trial. *Subst Abuse* 2009;30(4):295–305. doi:10.1080/08897070903250084

Brower KJ, Mudd S, Blow FC, Young JP, Hill EM. Severity and treatment of alcohol withdrawal in elderly versus young patients. *Alcohol Clin Exper Res* 1994;18(1), 196–201.

Burns DM Cigarette smoking among the elderly: Disease consequences and benefits of cessation. *Am J Health Promot* 2000;14(6):357–361.

Burke KC, Meek WJ, Krych R, Nisbet R, Burke JD.Jr. Medical services use by patients before and after detoxification from benzodiazepine dependence. *Psychiatr Serv* 1995;46(2):157–160.

Burnstein AH, Fullerton T, Clark DJ, Faessel HM. Pharmacokinetics, safety, and tolerability after single and multiple oral doses of varenicline in elder smokers. *J Clin Pharmacol* 2006;46(11):1234–1240. doi:10.1177/0091270006291837.

Carroll KM, Fenton LR, Ball SA, et al. Efficacy of disulfiram and cognitive behavior therapy in cocaine-dependent outpatients: A randomized placebo-controlled trial. *Arch Gen Psychiatry* 2004;61(3):264–272.

Carroll KM, Nich C, Ball SA, McCance E, Frankforter TL, Rounsaville BJ. One-year follow-up of disulfiram and psychotherapy for cocaine-alcohol users: Sustained effects of treatment. *Addiction* 2000;95(9):1335–1349.

Cawkwell BP, Blaum C, Sherman SE. Pharmacological smoking cessation therapies in older adults: A review of the evidence. *Drugs Aging* 2015;32(6):443–451.

Center for Substance Abuse Treatment. Expert Panel Clinical Guidelines on LAAM in Opioid Agonist Therapy. Technical Assistance Publication (TAP) Series. 2002. Rockville, MD: U.S. Dept. of Health and Human Services.

Center for Substance Abuse Treatment. Incorporating Alcohol Pharmacotherapies into Medical Practice. Treatment Improvement Protocol (TIP) Series #49. HHS Publication No. (SMA) 09-4380. 2009. Rockville, MD: Substance Abuse and Mental Health Services Administration.

Center for Substance Abuse Treatment. Substance Abuse Relapse Prevention for Older Adults: A Group Treatment Approach. DHHS Publication No. (SMA) 05-4053. 2005. Rockville, MD: Substance Abuse and Mental Health Services Administration.

Chang YP, Compton P, Almeter P, Fox CH. The effect of motivational interviewing on prescription opioids adherence among older adults with chronic pain. *Perspect Psychiatr Care.* 2014; doi:10.1111/ppc.12082. [Epub ahead of print.]

Chau DL, Walker V, Pai L, Cho LM. Opiates and elderly: Use and side effects. *Clin Interv Aging* 2008;3(2):273–278.

Colfax GN, Santos GM, Das M, et al. Mirtazapine to reduce methamphetamine use: A randomized controlled trial. *Arch Gen Psychiatry* 2011;68(11):1168–1175.

Coulton S, Watson J, Bland M, et al. The effectiveness and cost-effectiveness of opportunistic screening and stepped care interventions for older hazardous alcohol users in primary care (AESOPS)—a randomised control trial protocol. *BMC Health Serv Res* 2008;12(8):129.

Croissant B, Grosshans M, Diehl A, Mann K. Oxcarbazepine in rapid benzodiazepine detoxification. *Am J Drug Alcohol Abuse* 2008;34(5):534–540.

Cunningham PB, and Henggeler SW Engaging multiproblem families in treatment: Lessons learned throughout the development of multisystemic therapy. *Family Process* 1999;38(3):265–281.

Culberson J. Alcohol use in the elderly: Beyond the CAGE. Part 2: Screening instruments and treatment strategies. *Geriatrics* 2006;61(11):20–26.

Curran HB, Collins R, Fletcher S, Kee SC Y., Woods B, Iliffe S. Older adults and withdrawal from benzodiazepine hypnotics in general practice: Effects on cognitive function, sleep, mood, and quality of life. *Psychol Med* 2003;33:1223–1237.

Dackis CA. Recent advances in the pharmacotherapy of cocaine dependence. *Curr Psychiatry Rep* 2004;6(5):323–331.

Dackis CA, Kampman KM, Lynch KG, Pettinati HM, O'Brien CP. A double-blind, placebo-controlled trial of modafinil for cocaine dependence. *Neuropsychopharmacology* 2005;30(1):205–211.

Dackis CA, Kampman KM, Lynch KG, et al. A double-blind, placebo-controlled trial of modafinil for cocaine dependence. *J Subst Abuse Treat.* 2012;[Epub ahead of print.]

Dale LC, Glover ED, Sachs DP, et al. Buproprion for smoking cessation: Predictors of successful outcome. *Chest* 2001;119:1357–1364.

DasGupta K. Treatment of depression in elderly patients: Recent advances. *Arch Fam Med* 1998;7(3):274–280.

Denis C, Fatseas M, Lavie E, Auriacombe M. Pharmacological interventions for benzodiazepine mono-dependence management in outpatient settings. *Cochrane Database Syst Rev,* Issue 3, 2006;Art. No.: CD005194. doi:10.1002/14651858.CD005194.pub2

Digiusto E, Lintzeris N, Breen C, et al. Short-term outcomes of five heroin detoxification methods in the Australian NEPOD project. *Addict Behav* 2005;30(3):443–456.

Ebbert JO, Croghan IT, Sood A, Schroeder DR, Hays JT, Hurt RD. Varenicline and bupropion sustained-release combination therapy for smoking cessation. *Nicotine Tobacco Res* 2009;11(3):234–239.

Eisenberg MJ, Filion KB, Yavin D, et al. Pharmacotherapies for smoking cessation: A meta-analysis of randomized controlled trials. *CMAJ* 2008;179(2):135–144. doi:10.1503/cmaj.070256.

Elenbaas RM. Drug therapy reviews: Management of the disulfiram–alcohol reaction. *Am J Hosp Pharmacy* 1977;34(8):827–831.

Elkashef A, Rawson R, Anderson A, Li SH, Holmes T, Smith E, Ling W. Bupropion for the treatment of methamphetamine dependence. *Neuropsychopharmacology* 2008;33(5):1162–1170.

Elhassan A, Chow RD. Smoking cessation in the elderly. *Clin Geriatr* 2007;15(2):38–45.

Eyer F, Schreckenberg M, Hecht D, et al. Carbamazepine and valproate as adjuncts in the treatment of alcohol withdrawal syndrome: A retrospective cohort study. *Alcohol Alcoholism* 2011;46(2):177–184.

Fagerstrom KO, Schneider NG, Lunell E. Effectiveness of nicotine patch and nicotine gum as individual versus combined treatments for tobacco withdrawal symptoms. *Psychopharmacology* 1993;111:271–277.

Fink AF, Elliott MN, Tsai M, Beck JC. An evaluation of an intervention to assist primary care physicians in screening and educating older patients who use alcohol. *J Am Geriatr Soc* 2005;53(11):1937–1943. doi:10.1111/j.1532-5415.2005.00476.x

Fink A, Morton SC, Beck JK, et al. The Alcohol-Related Problems Survey: Identifying hazardous and harmful drinking in older primary care patients. *J Am Geriatr Soc* 2002;50:1717–1722.

Fiore MC, Jaen CR, Baker TB, et al. Clinical Practice Guidelines: Treating Tobacco Use and Dependence: 2008 Update. 2008. Rockville, MD: U.S. Department of Health and Human Services. Public Health Service.

Foy A, Kay J, Taylor A. The course of alcohol withdrawal in a general hospital. *Q J Med* 1997;90(4):253–261.

Galloway G, Buscemi R, Coule J, et al. A randomized, placebo-controlled trial of sustained-release dextroamphetamine for treatment of methamphetamine addiction. *Clin Pharmacol Ther* 2011;89(2):276–282.

Galanter M. *Network therapy for alcohol and drug abuse: a new approach in practice.* New York: Basic Books; 1993.

Garbutt JC, West SL, Carey TS, Lohr KN, Crews FT. Pharmacological treatment of alcohol dependence: A review of the evidence. *JAMA* 1999;281(14):1318–1325.

Glasner-Edwards S. Motivational interventions for substance abusers with psychiatric illness. In: Miles Cox W & Klinger E, Eds., *Handbook of motivational counseling: goal-based approaches to assessment and intervention with addiction and other problems,* 2nd ed. New York: John Wiley & Sons; 2011:329–348.

Glasner-Edwards S, Rawson R. Evidence-based practices in addiction treatment: Review and recommendations for public policy. *Health Policy* 2010;97(2–3):93–104.

Glass J, Lanctôt KL, Herrmann N, Sproule BA, Busto UE. Sedative hypnotics in older people with insomnia: Meta-analysis of risks and benefits. *BMJ.* 2005; doi:10.1136/bmj.38623.768588.47

Goodson CM, Clark BJ, Douglas IS. Predictors of severe alcohol withdrawal syndrome: A systematic review and meta-analysis. *Alcohol Clin Exper Res* 2014;38(10):2664–2677.

Grabowski J, Shearer J, Merrill J, Negus S. Agonist-like, replacement pharmacotherapy for stimulant abuse and dependence. *Addict Behav* 2004;29(7):1439–1464.

Hays JT, Croghan IT, Baker CL, Cappelleri JC, Bushmakin AG. Changes in health-related quality of life with smoking cessation treatment. *Eur J Public Health* 2012;22(2):224–229.

Heilig M, Thorsell A, Sommer WH, et al. Translating the neuroscience of alcohol into clinical treatments: From blocking the buzz to curing the blues. *Neurosci Biobehav Rev* 2010;35(2):334–344

Henningfield JE, Fant RV, Ruchhalter AG, Stitzer ML. Pharmacotherapy for nicotine dependence. *CA: Cancer J Clinicians* 2005;55(5):281–299.

Himmerich H, Nickel T, Dalal MA, Müller MB. Gabapentin treatment in a female patient with panic disorder and adverse effects under carbamazepine during benzodiazepine withdrawal [Article in German]. *Psychiatrische Praxis* 2007;34(2):93–94.

Hinkle CH, Castellon SA, Dickson-Fuhrman E, Daum G, Jaffe J, Jarvik L. Screening for drug and alcohol abuse among older adults using a modified version of the CGE. *Am J Addict* 2001;10:319–326.

Hirst A, Knight C, Hirst M, Dunlop W, Akehurst R. Tramadol and the risk of fracture in an elderly female population: A cost utility assessment with comparison to transdermal buprenorphine. *Eur J Health Econ* 2015;17(2):217–227.

Hughes JR, Stead LF, Lancaster T. Antidepressants for smoking cessation. *Cochrane Database Syst Rev* 2007;24(1), CD000031.

Hurt RD, Sachs DP, Glover ED, et al. A comparison of sustained-release bupropion and placebo for smoking cessation. *N Engl J Med* 1997;337:1195–1202.

Irvin JE, Bowers CA, Dunn ME, Wang MC. Efficacy of relapse prevention: A meta-analytic review. *J Consult Clin Psychol* 1999;67(4), 563–570.

Jackson H, Mandell K, Johnson K, Chatterjee D, Vanness DJ. Cost-effectiveness of injectable extended-release naltrexone compared with methadone maintenance and buprenorphine maintenance treatment for opioid dependence. *Subst Abuse* 2015;36(2):226–231.

Jayaram-Lindström N, Hammarberg A, Beck O, Franck J. Naltrexone for the treatment of amphetamine dependence: A randomized, placebo-controlled trial. *Am J Psychiatry* 2008;165(11):1442–1448.

Johnson BA, Ait-Daoud N, Bowden C, et al. Oral topiramate for treatment of alcohol dependence: A randomized controlled trial. *Lancet* 2003;361(9370):1677–1685.

Johnson BA, Ait-Daoud N, Wang XQ, et al. Topiramate for the treatment of cocaine addiction: A randomized clinical trial. *JAMA: Psychiatry* 2013;70(12):1338–1346. doi:10.1001/jamapsychiatry.2013.2295.

Jorenby DE, Leischow SJ, Nides MA, et al. A controlled trial of sustained-release bupropion, a nicotine patch, or both for smoking cessation. *N Engl J Med* 1999;340:685–691.

Joyce GF, Niaura R, Maglione M, et al. The effectiveness of covering smoking cessation services for Medicare beneficiaries. *Health Serv Res* 2008;43(6):2106–2123. doi:10.1111/j.1475-6773.2008.00891.x.

Kakko J, Svanborg KD, Kreek MJ, Heilig M. One-year retention and social function after buprenorphine-assisted relapse prevention treatment for heroin dependence in Sweden: A randomized, placebo-controlled trial. *Lancet* 2003;361(9358):662–668.

Kalapatapu RK, Lewis DK, Vinogradov S, Batki SL, Winhusen T. Relationship of age to impulsivity and decision making: A baseline secondary analysis of a behavioral treatment study in stimulant use disorders. *J Addict Dis* 2013;32(2):206–216.

Kampman KM, Pettinati H, Lynch KG, et al. A pilot trial of topiramate for the treatment of cocaine dependence. *Drug Alcohol Depend* 2004;75(3):233–240.

Kampman KM, Pettinati HM, Lynch KG, et al. A double-blind, placebo-controlled pilot trial of quetiapine for the treatment of Type A and Type B alcoholism. *J Clin Psychopharmacol* 2007;27(4):344–351.

Karp JF, Butters MA, Begley AE, et al. (2014). Safety, tolerability, and clinical effect of low-dose buprenorphine for treatment-resistant depression in midlife and older adults. *J Clin Psychiatry* 75(8):785–793.

Kasser C, Geller A, Howell E, Wartenberg A. *Detoxification: principles and protocols. Topics in addiction medicine.* Chevy Chase, MD: American Society of Addiction Medicine; 1997.

Kashner TM, Rodell DE, Ogden SR, Guggenheim FG, Karson CN. Outcomes and costs of two VA inpatient treatment programs for older alcoholic patients. *Hosp Commun Psychiatry* 1992;43(10):985–989.

Kiefer F, Jahn H, Tarnaske T, et al. Comparing and combining naltrexone and acamprosate in relapse prevention of alcoholism: A double-blind, placebo-controlled study. *Arch Gen Psychiatry* 2003;60(1):92–99.

Kiluk BD, Nich C, Babuscio T, Carroll KM. Quality versus quantity: Acquisition of coping skills following computerized cognitive-behavioral therapy for substance-use disorders. *Addiction* 2010;105(12):2120–2127.

Kiluk BD, Nich C, Carroll KM. Relationship of cognitive function and the acquisition of coping skills in computer assisted treatment for substance use disorders. *Drug Alcohol Depend* 2011;114(2–3):169–176.

Kleber HD. Detoxification from narcotics. In: Lowinson JH & Ruiz P, Eds., *Substance abuse: clinical problems and perspectives.* Baltimore, MD: Williams & Wilkins; 1981:317–338.

Kleykamp BA, Heishman SJ. The older smoker. *JAMA* 2011;306(8):876–877. doi:10.1001/jama.2011.1221

Klimas J, Tobin H, Field CA, et al. Psychosocial interventions to reduce alcohol consumption in concurrent problem alcohol and illicit drug users. *Cochrane Database Syst Rev,* 2014; (12). doi:10.1002/14651858.CD009269.pub3.

Kofoed LL, Tolson RL, Atkinson RM, Toth RL, Turner JA. Treatment compliance of older alcoholics: An elder-specific approach is superior to "mainstreaming." *J Stud Alcohol* 1987;48(1):47–51.

Kornitzer M, Boutsen M, Dramaix M, Thisjs J, Gustavsson G. Combined use of nicotine patch and gum in smoking cessation: A placebo-controlled trial. *Prevent Med* 1995;24(1):41–47.

Kosten TR, Kleber HD. Strategies to improve compliance with narcotic antagonists. *Am J Drug Alcohol Abuse* 1984;10(2):249–266.

Kraemer KL, Conigliaro J, Saitz R. Managing alcohol withdrawal in the elderly. *Drugs Aging* 1999;14:409–425.

Kranzler HR, Burleson JA, Korner P, et al. Placebo-controlled trial of fluoxetine as an adjunct to relapse prevention in alcoholics. *Am J Psychiatry* 1995;152(3):391–397.

Krupitsky E, Nunes EV, Ling W, Gastfriend DR, Memisoglu A, Silverman BL. Injectable extended-release naltrexone (XR-NTX) for opioid dependence: Long-term safety and effectiveness. *Addiction* 2013;108(9):1628–1637.

Krupitsky E, Nunes EV, Ling W, Illeperuma A, Gastfriend DR, Silverman BL. Injectable extended-release naltrexone for opioid dependence: A double-blind, placebo-controlled, multicentre randomised trial. *Lancet* 2011;377(9776):1506–1513.

Krystal JH, Cramer JA, Krol WF, Kirk GF, Rosenheck RA, Veterans Affairs. Naltrexone Cooperative Study 425 Group. Naltrexone in the treatment of alcohol dependence. *N Engl J Med* 2001;345(24):1734–1739.

Larney S, Bohnert AS, Ganoczy D, et al. Mortality among older adults with opioid use disorders in the Veteran's Health Administration, 2000–2011. *Drug Alcohol Depend* 2015;147:32–37.

Lemke S, Moos R. Treatment outcomes at 1-year and 5-years for older patients with alcohol use disorders. *J Subst Abuse Treat* 2003;24:43–50.

Lee S, Klein-Schwartz W, Welsh C, Doyon S. Medical outcomes associated with nonmedical use of methadone and buprenorphine. *J Emerg Med* 2013;45(2):199–205.

Leelahanaj T, Kongsakon R, Netrakom P. A 4-week, double-blind comparison of olanzapine with haloperidol in the treatment of amphetamine psychosis. *JMA Thailand* 2005;88(Suppl 3), S43–S52.

Levin FR, Mariani JJ, Specker S, et al. Extended-release mixed amphetamine salts vs placebo for comorbid adult attention-deficit/hyperactivity disorder and cocaine use disorder: A randomized clinical trial. *JAMA: Psychiatry* 2015;72(6):593–602. doi:10.1001/jamapsychiatry.2015.41

Ling W, Hillhouse M, Domier C, et al. Buprenorphine tapering schedule and illicit opioid use. *Addiction* 2009;104(2):256–265.

Littleton J. Acamprosate in alcohol dependence: How does it work? *Addiction* 1995;90(9): 1179–1188.

Malcolm R, Myrick H, Brady KT, Ballenger JC. Update on anticonvulsants for the treatment of alcohol withdrawal. *Am J Addict* 2001;10(Suppl), 16–23.

Mann K, Lehert P, Morgan MY. The efficacy of acamprosate in the maintenance of abstinence in alcohol-dependent individuals: Results of a meta-analysis. *Alcohol Clin Exper Res* 2004;28(1):51–63.

Mannelli P, Wu LT, Peindl KS, Swartz MS, Woody GE. Extended release naltrexone injection is performed in the majority of opioid-dependent patients receiving outpatient induction: A very low dose naltrexone and buprenorphine open label trial. *Drug Alcohol Depend* 2014;138:83–88.

Mason BJ, Goodman AM, Chabac S, Lehert P. Effect of oral acamprosate on abstinence in patients with alcohol dependence in a double-blind, placebo-controlled trial: The role of patient motivation. *J Psychiatr Res* 2006;40(5):383–393.

Mayo-Smith MF. Pharmacological management of alcohol withdrawal: A meta-analysis and evidence-based practice guideline. *JAMA* 1997;278(2):144–151.

McNeil JJ, Piccenna L, Ioannides-Demos LL. Smoking cessation—recent advances. *Cardiovasc Drugs Ther* 2010;24(4):359–367.

Meier P, Seitz HK. Age, alcohol metabolism, and liver disease. *Curr Opin Clin Nutr Metab Care* 2008;11:21–26.

Merrick EL, Horgan CM, Hodgkin D, et al. Unhealthy drinking patterns in older adults: Prevalence and associated characteristics. *J Am Geriatr Soc* 2008;56(2):214–223.

Menninger JA. Assessment and treatment of alcoholism and substance-related disorders in the elderly. *Bull Menninger Clin* 2002;66(2):166–183.

Miller WR. Motivational interviewing: Research, practice, and puzzles. *Addict Behav* 1996;21:835–842.

Molander L, Hansson A, Lunell E. Pharmacokinetics of nicotine in healthy elderly people. *Clin Pharmacol Ther* 2001;69(1):57–65. doi:10.1067/mcp.2001.113181

Monterosso JR, Flannery BA, Pettinati HM, et al. Predicting treatment response to naltrexone: The influence of craving and family history. *Am J Addict* 2001;10(3):258–268.

Moore AA, et al. Beyond alcoholism: Identifying older, at-risk drinkers in primary care. *J Stud Alcohol* 2002;63(3):316–324.

Moy P, Crome I, Fisher M. Systematic and narrative review of treatment for older people with substance problems. *Eur Geriatr Med* 2011;2:212–236.

Müller CA, Schäfer M, Schneider S, et al. Efficacy and safety of levetiracetam for outpatient alcohol detoxification. *Pharmacopsychiatry* 2010;43(5):184–189.

Myrick H, Malcolm R, Brady KT. Gabapentin treatment of alcohol withdrawal. *Am J Psychiatry* 1998;155(11):1632.

Myrick H, Malcolm R, Randall PK, et al. A double-blind trial of gabapentin versus lorazepam in the treatment of alcohol withdrawal. *Alcohol Clin Exper Res* 2009;33(9):1582–1588.

National Institute of Alcohol Abuse and Alcoholism (NIAAA) Helping patients who drink too much: A clinician's guide. October 2008 update: Prescribing medications for alcohol dependence. 2008. NIH Publication 07-3769. Retrieved from www.niaaa.nih.gov/guide.

National Institute on Drug Abuse (NIDA). Research Report Series: Prescription Drug Abuse. 2014. NIH Publication Number 15-4881. Accessed at: http://www.drugabuse.gov/publications/research-reports/prescription-drugs/trends-in-prescription-drug-abuse/older-adults on 04/15/16.

Nemes S, Rao PA, Zeiler C, Munly K, Holtz KD, Hoffman J. Computerized screening of substance abuse problems in a primary care setting: Older vs. younger adults. *Am J Drug Alcohol Abuse* 2004;30:627–642.

Newton TF, Kalechstein AD, Duran S, Vansluis N, Ling W. Methamphetamine abstinence syndrome: Preliminary findings. *Am J Addict* 2004;13(3):248–255.

Northrup TF, Stotts AL, Green C, et al. Opioid withdrawal, craving, and use during and after outpatient buprenorphine stabilization and taper: A discrete survival and growth mixture model. *Addict Behav* 2015;41:20–28.

Nunes EV, Krupitsky E, Ling W, et al. Treating opioid dependence with injectable extended-release naltrexone (XR-NTX): Who will respond? *J Addict Med* 2015;9(3):238–243.

O'Brien CP. Anticraving medications for relapse prevention: A possible new class of psychoactive medications. *Am J Psychiatry,* 2005;162(8):1423–1431.

O'Connell H, Chin AV, Cunningham C, et al. Alcohol use disorders in elderly people—redefining an age old problem in old age. *BMJ,* 2003;327:664–667.

O'Malley SS, Jaffe AJ, Chang G, Schottenfeld RS, Meyer RE, Rounsaville BJ. Naltrexone and coping skills therapy for alcohol dependence: A controlled study. *Arch Gen Psychiatry* 1992;49(11):881–887.

Oslin D, Liberto JG, O'Brien J, Krois S, Norbeck J. Naltrexone as an adjunctive treatment for older patients with alcohol dependence. *Am J Geriatr Psych* 1997;5(4):324–332.

Oslin D, Liberto JG, O'Brien J, Krois S. Tolerability of naltrexone in treating older, alcohol-dependent patients. *Am J Addict* 1997;6(3):266–270.

Oslin DW, Berrettini W, Kranzler H, et al. A functional polymorphism of the mu-opioid receptor gene is associated with naltrexone response in alcohol dependent patients. *Neuropsychopharmacology* 2003;28(8):1546–1552.

Oslin DW, Slaymaker VJ, Blow FC, Owen PL, Colleran C. Treatment outcomes for alcohol dependence among middle-aged and older adults. *Addict Behav* 2005;30(7):1431–1436.

Pani PP, Trogu E, Vacca R, Amato L, Vecchi S, Davoli M. Disulfiram for the treatment of co-caine dependence. *Cochrane Database Syst Rev* 2010;(1), CD007024.

Pergolizzi J, Boger RH, Budd K, et al. Opioids and the management of chronic severe pain in the elderly: Consensus statement of an International Expert Panel with focus on the six clinically most often used World Health Organization Step III opioids (buprenorphine, fentanyl, hydromorphone, methadone, morphine, oxycodone). *Pain Pract* 2008;8(4):287–313.

Pergolizzi J V Jr., Raffa RB, Taylor R, Jr., et al. An open-label pharmacokinetic study of oxymor-phone extended release in the presence of naltrexone in the older adult. *J Opioid Manag* 2012;8(6):383–393.

Petitjean SA, Dursteler-MacFarland KM, Krokar MC, et al. A randomized, controlled trial of combined cognitive-behavioral therapy plus prize-based contingency management for cocaine dependence. *Drug Alcohol Depend* 2014;145:94–100.

Petrakis IL, Carroll KM, Nich C, et al. Disulfiram treatment for cocaine dependence in methadone-maintained opioid addicts. *Addiction* 2000;95(2):219–228.

Pettinati HM, Volpicelli JR, Kranzler HR, Luck G, Rukstalis MR, Cnaan A. Sertraline treat-ment for alcohol dependence: Interactive effects of medication and alcoholic subtype. *Alcohol Clin Exper Res*, 2000;24(7):1041–1049.

Piper ME, Smith SS, Schalm TR, et al. A randomized placebo-controlled clinical trial of 5 smoking cessation pharmacotherapies. *Arch Gen Psychiatry* 2009;66:1253–1262.

Prochaska JO, DiClemente CC. Toward a comprehensive model of change. In: Miller WR & Heather N, Eds., *Treating addictive behaviors: processes of change.* New York: Plenum Press; 1986:3–27.

Prochazka AV, Weaver MJ, Keller RT, et al. A randomized trial of nortriptyline for smoking cessation. *Arch Intern Med* 1998;148(18):2035–2039.

Prochazka AV, Kick S, Steinbrunn C, et al. A randomized trial of nortriptyline combined with transdermal nicotine for smoking cessation. *Arch Intern Med* 2004;164:2229–2233.

Rabinowitz J, Cohen H, Atias S. Outcomes of naltrexone maintenance following ultra-rapid opiate detoxification versus intensive inpatient detoxification. *Am J Addict* 2002;11(1):52–56.

Raupach T, van Schayck CP. Pharmacotherapy for smoking cessation: Current advances and research topics. *CNS Drugs* 2011;25(5):371–382.

Rawson RA, Marinelli-Casey P, Anglin MD, et al. A multi-site comparison of psycho-social approaches for the treatment of methamphetamine dependence. *Addiction* 2004;99(6):708–717.

Rawson RA, McCann MJ, Flammino F, et al. A comparison of contingency management and cognitive-behavioral approaches for stimulant dependent individuals. *Addiction* 2006;101(2):267–274.

Resnick B, Junlapeeya P. Falls in a community of older adults: Findings and implications for practice. *Applied Nurs Res* 2004;17(2):81–91.

Rice C, Longabaugh R, Beattie M, Noel N. Age group differences in response to treatment for problematic alcohol use. *Addiction* 1993;88 (10):1369–1375.

Rickels K, DeMartinis N, Rynn M, Mandos L. Pharmacologic strategies for discontinuing benzodiazepine treatment. *J Clin Psychopharmacol* 1999;19(6 Suppl 2):12S–16S.

Roll JM, Petry NM, Stitzer ML, et al. Contingency management for the treatment of metham-phetamine use disorders. *Am J Psychiatry* 2006;163(11):1993–1999.

Rose JE, Herskovic JE, Behm FM, Westman EC. Precessation treatment with nicotine patch significantly increases abstinence rates relative to conventional treatment. *Nicotine Tobacco Res* 2009;11(9):1067–1075.

Rothrauff TC, Abraham AJ, Bride BE, Roman PM. Substance abuse treatment for older adults in private centers. *Subst Abuse* 2011;31(1):7–15. doi:10.1080/08897077.2011.540463

Rubio G, Bobes J, Cervera G, et al. Effects of pregabalin on subjective sleep disturbance symptoms during withdrawal from long-term benzodiazepine use. *Eur Addict Res* 2011;17(5):262–270.

Rubio G, Ponce G, Rodriguez-Jiménez R, Jiménez-Arriero MA, Hoenicka J, Palomo T. Clinical predictors of response to naltrexone in alcoholic patients: Who benefits most from treatment with naltrexone? *Alcohol Alcoholism* 2005;40(3):227–233.

Saitz R, O'Malley SS Pharmacotherapies for alcohol abuse: Withdrawal and treatment. *Med Clin N Am* 1997;81(4):881–907.

Satre DD, Knight BG, Dickson-Fuhrmann E, Jarvik LF. Predictors of alcohol-treatment seeking in a sample of older veterans in the GET SMART Program. *J Am Geriatr Soc* 2003;51:380–386.

Satre DD, Mertens JR, Arean PA, Weisner C. Five-year alcohol and drug treatment outcomes of older adults versus middle-aged and younger adults in a managed care program. *Addiction* 2004;99:1286–1297. doi:10.1111/j.1360-0443.2004.00831.x.

Schonfeld L, King-Kallimanis BL, Duchene DM, et al. Screening and brief intervention for substance misuse among older adults: The Florida BRITE project. *Am J Public Health* 2010;100(1):108–114.

Schweizer E, Rickels K, Case WG, Greenblatt DJ. Carbamazepine treatment in patients discontinuing long-term benzodiazepine therapy. Effects on withdrawal severity and outcome. *Arch Gen Psychiatry* 1991;48(5):448–452.

Sees KL, Delucci KL, Masson C, et al. Methadone maintenance vs. 180-day psychosocially enriched detoxification for treatment of opioid dependence: A randomized controlled trial. *JAMA*, 2000;283(10):1303–1310.

Shah SD, Wilken LA, Winkler SR, Lin SJ. Systematic review and meta-analysis of combination therapy for smoking cessation. *J Am Pharmaceut Assoc* 2003;48(5):659–665.

Shoptaw S, Kao U, Ling W. Treatment for amphetamine psychosis. *Cochrane Database Syst Rev,* 2009;(1), CD003026.

Schultz SK, Arndt S, Liesveld J. Locations of facilities with special programs for older substance abuse clients in the US. *Int J Geriatr Psych* 2003;18(9):839–843.

Sigmon SC, Bisaga A, Nunes EV, O'Connor PG, Kosten T, Woody G. Opioid detoxification and induction strategies: Recommendations for clinical practice. *Am J Drug Abuse* 2012;38(3):187–199.

Silagy C, Lancaster T, Stead L, Mant D, Fowler G. Nicotine replacement therapy for smoking cessation. *Cochrane Database Syst Rev* 2004; (3), CD000146.

Slemmer JE, Martin BR, Damaj MI. Bupropion is a nicotinic antagonist. *J Pharmacol Exper Ther* 2000;295(1):321–327.

Sommer BR, Fenn HH. Review of topiramate for the treatment of epilepsy in elderly patients. *Clin Interv Aging* 2010;5:89–99.

Sproule B, Brands B, Li S, Catz-Biro L. Changing patterns in opioid addiction: Characterizing users of oxycodone and other opioids. *Can Fam Physician* 2009;55(1):68–69.

Srisurapanont M, Jarusuraisin N. Naltrexone for the treatment of alcoholism: A meta-analysis of randomized controlled trials. *Int J Neuropsychopharmacol* 2005;8(2): 267–280.

Stead LF, Perera R, Bullen C, Mant D, Lancaster T. Nicotine replacement therapy for smoking cessation. *Cochrane Database Syst Rev* 2008;23(1), CD000146.

Stuppaeck CH, Pycha R, Miller C, Whitworth AB, Oberbauer H, Fleischhacker WW. Carbamazepine versus oxazepam in the treatment of alcohol withdrawal: A double-blind study. *Alcohol Alcoholism* 1992;27(2):153–158.

Sullivan JT, Sykora K, Schneiderman J, Naranjo CA, Sellers EM. Assessment of alcohol withdrawal: The revised Clinical Institute Withdrawal Instrument for Alcohol Scale (CIWA-Ar). *Br J Addict* 1989;84(11):1353–1357.

Taylor DHJr, Hasselblad V, Henley SJ, Thun MJ, Sloan FA. Benefits of smoking cessation for longevity. *Am J Public Health* 2002;92(6):990–996.

Thomas D. Is it useful to quit smoking in the elderly population? Yes! Smoking cessation is beneficial at any age [in French]. *La Presse Médicale* 2013;42(6 Pt 1):1019–1027. doi:10.1016/j.lpm.2013.02.320

Tiihonen J, Kuoppasalmi K, Föhr J, et al. A comparison of aripiprazole, methylphenidate, and placebo for amphetamine dependence. *Am J Psychiatry* 2007;164(1):160–162. Tipranavir Package Insert: http://bidocs.boehringer-ingelheim.com/BIWebAccess/ViewServlet.ser?docBase=renetnt&folderPath=/Prescribing+Information/PIs/Aptivus/10003515+US+01.pdf. Accessed June 27, 2012.

Vocci FJ, Montoya ID. Psychological treatments for stimulant misuse, comparing and contrasting those for amphetamine dependence and those for cocaine dependence. *Curr Opin Psychiatry* 2009;22(3):263–268.

Volkow ND, Li T.-K. Drug addiction: The neurobiology of behavior gone awry. *Neuroscience* 2004;5:963–970.

Volpicelli J, Rhines K, Rhines J, et al. Naltrexone and alcohol dependence: Role of subject compliance. *Arch Gen Psychiatry* 1997;54(8):737–742.

Weinbroum AA, Flaishon R, Sorkine P, Szold O, Rudick V. A risk-benefit assessment of flumazenil in the management of benzodiazepine overdose. *Drug Safety* 1997;17(3):181–196.

Weiss LM, Petry NM. Interaction effects of age and contingency management treatments in cocaine-dependent outpatients. *Exper Clin Psychopharmacol* 2011;19(2):173–181.

West SL, Garbutt JC, Carey TS, et al. Evidence Report No. 3. (AHCPR Pub. No. 99-E004). 1999. Rockville, MD: U.S. Department of Health and Human Services; Public Health Service, Agency for Health Care Policy and Research.

Wilde MI, Wagstaff AJ. Acamprosate. A review of its pharmacology and clinical potential in the management of alcohol dependence after detoxification. *Drugs* 1997;53(6):1038–1053.

Williams SH. Medications for treating alcohol dependence. *Am Fam Physician* 2005;72(9):1775–1780.

Wright C, Moore RD. Disulfiram treatment of alcoholism. *Am J Med* 1990;88(6):647–655.

Wu L-T, Blazer DG. Illicit and nonmedical drug use among older adults: A review. *J Aging Health* 2011;23(3):481–504.

Younger J, Parkitny L, McLain D. The use of low-dose naltrexone (LDN) as novel anti-inflammatory treatment for chronic pain. *Clin Rheumatol* 2014;33(4):451–459.

CHAPTER 11

# Technology-Based Interventions for Late-Life Addiction

*Esra Alagoz, Kim Johnson, Andrew Quanbeck, and David Gustafson, Jr.*

## Introduction

Late-life addiction has been a neglected topic in the field of substance-use disorders research. Considering the aging of the baby-boomer generation defined as those born between 1946 and 1964), the decline in fertility rates, and increases in life expectancy, substance-use disorders (SUDs) among individuals aged 65 and over will continue to become more prevalent. According to the statistics from the Department of Health and Human Services (2012), the older population numbered 43.1 million in 2012, with a 21% increase since 2002. Late-life addiction currently affects about 15% of this population. The number of older adults with SUD is expected to double by 2020 (Gfoerer et al. 2003), with an estimated 4.4 million older adults who will need treatment for substance-use problems. These numbers emphasize the increasing demands that will be placed in the next decade on the substance-abuse treatment systems designed specifically for this population.

Emerging technologies offer significant opportunities to advance the treatment and recovery management of SUDs. Recent studies in technology-based interventions for addiction treatment and recovery demonstrate promising results (Gustafson et al. 2014, Gustafson et al. 2011, Marsch et al. 2012, Carroll et al. 2008). Interactive web and mobile technologies for the practice of medicine and public health ("e-health") provide personalized screening and assessment tools easily accessible to physicians and other providers. Current research supports the benefits of web-based personalized screening in addiction treatment (Sinadinovic et al. 0000, Johnon et al. 2013). Such technology could significantly enhance SUD screening practices among older adults if adapted to this population's needs. In addition, the digital technologies, including videoconferencing and telephone-based interactive voice response, may also serve to improve the cost-effectiveness of an intervention by offering ongoing support after the patient has completed treatment. These systems can serve an important role in assisting patient self-management and psychosocial support (Bickel et al. 2011) to ensure effective aftercare.

Designing technology-based interventions for late-life addiction requires tailoring these technologies to the unique characteristics of this population. Research suggests that SUDs in older adults are under-detected and usually misdiagnosed due to reasons such as inefficient age-appropriate screening instruments, comorbid physical or psychiatric conditions, and atypical presentations of SUD at this age (O'Connell et al. 2003). Healthcare workers' attitudes towards older patients (e.g., lower degree of suspicion during assessments, assigning different quality-of-life standards, stereotyping based on age and socioeconomic status) can also lead to misdiagnosis and thus lack of treatment.

Studies examining technology-based interventions for older adults have been scarce. Although these interventions can be highly efficient and cost-effective (Marsch et al. 2012, Olmstead et al. 2010, Gibbons et al. 2008, Marsch 2012) in healthcare settings, the challenges to implementation and sustainability that are specific to unique characteristics of this population include age-related changes such as declines in color sensitivity, perception of high-frequency tones, and slower response times (Ijsselsteijn et al. 2007) may discourage the integration of technology-based interventions into existing healthcare processes.

This chapter aims to explore the use of technology-based interventions for late-life addiction, examine the design adaptations of using technology for elderly population, and discuss ways to overcome possible challenges that might be encountered during treatment and recovery. In the following sections, we will first briefly describe the addiction treatment of older adults, including the risk factors, the reasons why addiction in this population usually goes unrecognized, and how older adults respond to treatment. The next section will explore the technologies that are designed to assist with addiction treatment in general. We will further discuss how these technologies can be adopted to older populations. This section is designed to depict (a) technologies that support healthcare providers and (b) patient-centered technologies for addiction treatment. Then we will elaborate on the opportunities and challenges in using for addiction treatment in older adults and give examples from our design process of ElderTree, an interactive health technology designed for older adults, and list implications of designing addiction treatment systems specifically for older adults.

## Addiction Treatment in Older Adults

Although there is a growing need for addiction treatment for people over 65 for both alcohol and drug-use disorders, treatment admissions for people over 65 with alcohol-use disorders in the United States and Europe have decreased slightly, and admissions for people over 65 with drug-use disorders have increased very slightly (Wang et al. 2013). As the cohort of baby boomers ages, they continue to use alcohol and drugs at a higher rates than previous cohorts (Blow et al. 2007). Furthermore, as aging leads to reduced ability to metabolize alcohol, greater probability of being on medications that may interact with alcohol and illegal drugs, and increased risk for comorbidities, there may be a greater risk of late-onset substance-use disorders that need to be treated due to the continued use of alcohol and drugs for people over 65 (Caputo et al. 2012).

Addiction in older adults most often goes unrecognized. There are multiple reasons that healthcare providers—and family members—overlook the symptoms. One of the most common reasons for underdiagnoses of problem drinking, for example, is that patients are not drinking any more than they usually drink. However, as people age, the ways their bodies metabolize alcohol also change due to the decrease in body water and in the gastric alcohol dehydrogenase enzyme, which is responsible for breaking down alcohols in the body (Center for Substance Abuse Treatment 1998)that might lead to intoxication. Additionally, the way prescription drugs—especially psychoactive drugs, as these have the most potential for misuse—interact with alcohol can create more serious problems that would lead to adverse drug reactions. Prejudice regarding the treatment of addiction in older adults is another reason for misdiagnoses of addiction at older age. Research demonstrates that doctors neglect to ask older patients about drinking, assuming that they would not change after that age (Sharp et al. 2011). However, Oslin and colleagues (2005) note that older people respond better to addiction treatment than younger people, as they are more likely to attend therapy sessions and less likely to relapse.

Older adults in addiction treatment have been characterized as either early onset—those whose SUD has been chronic or recurrent since an early age—or late onset, those whose continued use of alcohol or recent use of prescription medications has led to disordered use later in life (Wadd et al. 2011). While treatment is effective for both groups, the later onset group has been shown to have better outcomes (Schutte et al. 1994).

Treatment has been shown to be at least as effective, and in some studies, more effective for older people than for younger populations, whether it is are offered in mixed-age settings or age-specific groups (Oslin et al. 2002, Lemke et al. 2003, Satre et al. 2004). Older people tend to have better adherence to treatment protocols in terms of both medication adherence and attendance at counseling sessions (Oslin et al. 2002), which may account for more posi-tive outcomes post-treatment. Older women are more susceptible to late-onset SUDs via use of alcohol and prescription medication due to reasons such as genetic predisposition or environmental stress (Tuchman 2010), but they are also more responsive to treatment and have better outcomes than older men (Lemke et al. 2003). A review of treatment effectiveness literature completed in 2013 (Kuerbis et al. 2013, found that research on the effectiveness of specific treatments for older adults was lacking, but that, in general, treatment was at least as effective for older adults as for young adults and that, as with other age groups, spending a longer time in treatment, regardless of treatment setting, and age-specific treatment both enhance outcomes.

Because time in treatment is important regardless of level of care or treat-ment setting, and because age-specific treatment seems to enhance the effect of treatment for older adults (Wadd et al. 2011), technology may provide a vehicle through which effective treatment can be provided despite mobility issues, low numbers of older adults needing treatment in a specific geographic area, and other issues that limit the ability to offer age-specific addiction treat-ment to older populations.

## Technologies for Addiction Treatment

### TECHNOLOGIES THAT SUPPORT HEALTHCARE PROVIDERS

*Electronic Health Records*
Electronic health records (EHR) are one of the most frequently adopted tech-nologies in healthcare on account of the Health Information Technology for Economic and Clinical Health Act (HITECH), which authorizes incentive payments to clinicians and hospitals if they implement EHRs and use them ex-tensively to achieve improvements in their institution (Blumenthal et al. 2010). A set of objectives, such as entering patient information, putting in medication orders, and keeping an active medication and allergies list in EHRs, has to be attained to qualify for incentive payments; in other words, to be "meaning-ful users." One of the strengths of EHRs is that the EHR system software in-cludes automatic checks for drug–drug and drug–allergy interactions. These checks then can be used to alert the providers if a newly prescribed medication could interfere with other medications that the patient is on. This feature is especially important for older adult patients, as they are frequently on mul-tiple prescription medicines, and mixing medications could lead to adverse ef-fects. Studies investigating the relationship between advanced EHR use and clinical quality of care demonstrated a positive correlation (Jarvis et al. 2013. Additionally, EHR-based surveillance of chronic diseases such as diabetes

and addiction has been found to be a useful resource for both researchers and physicians in determining pre-disease characteristics by studying the records retrospectively or prospectively (Pearson et al. 2011).

## Communication tools

Patient–provider communication plays a crucial role in healthcare delivery. With the development of new technologies, several communication tools have emerged that offer alternative platforms for patient–provider communication outside the clinics. Today, telehealth services offer many sophisticated tools, including short message service (SMS), email, teleconferencing, and video-conferencing. These communication systems are typically used for checkups, consultation, and behavioral health management. They are also successfully used in home care settings. For instance, an integrated telehealth intervention (Integrated Telehealth Education and Activation of Mood: I-TEAM) to treat chronic illness and depression in geriatric home care patients has been found to offer support for clinical decision-making for both the providers and patients. I-TEAM also provides a system to continuously monitor physical and mental health status (Gellis et al. 2014). The participants were very satisfied with I-TEAM due to the quicker treatment times compared to the face-to-face settings. However, integrating telehealth systems into healthcare delivery increases system complexity, presenting major challenges such as security, networking interoperability, and technology management (Ackerman et al. 2010), which need to be accounted for.

## Monitoring Tools

Because alcohol is partially eliminated transdermally (Swift 2003), it can be measured using transdermal alcohol-monitoring systems—special devices for assessing the alcohol level in body. While there are transdermal alcohol-monitoring systems that can be utilized to track alcohol use remotely, they are too large and uncomfortable for use in any population not mandated to wear them (Barnett et al. 2011). Therefore, an improved design may make them more valuable in a different treatment population where they could be used to help patients resist the urge to use, and to alert family members or caregivers to dangerous levels of use. No such device has been developed to monitor use of other drugs besides alcohol, though existing sensors could be used to monitor for symptoms of drug use such as increased or decreased heart rate and pupil dilation. These tools could help patients, families, and caregivers monitor for symptoms or alcohol or drug use that may result in danger to the patient, and intervene quickly.

Other remote electronic-monitoring technologies have been studied as assistive devices for elderly adults, with mixed results (Blaschke et al. 2009).

Studies have assessed the value of wearable devices, sensors placed in the environment, and complete home systems that are often called "smart homes" (Rashidi et al. 2013). Various devices have been successfully employed to measure gait impairment (Mudge et al. 2007), social interaction (Sung et al. 2005), and activity levels (Yang et al. 2010). Two main issues that are raised in research studies related to these technologies are patients' unwillingness to use them (Kang et al. 2010), and some overly complex, difficult-to-use designs (Vastenburg et al. 2008). Although no studies have been conducted as of this writing, these technologies could potentially be repurposed to support an older person with his/her early recovery from SUDs. Tools that have been utilized to assess social interaction, for example, could be used to assess a patient's level of participation in self-help activities and/or engagement in social activity that is supportive of recovery. If social interaction is low for a pre-set period of time, recommendations for improving social contact could be provided via text messaging or calendaring.

### Dashboards and Decision support systems

Computer-based clinical decision-support systems have been shown to be effective in improving healthcare delivery (Kawamoto et al. 2005). On the other hand, clinical decision-support systems are successful only if they provide treatment recommendations that are offered during the routine provision of care and their use is part of the usual work flow of patient care. There is evidence that decision-support systems improve the medication prescription in older adults (Martin et al. 2012), and they are effective in identifying patients who would benefit from more intensive case management post-discharge from hospitalization (Bowles et al. 2014). Decision-support systems have also been used to train residents in providing geriatric care specifically to prevent falls, and assess for vision issues and dementia (Litvin et al. 2012). In terms of addiction treatment-decision support, there is currently very little available. A recent study assesses the predictive validity of an electronic assessment tool using the American Society of Addiction Medicine (ASAM) criteria and finds that it is a valid tool for predicting the required level of care (Stallvik et al. 2014). On the other hand, there are no other decision-support systems currently tested for the treatment or monitoring of SUDs once they have been identified.

## PATIENT-CENTERED TECHNOLOGIES
## FOR ADDICTION TREATMENT

Research highlighting the use of technology to deliver addiction treatment services has been expanding in recent years. A 2014 special issue of the *Journal of Substance Abuse Treatment* was dedicated to studies on technologically mediated ways to deliver evidence-based treatments for addiction. Articles featured in that special issue considered a variety of topics, including brief interventions, behavior therapy, medication adherence tools, and HIV-prevention interventions (Marsch et al. 2014). These interventions have been deployed using a variety of technology platforms (mobile, web, videoconferencing, and phone-based interactive voice response) and tested in different populations (including adults, adolescents, criminal justice, and post-partum women) (Marsch et al. 2014). However, no such systems have been specifically developed for the treatment of addiction in older adults.

There is a large number of combinations of interventions, technology platforms, and populations that might be surveyed in any literature review on technology use for addiction treatment, and the field increasingly recognizes the potential for technology to deliver evidence-based addiction treatment efficiently and effectively. Increasingly, mobile phones and touch-screen–enabled tablets are becoming the dominant platforms for developing and delivering e-health interventions. These types of devices have become the preferred choices for e-health developers for several reasons: First, ownership of mobile phones and tablets is increasing steadily across all age groups, owing in part to their relatively low cost. Although the elderly have been slower to adopt mobile phones and tablets than their younger counterparts, adoption rates are increasing quickly, and the trend shows no sign of reversing. Thus, mobile devices provide nearly universal access to e-health interventions. Secondly, the touch-screen user interface found in these devices make them easier to use than mouse-controlled computer screens for inexperienced users and those with physical impairments. E-health interventions can be optimized for viewing on different devices to ensure usability for various populations such as those with visual impairments.

In order to demonstrate the potential that technology could hold for the treatment of addiction in the elderly, we highlight a 2014 literature review of mobile-phone–based systems for treatment of alcohol-use disorders. The literature review revealed that 14 such systems have been developed since 2007. These systems were classified into four categories:

1. Text-messaging monitoring and reminder systems that primarily use the mobile phones' text-messaging capabilities to monitor alcohol use or remind the user to report their alcohol consumption;
2. Text-messaging intervention systems that, in addition to monitoring alcohol use, deliver text messages that are intended to promote abstinence and recovery;
3. Comprehensive recovery management systems that use the internal sensors (e.g., monitoring of GPS coordinates) and other computer-like

capabilities of modern smartphones to deliver multifaceted messages and interventions; and

4. Game-based systems that engage the user through game playing (Quanbeck et al. 2015).

This literature review found that systems that rely primarily on texting for monitoring and intervention have the advantages of being inexpensive, widely available, and easy to operate for both senders and receivers of text messages. The main disadvantage of texting-based systems to date is that the evidence for their effectiveness is limited, and there is no evidence at all that such systems have been found useful or effective for the treatment of addiction in older adults.

Monitoring and reminder systems that use mobile phones' text-messaging feature are shown to have high response rates among patients. For example, the response rate for collecting data on patients' drinking was reported to be 84.4% (Kuntsche et al. 2009), and the response rate for a brief alcohol intervention in the form of a questionnaire was 88% (Irvine et al. 2012). On the other hand, reminder systems that focus on monitoring consumption are found to be ineffective in reducing alcohol use. Agyapong and colleagues (Agyapong et al. 2012) employed personalized supportive text messages (rather than basic reminders) to patients with alcohol-use disorders and comorbid depression. The results after three months demonstrated a reduction in depression and better cumulative abstinence. Surprisingly, six-month outcomes of the same study demonstrated no statistically significant difference in depression and better cumulative abstinence, implying that the effects of supportive text-messaging were not sustained after three months (Agyapong et al. 2013). It should also be noted that these systems were tested on adults of all ages, and some focused mainly on college students. Thus, the applicability and potential usefulness of text-messaging for the treatment of addiction in the older adults should be reconsidered while adapting it to this population.

Comprehensive recovery management systems that utilize the capabilities of smartphones such as location-monitoring through GPS and interactive multimedia applications tailored to the needs of individuals have been found to be effective in reducing the risky drinking days. Location-Based Monitoring and Intervention System for Alcohol Use Disorders (LBMI-A) (Dulin et al. 2014) and Addiction–Comprehensive Health Enhancement Support System (A-CHESS) (Gusfason et al. 2014) are two prominent systems that are designed to deliver recovery management. In particular, A-CHESS, a comprehensive system that is designed to assist patients after treatment, has had the strongest and longest lasting effects, including a reduction in heavy-drinking days of 57% compared with a control group (Gustafson et al. 2014). LBMI-A, with a different target audience from A-CHESS (people with alcohol-use disorders who were not engaged in another form of treatment) also demonstrated promising early results, with a reduction in hazardous drinking days by 60% over the course of six weeks. However, the enhanced features and effectiveness of these comprehensive systems are associated with increased costs. Owning and operating a smartphone still is more expensive than owning and operating a standard cellular phone. Furthermore, comprehensive systems such as A-CHESS and LBMI-A are similarly expensive to develop, operate, and maintain. However, a recent survey regarding the technology acceptance of older adults indicates that the majority of older adults' attitudes were positive towards technology if they believed that the benefits of using technology would outweigh the cost (Mitzner et al. 2010).

## Opportunities and Challenges in Using Technology for Addiction Treatment in Older Adults

Although research on the use of technology for addiction treatment is developing quickly, to our knowledge, there have not been any studies that directly investigated the use of technology for treatment of addiction specifically in older adults. Considering the advancements in e-health and how well e-health technologies have been received by older adults in terms of home care and self-management, research needs to focus on designing technologies for addiction treatment at older ages. Before discussing the age-related accommodations that should be considered while designing for this specific demographic, it is important to point out how e-health would be beneficial to addiction treatment in older adults. As discussed earlier, the reasons for drug or alcohol use that begins at older age appear fundamentally different from the reasons of SUDs started at earlier age. There is evidence that social isolation at later ages, losing loved ones, and changes in lifestyle after retirement may contribute to heavier alcohol consumption. Additionally, misuse or abuse of prescription drugs to alleviate chronic pain or insomnia may lead to addiction (Wu et al. 2011). Designing technologies to treat addiction in the older adults poses unique challenges. About 75% of people 65 and older have two or more chronic conditions that significantly affect their well-being, and older adults often face existential challenges related to engagement and life-management. People 65 and older also are less likely to use technology. One study found that older adults used email, the Internet, and cell phones significantly less than those middle-aged and younger (Weinberg et al. 1998), and smartphone penetration is lowest among those 65 and older. Although smartphone penetration is changing swiftly (e.g., from 13% penetration among

Americans 65 and older in 2012 to 18% in 2013) (Smith 2012), problems such as dimming eyesight and tremors make it hard for many older adults to touch small buttons on small screens or use a mouse. Technology for older adults must address these issues.

E-health systems that are developed to assist older adults with everyday tasks (e.g., driving, taking medications, etc.) or create possibilities to socialize with others (through forums, bulletin boards, and daily messages) would support older adults to be more involved in communal activities, which in turn would decrease the risks of hazardous drinking or substance-use disorders that might be caused by social isolation or depression. Such a project has been in development by Gustafson et al. (Gustafson Sr. et al. 2014) through a National Institutes of Health (NIH) grant since the end of 2010. ElderTree is an interactive health technology designed specifically for older adults and their family caregivers to improve older adult quality of life and address challenges they face in maintaining their independence, such as loneliness and isolation, falling, managing medications, driving and transportation, and the need for services in the home.

## Lessons Learned from the ElderTree Experience

Our research group has learned several important lessons as part of the development of ElderTree. While not specifically designed for addiction treatment in this demographic, these guidelines will probably be relevant for any technology developed for use by older adults. We found out that technology must give users ways to relate to and help others. Previous research supports that using the Internet for communication is associated with reduced loneliness in older adults (Sum et al. 2008). The risk of social isolation is a serious concern for this age group, while it is also a risk factor for increased alcohol consumption and SUDs in older age. Therefore, the social connecting piece of ElderTree has become the focal point of the system. It has also been the most popular tool of ElderTree, both with active users that post at least once a day, and with "lurkers" who mostly read the entries and only participate in discussions occasionally. The communication format is asynchronous, with a personalized alert system whenever the users get a new message. There are many topics that users can contribute to (just chatting, religion/spirituality, healthy living, etc.) that have been narrowed down from myriad topics by the technical staff, based on the most popular and active discussions. The users can also participate in regional discussion groups. However, because of online security issues, their online profile is restricted to their username and personal interests. This is a major concern for older adults. They value a "walled garden" that is free from advertising. To develop trust in technology, older adults need to feel confident that they will not be scammed through use of technology.

Actively involving older adults in system development is essential to ensure that the technology meets users' needs and is tailored to their capabilities. During the development phase of ElderTree, we were constantly working to understand the needs of our customers. This included traditional methods of gathering customer feedback like conducting focus groups, one-on-one interviews, and usability testing, as well as less traditional approaches like creating and teaching courses at a local senior center on computers and the Internet. We adopted an iterative design approach, conducting short pilot tests of the system, gathering feedback, implementing changes and testing again. In the end, we conducted five pilot tests involving over 300 older adults.

Throughout this process, we had to balance the amount of features with the simplicity of the system. Consistently, feedback from our customers was a desire for simplicity, not more features. Special attention was paid to providing a simple user interface that met basic accessibility guidelines (e.g., 7:1 contrast ratio, large font sizes). We reduced distractions or clutter on the screen and tried to adopt a philosophy of providing the user only one task per web page.

Successive iterations of ElderTree included adding information and resources on fall-prevention, medication-management and driving, testing and ultimately removing a personal calendar system, and replacing a dashboard-style home page with a simple, graphic home page that would not overwhelm the older adult with information. While the rapid proliferation of technology offers myriad features and functions, older adults favor a simple interface with fewer choices. Recent studies that investigate the potential of ambient displays for a smooth integration of social networking sites into older adults' everyday lives present supporting evidence for this argument (Cornejo et al. 2010). Focusing on the important elements of the system and making the technology simple to use has been of paramount importance and one that ElderTree designers keep being challenged with.

One of the key barriers to adoption of technology for older adults is accessibility of the system. Systems designed for the elderly have to address issues of accessibility like compromised vision and motor dexterity. Throughout the development process, we found no magic bullet when it came to the most accessible hardware. Each device we tested (tablets, laptops, desktops, large touchscreen desktops) presented some issue of accessibility. Some users preferred tablets; others, desktops. Some users liked using a mouse, while others preferred gesture-based interaction. We ultimately settled on using a responsive design approach, which allows the customer to use whichever system they are most comfortable with, whether that be a phone, tablet, laptop, or desktop (Figure 11.1).

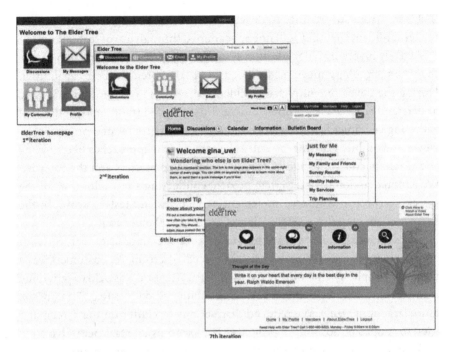

*Figure 11.1*  Screenshots from the iteration process.

What is unique about ElderTree is the coaching aspect that is offered throughout the system. Currently, there are four coaches actively involved in ElderTree. A falls-prevention coach, a diabetes diet coach, a caregiving coach, and a technology coach follow and respond to questions and comments on the forum, post "active living tips" that would support participants in being more independent, and offer consultation to the users. ElderTree includes an "Ask a Coach" tab on the opening page so that it is easily accessible to users.

Based on the preliminary results of our research, technology coaching has already yielded constructive results. Previous use of technology is not a prerequisite for this project. Therefore, participants have had a varying range of experience using technology and social media. Specifically, users who are new to social media benefit the most from personalized technology coaching. For many of these participants, ElderTree has been a *stepping-stone* by which they could increase their comfort with technology and start using other popular social media tools such as Facebook to share media and connect with their friends and family members. However, the advertisement-free, secure, and personalized (for older aged people) environment that ElderTree offers has been an attractive element that appeals to the target audience. ElderTree also promotes the participation of family and friends. The users can invite family members to ElderTree by sending a system-generated email to their email addresses. They would be directed to a "Family and Friends" discussion group on the website much like any other forum discussion. However, their participation is limited to this tab only, and they would not be able to access any other areas of the site.

In an effort to make the features more engaging, we investigated gamification (i.e. the application of gaming techniques to nongaming contexts to encourage engagement) techniques that might appeal to our users. Currently, the site offers "ratings" on the usefulness of active living tips that are posted by the coaches. Participants can give the tips a "thumbs up" to indicate their helpfulness. We restricted the rating to posts by coaches so that the participants do not get offended or refrain from posting their experiences for fear of getting negative reaction.

One issue we were not expecting concerned Internet etiquette. For many of our users, this was the first time they had participated in an online discussion group. Communicating electronically is very different from face-to-face communication. Social graces common in face-to-face communication aren't necessarily found on the Internet. It's also difficult to always know the author's intent with online communication. Educating users on our discussion group guidelines has been an ongoing effort.

## Conclusion

Addiction treatment in the older population is becoming more important than ever, due to an aging population and an increasing rate of SUDs in this population. On the other hand, surprisingly, treatment admissions for older people are decreasing for several reasons, such as an SUD diagnosis that goes unrecognized in the older patient, and social stigma for diagnosing and treating older adults with SUDs. One emerging area in treatment that may be effective in addiction treatment in older patients is the use of new technologies such as electronic health records, dashboards, communication tools, and new-generation monitoring devices.

On the other hand, older patients have several unique features that require special attention in utilizing new technologies for addiction treatment:

- Their mobility levels are limited. Communication tools and monitoring devices that would reduce the hospital visits for older adults will continue to be an essential asset.
- The reasons for SUDs in older patients are fundamentally different than for younger patients. It is important to customize the technologies to the special needs of this population.

- Older adults are less likely to adopt new technologies into their everyday lives. The implementation process should be well-thought-out and supported with coaching services.
- Ease of use is very critical.

To this end, there is a strong need for research on customizing these new technologies for the elderly population, because no study has focused specifically on using technology for addiction treatment in older population. Along with the unique features of older population listed above, the lessons learned during our research group's development of ElderTree, an interactive health technology designed for older populations, may also help other researchers considering studying this problem. Note that while ElderTree was not specifically designed for addiction treatment, we believe some of our findings may easily be valid for addiction treatment as well:

- Older patients put significant emphasis on online environments that are insulated from commercial interference (advertisements).
- Mobile phone–based systems may not be preferred by the older patients with vision and motor issues. Designs considering these issues would be more successful in reaching out to older patients.
- One-to-one technology coaching is critical for older users who are new to the social media.
- Gamification may be helpful in increasing the engagement of the older users.

In conclusion, we foresee great promise in the use of emerging technologies for addiction treatment in older patients. Considering that the older population is growing over time, the economic and social impacts of any improvement in addiction treatment in this population would be even higher in the future. We believe the opportunities and challenges that are outlined in this chapter may provide a good roadmap for researchers considering research in this area.

# References

Ackerman MJ, et al. Developing next-generation telehealth tools and technologies: patients, systems, and data perspectives. *Telemed J E-Health* 2010;16(1):93–95.

Agyapong VI, McLoughlin DM, Farren CK. Supportive text messaging for depression and comorbid alcohol use disorder: Single-blind randomised trial. *J Affect Disord* 2012;141(2–3):168–176.

Agyapong VI, McLoughlin DM, Farren CK. Six-months outcomes of a randomised trial of supportive text messaging for depression and comorbid alcohol use disorder. *J Affect Disord* 2013;151(1):100–104.

Barnett NP, et al. Contingency management for alcohol use reduction: A pilot study using a transdermal alcohol sensor. *Drug Alcohol Depend* 2011;118(2):391–399.

Bickel WK, Christensen DR, Marsch LA. A review of computer-based interventions used in the assessment, treatment, and research of drug addiction. *Subst Use Misuse* 2011;46(1):4–9.

Blaschke CM, Freddolino PP, Mullen EE. Ageing and technology: A review of the research literature. *Br J Social Work* 2009;39(4):641–656.

Blow FC, Serras AM, Barry KL. Late-life depression and alcoholism. *Curr Psychiatry Rep* 2007;9(1):14–19.

Blumenthal D, Tavenner M. The "meaningful use" regulation for electronic health records. *N Engl J Med* 2010;363(6):501–504.

Bowles KH, Hanlon A, Holland D, Potashnik SL, Topaz M. Impact of discharge planning decision support on time to readmission among older adult medical patients. *Prof Case Manag* 2014;19(1):29–38.

Caputo F, et al. Alcohol use disorders in the elderly: A brief overview from epidemiology to treatment options. *Exper Gerontol* 2012;47(6):411–416.

Carroll K, et al. Computer-assisted delivery of cognitive-behavioral therapy for addiction: A randomized trial of CBT4CBT. *Am J Psychiatry* 2008;165(7):881–888.

Center for Substance Abuse Treatment. Substance Abuse Among Older Adults. 1998. Rockville, MD: Substance Abuse and Mental Health Services Administration (U.S.).

Cornejo R, Favela J, Tentori M. *Ambient displays for integrating older adults into social networking sites, in collaboration and technology.* New York: Springer; 2010:321–336.

Dulin PL, Gonzalez VM, Campbell K. Results of a pilot test of a self-administered smartphone-based treatment system for alcohol use disorders: Usability and early outcomes. *Subst Abuse* 2014;35(2):168–175.

Gellis ZD, Kenaley BL, Have TT. Integrated telehealth care for chronic illness and depression in geriatric home care patients: The Integrated Telehealth Education and Activation of Mood (I-TEAM) study. *J Am Geriatr Soc* 2014;62(5):889–895.

Gfroerer J, et al. Substance abuse treatment need among older adults in 2020: The impact of the aging baby-boom cohort. *Drug Alcohol Depend* 2003;69(2):127–135.

Gibbons MC, Strachan DD. *eHealth solutions for healthcare disparities.* New York: Springer; 2008.

Gustafson DH, et al. Explicating an evidence-based, theoretically informed, mobile technology-based system to improve outcomes for people in recovery for alcohol dependence. *Subst Use Misuse* 2011;46(1):96–111.

Gustafson DH, McTavish, F.M., Chih MY, et al. A smartphone application to support recovery from alcoholism: A randomized controlled trial. *JAMA: Psychiatry* 2014;71(5):566–572.

Gustafson DHSr, McTavishet F, Gustafson DHJr.al. (2015). The effect of information and communication technology (ICT) on older adults' quality of life: study protocol for a randomized trial. *Trials* 2015;16:191.

Ijsselsteijn W, Nap HK, de Kort Y, et al. (2007). Digital game design for elderly users. In *Proceedings of the 2007 Conference on Future Play.* Toronto, ON, Canada, ACM Digital Library, pp. 17-22. Available at: http://dl.acm.org/citation.cfm?doid=1328202.1328206. Accessed on May 7, 2016.

Irvine, L. Falconer DW, Jones C, et al. Can text messages reach the parts other process measures cannot reach? An evaluation of a behavior change intervention delivered by mobile phone. *PloS One* 2012;7(12):e52621.

Johnson N, et al. The Hospital Outpatient Alcohol Project (HOAP): Protocol for an individually randomized, parallel-group superiority trial of electronic alcohol screening and brief intervention versus screening alone for unhealthy alcohol use. *Addict Sci Clin Pract* 2013;8(1):1–7.

Kang HG, et al. In situ monitoring of health in older adults: Technologies and issues. *J Am Geriatr Soc* 2010;58(8):1579–1586.

Kawamoto K, et al. Improving clinical practice using clinical decision support systems: A systematic review of trials to identify features critical to success. *BMJ* 2005;330(7494):765.

Kuerbis A, Sacco P. A review of existing treatments for substance abuse among the elderly and recommendations for future directions. *Subst Abuse Res Treat* 2013;7, 13.

Lemke S, Moos RH. Outcomes at 1 and 5 years for older patients with alcohol use disorders. *J Subst Abuse Treat* 2003;24(1):43–50.

Litvin CB, Davis KS, Moran WP, Iverson PJ, Zhao Y, Zapka J. The use of clinical decision-support tools to facilitate geriatric education. *J Am Geriatr Soc* 2012;60(6):1145–1149.

Marsch LA. Leveraging technology to enhance addiction treatment and recovery. *J Addict Dis* 2012;31(3):313–318.

Marsch LA, Dallery J. Advances in the psychosocial treatment of addiction: The role of technology in the delivery of evidence-based psychosocial treatment. *Psychiatr Clin N Am* 2012;35(2):481.

Martin M, Goldstein MK. (2012). Computer-based clinical decision support systems in the care of older patients. In JM Holroyd-Leduc M, Reddy M. (Ed.), *Evidence-Based Geriatr Med* (pp. 13–24). Oxford, UK: Blackwell Publishing Ltd.

Mitzner TL, et al. Older adults talk technology: Technology usage and attitudes. *Computers Hum Behav* 2010;26(6):1710–1721.

Mudge S, Stott NS. Outcome measures to assess walking ability following stroke: A systematic review of the literature. *Physiotherapy* 2007;93(3):189–200.

O'Connell H, et al. Alcohol use disorders in elderly people—redefining an age old problem in old age. *BMJ* 2003;327(7416):664–667.

Olmstead TA, Ostrow CD, Carroll KM. Cost-effectiveness of computer-assisted training in cognitive-behavioral therapy as an adjunct to standard care for addiction. *Drug Alcohol Depend* 2010;110(3):200–207.

Oslin DW, Pettinati H, Volpicelli JR. Alcoholism treatment adherence: Older age predicts better adherence and drinking outcomes. *Am J Geriatr Psych* 2002;10(6):740–747.

Pearson JF, Brownstein CA, Brownstein JS. Potential for electronic health records and online social networking to redefine medical research. *Clin Chem* 2011;57(2):196–204.

Quanbeck A, Chi M-Y, Isham A, et al. Mobile delivery of treatment for alcohol use disorders: A review of the literature. *Alcohol Res* 2015;36(1): 111-22.

Rashidi P, Mihailidis A. A survey on ambient-assisted living tools for older adults. *IEEE J Biomed Health Inform* 2013;17(3):579–590.

Satre DD, et al. Five-year alcohol and drug treatment outcomes of older adults versus middle-aged and younger adults in a managed care program. *Addiction* 2004;99(10):1286–1297.

Schutte KK, Brennan PL, Moos RH. Remission of late-life drinking problems: A 4-year follow-up. *Alcohol Clin Exper Res* 1994;18(4):835–844.

Sharp L, Vacha-Haase T. Physician attitudes regarding alcohol use screening in older adult patients. *J Applied Gerontol* 2011;30(2):226–240.

Sinadinovic K, et al. Targeting individuals with problematic alcohol use via web-based cognitive-behavioral self-help modules, personalized screening feedback or assessment only: A randomized controlled trial. *Eur Addict Res* 2014;20(6):305–318.

Smith A. Nearly half of American adults are smartphone owners. Pew Research Center. Internet, *Science & Tech*, March 1, 2012. http://www.pewinternet.org/2012/03/01/nearly-half-of-american-adults-are-smartphone-owners/. Accessed on March 17, 2016.

Stallvik M, Gastfriend DR. Predictive and convergent validity of the ASAM criteria software in Norway. *Addict Res Theory* 2014;22(6):515–523.

Sum S, et al. Internet use and loneliness in older adults. *Cyberpsychol Behav* 2008;11(2):208–211.

Sung M, Marci C, Pentland A. Wearable feedback systems for rehabilitation. *J Neuroengineer Rehabil* 2005;2: 17.

Swift R. Direct measurement of alcohol and its metabolites. *Addiction* 2003;98(s2):73–80.

Tuchman E. Women and addiction: The importance of gender issues in substance abuse research. *J Addict Dis* 2010;29(2):127–138.

Vastenburg MH, et al. *Designing acceptable assisted living services for elderly users, in ambient intelligence.* New York: Springer; 2008:1–12.

Wang Y-P, Andrade LH. Epidemiology of alcohol and drug use in the elderly. *Curr Opin Psychiatry* 2013;26(4):343–348.

Weinberg NZ, et al. Adolescent substance abuse: A review of the past 10 years. *J Am Acad Child Adolesc Psychiatry* 1998;37(3):252–261.

Wu L-T, Blazer DG. Illicit and nonmedical drug use among older adults: A review. *Journal of Aging and Health* 2011;23(3):481–504.

Yang C-C, Hsu Y-L. A review of accelerometry-based wearable motion detectors for physical activity monitoring. *Sensors* 2010;10(8):7772–7788.

CHAPTER 12

# Conclusion

*Maria A. Sullivan*

We have reviewed the available literature on alcohol and substance-use disorders (SUDs) in older adults, a topic that to date has received relatively little attention. Late-life addiction currently affects about 15% of the population, and the number of older adults with SUD is expected to reach 4.4 million by 2020 (Gfroerer et al. 2003). However, addiction in older adults very often remains unrecognized. There are several reasons for this clinical misperception, including social biases about the elderly. Family members and providers carry unexamined biases that older adults do not suffer from alcohol use disorder (AUD) or use illicit drugs, or that they should be allowed to engage in whatever behaviors they choose, at their age. Other challenges to accurate diagnosis include a paucity of behavioral disturbances or social "red flags" typically seen in younger adults with addiction (Graham 1986), age-related metabolic changes that lead to negative consequences from "drinking the same amount as usual," and patterns of inappropriate prescribing of benzodiazepines and opioids to address untreated anxiety and mood conditions in late life. Physicians and other healthcare providers often neglect to ask older patients about alcohol use, assuming that older patients will not change their patterns of use (Sharp et al. 2011). However, research suggests the contrary: older individuals respond better than younger people to treatment, as they are more likely to adhere to medication and attend therapy sessions, and thus less likely to relapse. This encouraging finding has been demonstrated both for the treatment of alcohol dependence (Oslin et al. 2005) as well as for SUDs in older adults, regardless of treatment setting (Kuerbis et al. 2013).

Reasons for an increase in addiction in later life include expanding numbers of both early-onset and late-onset addiction in older patients. The aging baby-boomer cohort has had an unprecedented exposure to drugs and alcohol, and as these individuals age, they continue to use these substances at higher rates than previous cohorts did (Blow et al. 2007). Older women appear particularly susceptible to late-onset SUDs because of genetic vulnerability or environmental stress (Tuchman et al. 2010), but they also tend to have better treatment outcomes than older men (Lemke et al. 2003).

## Epidemiology

Alcohol is the most frequently used drug in older adults. Older adults drink less alcohol than younger adults, yet a significant portion of older individuals who use alcohol exhibit harmful drinking behavior. The Substance Abuse and Mental Health Services Administration (SAMSHA) recommends no more than one drink per day in older men, and lower limits in older women. DSM criteria are difficult to apply to older adults, lack sensitivity for older adults, and should not be the only measure used when assessing unhealthy alcohol use (TIP #26, SAMHSA 2008). A panel of the U.S. Department of Health and Human Services has suggested using the terms "at-risk" and "problem drinkers" when describing alcohol use in older adults. At-risk drinkers engage in drinking in a manner that carries the potential for future problems. Problem drinkers include those who use alcohol heavily, have experienced problems related to alcohol, or who meet criteria for alcohol abuse or dependence (TIP #26, SAMHSA 2008).

While rates of substance use in older adults are lower than in younger or middle-age adults, they are nevertheless believed to be substantial, in spite of the limited epidemiological data available; much of the current information is extrapolated from studies of younger and middle-aged adults and applied to older adults. In conjunction with alcohol and cannabis, the substances most commonly used by older adults are nicotine and stimulants. Epidemiological data on cannabis, tobacco, and cocaine use are primarily limited to large national surveys; few studies have examined clinical subpopulations, or considered medical or psychiatric comorbidity, and other demographic features.

Based on patterns of marijuana use by aging baby boomers, Colliver et al. (2006) projected that 2.9% of older adults would be past-year marijuana users by 2020. Political and social forces that have led to the medicalization of marijuana in nearly half of all U.S. states also serve to increase late-life marijuana use. Older adult cigarette smokers, like older cannabis users, are often long-term, heavy smokers who are physiologically dependent and most at risk of developing serious medical consequences (Hall et al. 2009). After cannabis, cocaine is the second most common illicit drug of abuse used by older adults. Despite prevailing misconceptions about the "rarity" of SUDs in older adults, epidemiological evidence suggests that millions of adults over age 50 use marijuana or cocaine, in addition to tobacco.

Prescription drug abuse involving opioids and benzodiazepines is an issue of particular relevance to the older population, yet there has been little direct examination of this issue to date. Adults aged 65 and older account for 13% of the U.S. population but currently use one-third of all medications prescribed in the United States [National Institute on Drug Abuse (NIDA) 2014]. Aging substance-abusing patients carry a much higher disease burden than the non-substance-abusing population, including those who also receive opioid treatment for chronic pain (Patterson and Jeste 1999, Parikh and Chung 1995). Opioids are the largest class of medications abused non-medically. While illicit opioid use has a lower prevalence in the elderly compared to younger cohorts (Denisco et al. 2008), opioid misuse is likely to rise in the future with the expansion of the elderly population and pain conditions (Becker et al. 2008).

Similarly, sedative-hypnotic-use disorder is a serious and often disguised problem in the elderly. The American Geriatrics Society's "Choosing Wisely" initiative cautions against the use of any benzodiazepines or other sedative-hypnotics as initial treatment in older adults, yet benzodiazepines are the most frequently prescribed drugs in the elderly for both insomnia and anxiety. Studies have indicated that older patients disproportionately experience adverse events with benzodiazepines, such as falls and cognitive deficits. They also have difficulty reducing or stopping long-term use without experiencing rebound effects such as anxiety and insomnia. Sedative-hypnotic-use disorders among older adults are increasing in prevalence and warrant heightened clinical attention and active management.

The prevalence of benzodiazepine use is twice as high among older females as among older males (Olfson 2015, Bogunovic 2004). This finding may reflect the lower rates of alcohol-use disorders among older women compared to older men, as well as a bias among healthcare providers to overlook aberrant drug-taking behaviors in older women (Bogunovic 2004). In addition to high rates of insomnia, increased rates of anxiety and mood disorders among women may mediate an increased likelihood of developing benzodiazepine abuse or dependence in later life, particularly if these disorders remain untreated. Benzodiazepine-use disorder is a serious problem in the elderly, but further research is needed to better understand the risk factors and potential markers for benzodiazepine-use disorder in older adults. Clinicians should be alert to the risks associated with benzodiazepine misuse in this population in order to develop strategies for prevention, detection, and treatment.

Mortality data from the Drug Abuse Warning Network (DAWN) indicate that the rate of drug-related deaths among adults age 55 and over increased from 49.5 per 1 million population in 2003 (DAWN 2003) to 66 per million in 2007 (DAWN 2007). Impacting this death rate is the concurrent prescribing of benzodiazepines in the elderly (Jones et al. 2012). Benzodiazepine use increases steadily with age, exceeding 8% in those 65–80 (Olfson et al. 2015). Used principally for insomnia and/or anxiety, they are much more likely to be prescribed for women than for men. Combined use of benzodiazepines with opioid pain relievers (or alcohol) significantly increases the risk of inpatient admission or death. Risk factors for prescription pain medication misuse and/ or opioid-use disorders in the elderly include being female, having a personal or family history of substance abuse, having comorbid psychiatric disorders such as Cluster B personality disorders, having multiple medical problems, and having chronic pain (American Geriatrics Society 2009).

## Presentation and Diagnosis

Alcohol use is associated with significant morbidity in older adults. Alcohol-related hospitalizations in older adults occur with similar frequency to hospitalization rates for myocardial infarction: 54.7 per 10,000 in men and 14.8 per 10,000 in women (Adams 1993). In terms of neurological sequelae, heavy alcohol use has been linked, not only to alcohol-related dementia (ARD), but also to vascular dementia and mixed dementia subtypes. There is evidence of memory and executive function impairment in those not specifically diagnosable with ARD who use alcohol excessively (Sinforiani 2010). Gastrointestinal effects may include gastritis, gastro-esophageal reflux disease (GERD), and fatty liver progressing to alcoholic hepatitis and finally cirrhosis. Alcohol can also result in malnutrition, weight loss, and vitamin and mineral deficiencies (Chase 2005). Cardiovascular complications include cardiomyopathy, hypertension, and arrhythmias, while pulmonary risks include worsening sleep apnea and aspiration pneumonia. Of particular relevance to the elderly, alcohol can also lead to an increased risk of fractures due to gait instability, osteoporosis, and decreased total muscle mass. Bone marrow stem cell suppression can lead to anemia and increased risk of infections and bleeding. Chronic alcohol use is also associated with an increased risk of a variety of cancers, including pharyngeal, esophageal, and breast cancer. In addition, older adults with AUD have been found to have increased rates of depression, anxiety, and insomnia. In addition, since more than 90% of older adults use prescription medications, the risk of drug–alcohol interactions is high in this population. Such reactions may include increased blood alcohol levels, increased or decreased prescription drug metabolism, increased risk of hepatic toxicity, and an exacerbation of side effects such as gastrointestinal bleeding, hypotension, and sedation. Thus, it is important for clinicians to consult web-based resources and desk references to check for drug interactions when prescribing for older patients who regularly use alcohol.

Older adults with SUD have high rates of comorbid medical and psychiatric disorders (21–66%; Blow et al. 2014). The most prevalent psychiatric diagnoses in the elderly include depression, generalized anxiety disorder, alcohol dependence, dementia, and bipolar disorder (Seby et al. 2011). Dementia is significantly more common among elderly with alcohol use than for non-drinkers (Caputo et al. 2012). We have seen that, while alcohol and psychoactive medications are the substances most frequently used among older adults, the prevalence of illegal drug use is increasing as the baby-boomer generation is aging, as they are more likely than past generations to have used illicit substances during their youth (Koechl et al. 2012). The clinical indicators of substance use can be misinterpreted as indicative of other common medical or psychiatric conditions among older adults, making diagnosis more challenging (Mulinga 1999, Lang et al. 2007). In addition, social stereotypes, such as the false perception that older adults do not suffer from SUDs, also contribute to misidentification of such conditions by families and healthcare providers (Naik et al. 1994). Furthermore, older adults may show fewer of the behavioral "red flags" typically seen in younger adults with addictions (Graham 1986).

In particular, substance use in older women is often undetected and untreated by clinicians. It is, therefore, important to screen older women regularly for alcohol and prescription drug use and abuse, to ask screening questions in a non-judgmental manner, to be sensitive to potential slower processing times, and to make use of collateral information from family/caregivers when possible. Motivational brief interventions and therapies can be effective in older adults and should be utilized when risky use is identified. Finally, individualizing treatment plans with age-appropriate content is essential when treating older men and women with SUDs.

While some elderly patients present with AUD or SUD that is a continuation of an early-onset problem, others develop an alcohol or substance disorder only later in life. Many older individuals may begin to experience adverse effects from a stable level of alcohol or drug use that had not previously caused apparent harm, as a consequence of reduced metabolism or other age-related vulnerabilities. In general, SUDs in older individuals may often present in subtle and atypical ways. Helpful strategies to overcome barriers to diagnosis and treatment of SUDs in later life include systematic screening using validated instruments, patient education regarding the impact of psychoactive substances on aging patients' health, and cautious prescribing practices.

Because of the increased risks to health posed by alcohol in the older population, it is essential to screen for AUD in primary care, emergency, and specialty clinic settings using tools tailored for older adults such as the SMAST-G. The value of self-report measures for alcohol-use disorder is underappreciated and underutilized by most primary care physicians; fewer than 10% of adults over 65 years old receive validated screening measures such as the CAGE or short MAST-G (McKnight-Eily 2014). Traditional biomarkers (e.g., Mean Corpuscular Volume (MCV), Gamma Glutamyl Transpeptidase (GGT), Aspartate aminotransferase (AST) and Alanine transaminase (ALT)) are unreliable in the elderly, but ethylglucuronide (EtG), a metabolite of alcohol detected in urine, appears to be the most reliable biomarker for alcohol use in older adults.

It is important to consider that an SUD may present differently in older adults, due to their diminished social responsibilities and retirement. DSM-5 criteria may not be sensitive enough to detect substance misuse in this population; addiction researchers have recommended a two-tier stratification of substance use in older adults: at-risk (any use of an illicit drug) vs. problem use (substance use that results in social, medical, or psychological consequences, regardless of quantity or frequency of use or whether DSM criteria are met) (Kuerbis et al. 2014). Older adults with SUDs may also present with cognitive changes, confusion, or falls, all of which have a broad differential diagnosis.

## Screening and Treatment

While guidelines are lacking for screening procedures and treatment approaches directed at SUD in older patients, increasing numbers of older adults are seeking treatment for drug and alcohol use (Wu et al. 2011). One promising approach to treatment interventions appears to be integrating these into primary care for the elderly (Fink et al. 2005, Bartels et al. 2004). Fortunately, the research literature to date has suggested that treatment outcomes in this population are as good as, if not better than, in younger adults treated for SUD (Oslin et al. 2005, Lemke and Moos 2003, Blow et al. 2000).

Existing research supports the benefits of developing and implementing elder-specific SUD treatment centers or tracks within general treatment programs. Features of treatment tailored to the needs of older individuals may include: behavioral programs with a focus on the biological, psychological, and social aspects of aging, adjusting medications due to metabolic differences, or consideration of drug–drug interactions in light of the high prevalence of polypharmacy. Particularly relevant to older patients are cognitive-behavioral therapy (CBT) skills that take into account issues of cognitive impairment common in later life, as these may reduce the ability to acquire positive coping skills. Motivational interviewing (MI) has also been found to be a successful strategy in older adults (Chang et al. 2014), as has family therapy tailored to the needs of older adults (e.g., including adult children, spouses, or siblings). And finally, working with older adults may necessitate addressing specific treatment barriers such as medical comorbidity, ageism, and transportation issues, as well as integrating other relevant therapeutic issues such as loss, grief, isolation, or concerns about poor health [Center for Substance Abuse Treatment (CSAT) 2004].

Brief interventions for substance misuse in older adults are an important type of structured intervention for those whose SUD has previously gone unrecognized or undertreated. Potential goals of brief interventions for SUD include harm reduction, cessation, or facilitating entry into treatment. These brief interventions may take the form of brief advice, a motivational conversation, or a structured intervention. SUD interventions in older adults should take into account the high likelihood that prescription drugs are being used. Seeking alternatives to chronic pain relief and addressing problems that perpetuate or exacerbate SUD (e.g., alcohol misuse, insomnia, mental health problems) should be included in such interventions. An important consideration when designing multi-session brief interventions for older adults is limited mobility or transportation (Cooper 2012); alternate methods of delivering additional sessions may be needed, such as by telephone or in-home visits. Interventionists working with older adults should have a non-judgemental attitude toward substance misuse and a nonconfrontational style (Wu et al. 2011). Preliminary research suggests that some brief interventions are effective at reducing tobacco, alcohol, and substance misuse in older adults, but it is unclear if these result in sustained abstinence. There is still a need for more robust clinical trials of brief interventions for substance misuse in older adults, particularly with regard to illicit drugs.

Older women may be an especially vulnerable population, with unique risk factors and medical and psychiatric comorbidities. Owing to their longer life expectancies than men, and consequent higher likelihood of living alone, being widowed, or suffering financial troubles, older women may be at a greater risk for SUDs than older men (Blow and Barry 2002, National Center on Addiction and Substance Abuse Columbia 1998). Numerous studies have documented that older women are more likely than older men to be exposed to psychoactive prescription drugs with abuse potential, particularly benzodiazepines (Simoni-Wastila et al. 2004, Blow and Barry 2002). Finally, biological and physiological changes that occur with age (e.g., reductions in total body water and falling levels of alcohol dehydrogenase), some of which are more prominent in older women than in older men, function as risk factors for intoxication and adverse effects (Blow and Barry 2002, Brady 1999). In addition, women of all ages are more likely to have affective illness or anxiety disorders, which are independent risk factors for substance misuse. Thus, healthcare providers need to be aware of the potential for comorbid affective illness when screening and treating older women with SUDs.

Several risk assessment tools have been developed to help evaluate the likelihood of opioid misuse. While the Opioid Risk Tool (ORT) and Opioid Assessment for Patients with Pain–Revised (SOAPP-R) are helpful questionnaires to assess initial risk, the Pain Medication Questionnaire (PMQ) also appears to be useful for screening community-dwelling elderly for pain medication misuse (Park et al. 2010). Chronic pain is very common in the elderly, with an estimated prevalence of 45–85% in those 65 and older (Krueger et al. 2008, Sjogren et al. 2009). One in four elderly individuals receives opioids for chronic pain (Solomon et al. 2006). Pain detection in older patients is complicated by cognitive decline, communication difficulties, and cultural factors such as stoicism (Molton and Terrill 2014, Dowling et al. 2008). Although undertreatment of pain in the elderly is a concern, misuse and non-medical use of prescription pain medications is a significant emerging issue in the elderly (Wang and Andrade 2013). Risk stratification for opioid use in the elderly should become standard practice, as should routine screening for opioid misuse and opioid-use disorders in the elderly. Among the risk factors for prescription opioid misuse in the elderly arebeing female, having a personal or family history of substance abuse, having comorbid psychiatric disorders such as Cluster B personality disorders, having multiple medical problems, and having chronic pain (American Geriatric Society 2009). Evidence-based treatment approaches for OUD in the elderly include closely monitored methadone, buprenorphine with its superior safety profile, and oral or injection naltrexone (if the chronic pain syndrome can be managed without opioid analgesics). CBT, relapse prevention, and 12-Step programs are effective nonpharmacological strategies. Group interventions involving age-appropriate cohorts are most likely to succeed at engaging older patients in treatment. Supportive approaches that avoid confrontation should focus on cohort issues such as loss, medical or psychiatric comorbidities, and social isolation in the elderly patient.

Emerging interactive web and mobile technologies for the practice of medicine and public health ("e-health") offer significant opportunities to advance the treatment and recovery management of SUDs (Sinadinovic et al. 2014). Sincetime in treatment is important regardless of the level of care or treatment setting, and because age-specific treatment seems to enhance the effect of treatment for older adults (Wadd et al. 2011), technology (e.g., personalized screening, assessment, communication tools, and new-generation monitoring devices) may provide a vehicle through which effective treatment can be provided despite reduced mobility, low numbers of older adults needing treatment in a specific geographic area, and other issues that limit the ability to offer age-specific addiction treatment to older populations.

Brief interventions have been shown to be effective for hazardous use in this population, and medication management should be discussed with individuals who may benefit from these. More research is needed regarding evidence-based practices in identification and treatment of hazardous and harmful alcohol use in older adult populations. Assessment and tailoring treatment to the patient's individual risk factors in a non-judgemental and collaborative way is the single most important intervention to prevent harm from alcohol use in this population.

We have seen that, in spite of growing epidemiological evidence from population-based surveys that alcohol and substance use are significant and increasing problems in the older adult population, there is a dearth of evidence-based research in this area due to the exclusion of older adults based on age and co-occurring medical disorders from clinical research studies on SUDs, as well as widespread misconceptions about substance use in this population. There are important clinical gaps in our understanding of risk factors, identifying features, and response to treatment for individuals who develop a SUD later in life or who persistently use substances throughout their lives. Under-explored areas of research include identification of, and age-appropriate treatment interventions for, older populations.

## Summary

Successful identification and management of alcohol and SUDs in older patients requires that clinicians be alert to the need to screen for these often undetected conditions. While alcohol is the most frequently used drug in this population, rates of cannabis and cocaine use are also rising. Relying on standard DSM criteria may result in a failure to detect an SUD that presents with cognitive symptoms or physical injury, as well as the absence of work or social consequences. It is important to set aside social biases and misperceptions that can blind a clinician to the presence of prescription or illicit substance use in the older individual. As with younger populations, older individuals can benefit from the application of risk-stratification measures. Validated screening measures can be an important diagnostic tool, and the presence of anxiety or affective disorders should raise concern about heightened risk for alcohol or substance use. Older women in particular are a group vulnerable to prescription misuse, especially benzodiazepines and opioid painkillers. Brief interventions appear promising in older individuals, and barriers to treatment which may need to be addressed include medical comorbidity and practical concerns such as transportation. Newer technologies for communication and patient monitoring may also prove helpful in ensuring effective treatment for some older patients. It is recommended that older individuals be referred to treatment settings that offer age-appropriate group therapy and nonconfrontational individual therapy focusing on late-life issues of loss and sources of social support. Older adults also deserve to be given full consideration for the potential benefits of medication management for alcohol or SUD. Although research to date has been limited in this population, treatment outcomes for SUD have been found to be superior in older adults compared to younger or middle-aged adults. This encouraging finding seems to reflect older patients' better adherence and consequently lower relapse rates.

Demographic changes and the arrival of the baby-boomer cohort into older age have highlighted that addiction is under-recognized and under-treated in later life. As the general population continues to age, understanding how to address the unique concerns of older adults with alcohol, substance, or prescription-use disorders will become an increasingly important issue for clinicians. Ongoing and future research will guide new methods of assessing SUDs and implementing effective treatments in the older population. We anticipate that this text will serve as a useful introduction for clinicians who will encounter such patients in the primary or specialty care setting. It is hoped that the recommendations provided here will help to enhance clinical focus on this issue and guide useful and timely clinical interventions for the at-risk or substance-abusing older patient.

# References

Adams WL, Yuan Z, Barboriak JJ, Rimm AA. Alcohol-related hospitalizations of elderly people. Prevalence and geographic variation in the United States. *JAMA* 1993;270(10):1222–1225.

American Geriatrics Society. Panel on the Pharmacological Management of Persistent Pain in Older Persons. Pharmacological management of persistent pain in older persons. *J Am Geriatr Soc* 2009;57:1331–1346.

Becker WC, Sullivan LE, Tetrault JM, et al. Non-medical use, abuse and dependence on prescription opioids among U.S. adults: Psychiatric, medical and substance use correlates. *Drug Alcohol Depend* 2008;94:38–47.

Blow FC, Barry K. Treatment of older adults. In: Ries RF, Fiellin DA, Miller SC, Saitz R, Eds., *The ASAM principles of addiction medicine,* 5th ed. Chevy Chase, MD: American Society of Addiction Medicine; 2014:470–492.

Blow FC, Barry KL. Use and misuse of alcohol among older women. *Alcohol Res Health* 2002;26:308–315.

Blow FC, Serras AM, Barry KL. Late-life depression and alcoholism. *Curr Psychiatry Rep* 2007;9(1):14–19.

Bogunovic OJ, Greenfield S. Practical geriatrics: Use of benzodiazepines among elderly patients. *Psychiatr Serv* 2004;55(3):233–235.

Brady K. T., Randall CL. Gender differences in substance use disorders. *Addict Disord* 1999;22(2):241–252.

Caputo F, Vignoli T, Leggio L, Addolorato G, Zoli G, Bernardi M. Alcohol use disorders in the elderly: A brief overview from epidemiology to treatment options. *Exper Gerontol* 2012;47(6), 411–416.

Chase V, Neild R, Sadler C, Batey R. The medical complications of alcohol use: Understanding mechanisms to improve management. *Drug Alcohol Rev* 2005;24(3):253–265. doi:10.1080/09595230500167510

Colliver JD, Compton WM, Gfroerer JC, Condon T. Projecting drug use among aging baby boomers in 2020. *Ann Epidemiol* 2006;16(4):257–265.

Cooper L. Combined motivational interviewing and cognitive-behavioral therapy with older adult drug and alcohol abusers. *Health & Social Work* 2012;37(3):173–179.

Dowling GJ, Weiss SR, Condon TP. Drugs of abuse and the aging brain. *Neuropsychopharmacology* 2008;33:209–218.

Drug Abuse Warning Network. Area Profiles of Drug Related Mortality. 2003. At http://dawninfo.samhsa.gov/files/ME2003/ME report 2003 Profiles B.pdf. Accessed October 20, 2014.

Drug Abuse Warning Network. Area Profiles of Drug Related Mortality. Profiles B. 2007. At http://dawninfo.samhsa.gov/files/ME2007/ME Accessed October 20, 2014.

Fink A, Elliott MN, Tsai M, Beck JG. An evaluation of an intervention to assist primary care physicians in screening and educating older patients who use alcohol. *J Am Geriatr Soc* 2005;53(11): 1937-43.

Gfroerer J, Penne M, Pemberton M, Folsom R. Substance abuse treatment need among older adults in 2020: The impact of the aging baby-boom cohort. *Drug Alcohol Depend* 2003;69(2):127–135.

Graham K. Identifying and measuring alcohol abuse among the elderly: Serious problems with existing instrumentation. *J Stud Alcohol* 1986;47(4):322–326.

Hall SM, Humfleet GL, Munoz RF, Reus VI, Robbins JA, Prochaska JJ. Extended treatment of older cigarette smokers. *Addiction* 2009;104(6):1043–1052.

Koechl B, Unger A, Fischer G. Age-related aspects of addiction. *Gerontology* 2012;58(6): 540–544.

Krueger AB, Stone AA. Assessment of pain: a community-based diary survey in the USA. *Lancet* 2008;371:1519–1525.

Kuerbis A, Sacco P, Blazer DG, Moore AA. Substance abuse among older adults. *Clin Geriatr Med* 2014;30(3):629–654.

Mulinga JD. Elderly people with alcohol-related problems: Where do they go? *Int J Geriatr Psych* 1999;14(7):564–566.

Lang I, Guralnik J, Wallace RB, Melzer D. What level of alcohol consumption is hazardous for older people? Functioning and mortality in U.S. and English national cohorts. *J Am Geriatr Soc* 2007;55(1):49–57.

Lemke S, Moos RH. Outcomes at 1 and 5 years for older patients with alcohol use disorders. *J Subst Abuse Treat* 2003;24(1):43–50.

McKnight-Eily LR, Liu Y, Brewer RD, et al. Vital signs: Communication between health professionals and their patients about alcohol use: 44 states and the District of Columbia, 2011. *MMWR: Morb Mortal Weekly Rep* 2014;63(1):16–22.

Molton IR, Terrill AL. Overview of persistent pain in older adults. *Am Psychologist* 2014;67:197–207.

Naik PC, Jones RG. Alcohol histories taken from elderly people on admission. *BMJ* 1994;308 (6923):248.

National Center on Addiction and Substance Abuse (Columbia University). *Under the rug: substance abuse and the mature woman.* New York: National Center on Addiction and Substance Abuse at Columbia University; 1998.

Olfson M, King M, Schoenbaum M. Benzodiazepine use in the United States. *JAMA Psychiatry* 2015;72:136–142.

Oslin, DW, Slaymaker VJ, Blow FC, Owen PL, Colleran C. Treatment outcomes for alcohol dependence among middle-aged and older adults. *Addict Behav* 2005;30(7):1431–1436.

Parikh SS, Chung F. Postoperative delirium in the elderly. *Anesth Analg* 1995;80:1223–1232.

Park J, Clement R, Lavin R. Factor structure of pain medication questionnaire in community-dwelling older adults with chronic pain. *Pain Pract* 2010;11:314–324.

Patterson TL, Jeste DV. The potential impact of the baby-boom generation on substance abuse among elderly persons. *Psychiatr Serv* 1999;50:1184–1188.

Seby K, Chaudhury S, Chakraborty R. Prevalence of psychiatric and physical morbidity in an urban geriatric population. *Ind J Psychiatry* 2011;53(2):121–127.

Sharp L, & Vacha-Haase T. Physician attitudes regarding alcohol use screening in older adult patients. *J Appl Gerontol* 2011;30(2):226–240.

Sinadinovic K., Wennberg P, Johansson M, Berman AH. Targeting individuals with problematic alcohol use via web-based cognitive-behavioral self-help modules, personalized screening feedback or assessment only: A randomized controlled trial. *Eur Addict Res* 2014;20(6):305–318.

Simoni-Wastila L, Ritter G., Strickler G. Gender and other factors associated with the non-medical use of abusable prescription drugs. *Subst Use Misuse*, 2004;39(1):1–23.

Sinforiani E, Zucchella C, Pasotti C, Casoni F, Bini P, Costa A. The effects of alcohol on cognition in the elderly: From protection to neurodegeneration. *Funct Neurol* 2010;26(2):103–106.

Sjogren P, Ekholm O, Peuckmann V, Gronbaek M. Epidemiology of chronic pain in Denmark: An update. *Eur J Pain* 2009;13:287–292.

Solomon DH, Avorn J, Wang PH, et al. Prescription opioid use among older adults with arthritis or low back pain. *Arch Rheumat* 2006;55:35–41.

SAMHSA. Substance Abuse Among Older Adults: TIP #26. HHS Publication No. (SMA) 12-3918. 2008. Rockville, MD: Substance Abuse and Mental Health Services Administration. Available at: http://store.samhsa.gov/product/TIP-26-Substance-Abuse-Among-Older-Adults/SMA12-3918. Accessed February 14, 2015.

Tuchman E. Women and addiction: The importance of gender issues in substance abuse research. *J Addict Dis* 2010;29(2):127–138.

Wadd S, Forrester D. Alcohol problems in old age. *Generations Review*, July 2011. Available at http://www.britishgerontology.org/DB/gr-editions-2/generations-review/alcohol-problems-in-old-age.html. Accessed on March 17, 2016.

Wang Y-P, Andrade H. Epidemiology of alcohol and drug use in the elderly. *Curr Opin Psychiatry* 2013;26:343–349.

Wu LT, Blazer DG. Illicit and nonmedical drug use among older adults: A review. *J Aging Health* 2011;23(3):481–504.

# INDEX